AF213406

Weight Management

Edited by Hubertus Himmerich

Published in London, United Kingdom

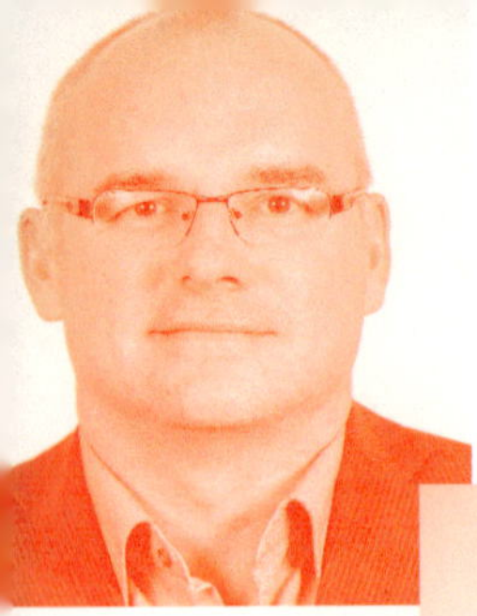
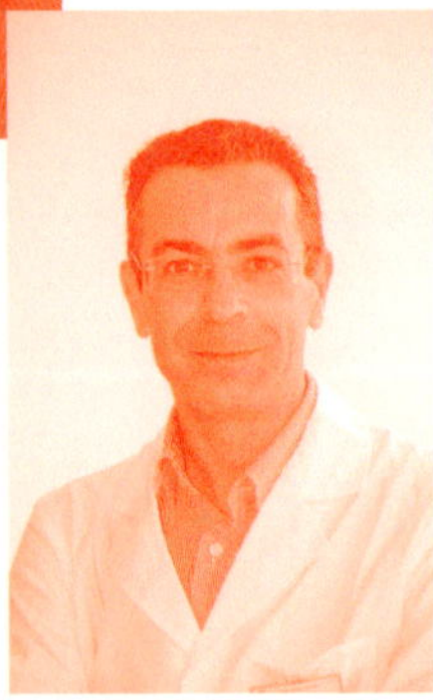
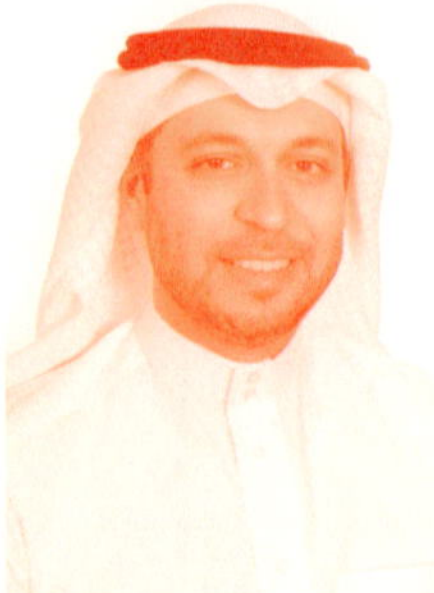
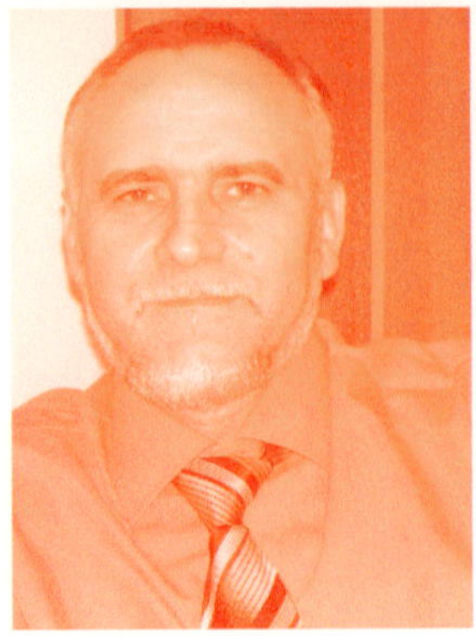
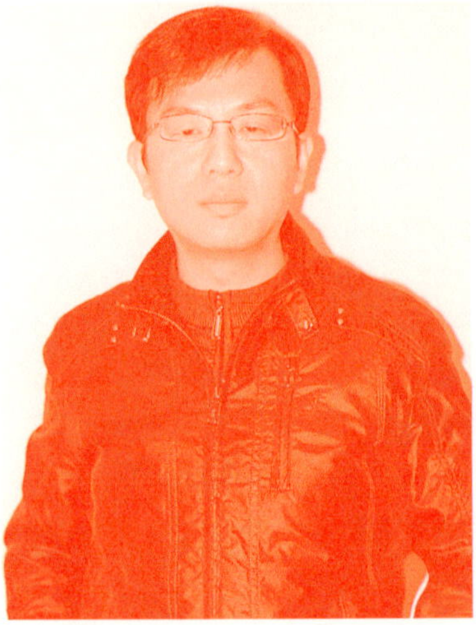
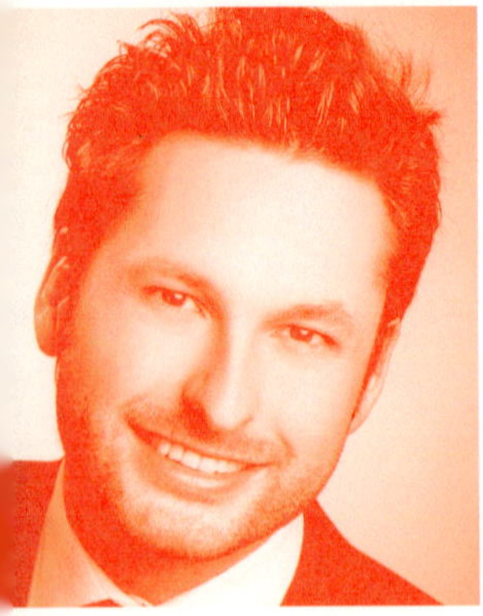
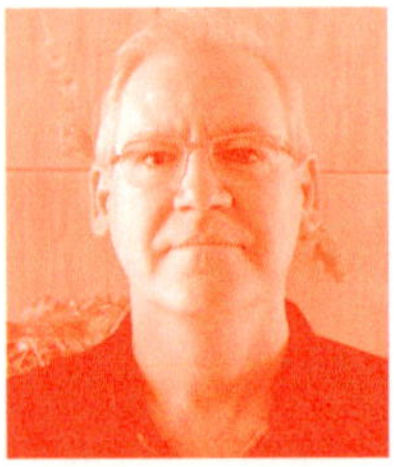

IntechOpen

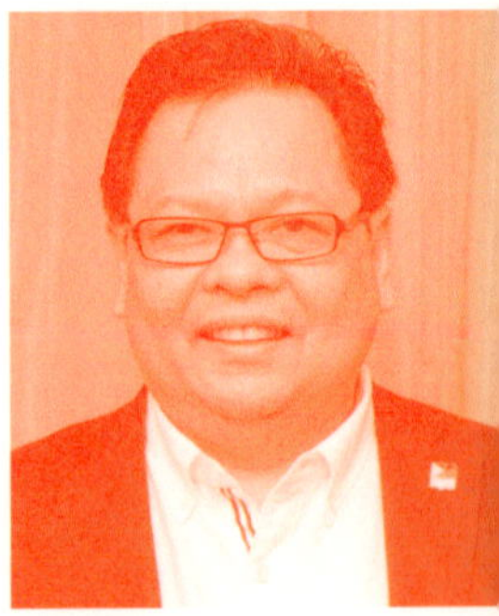
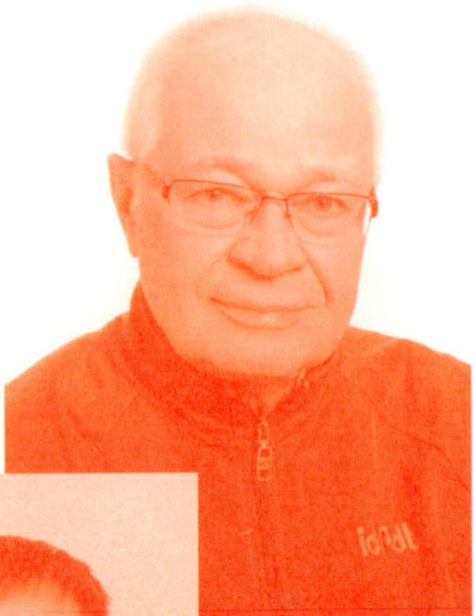
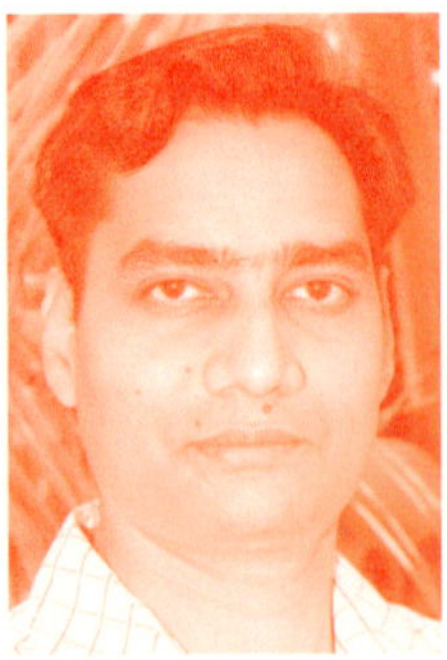
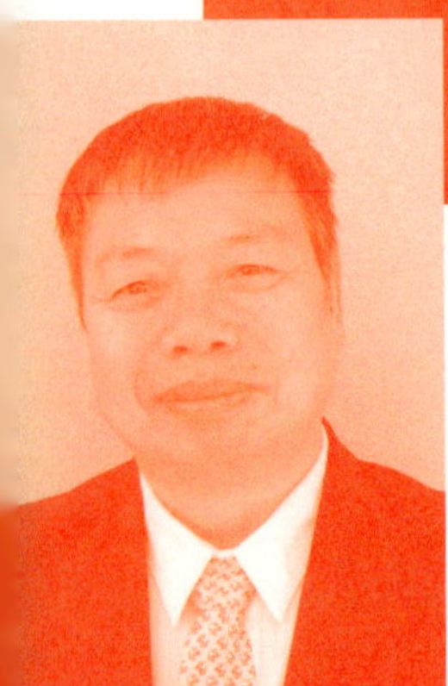
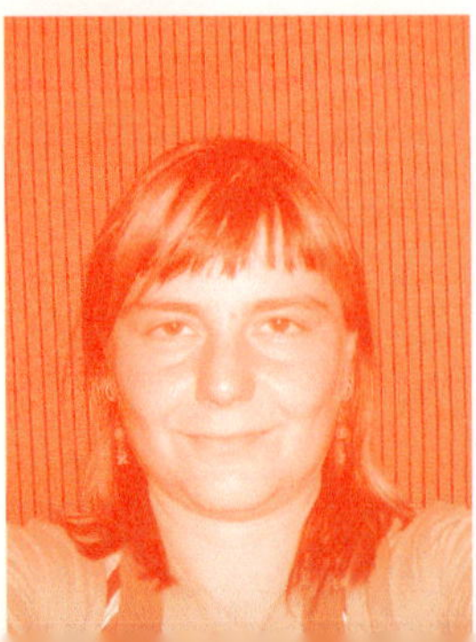
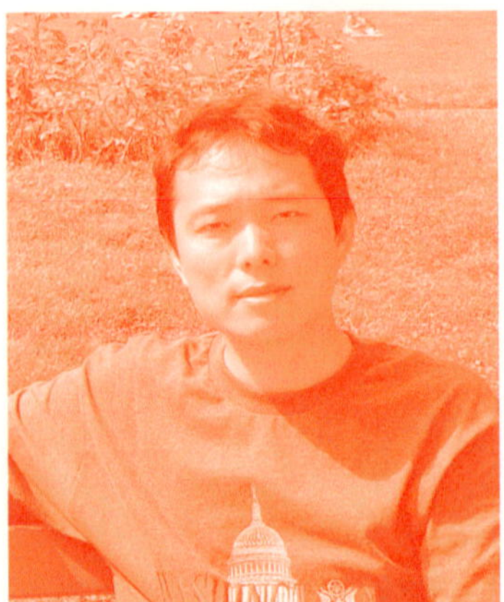

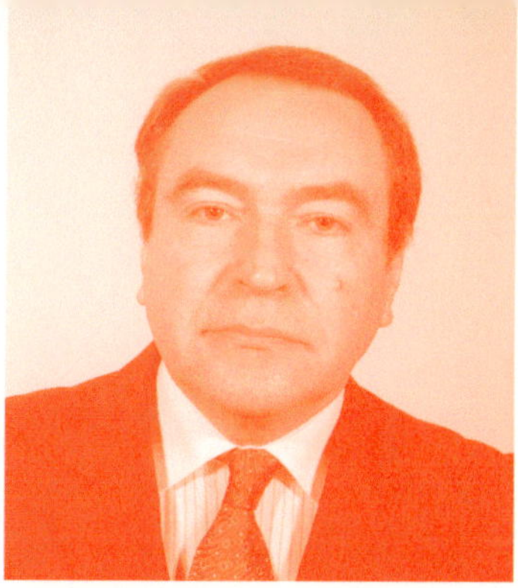
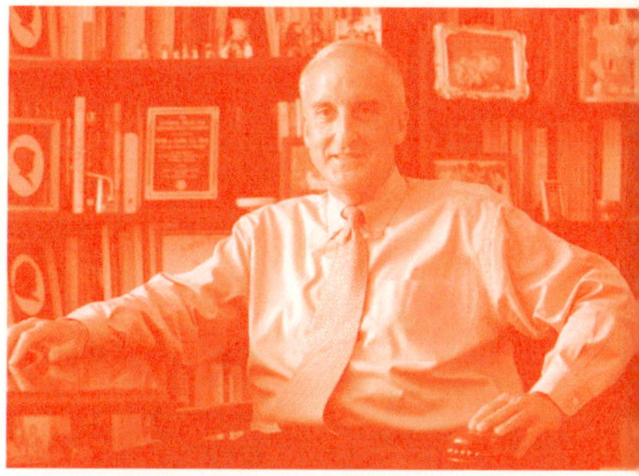
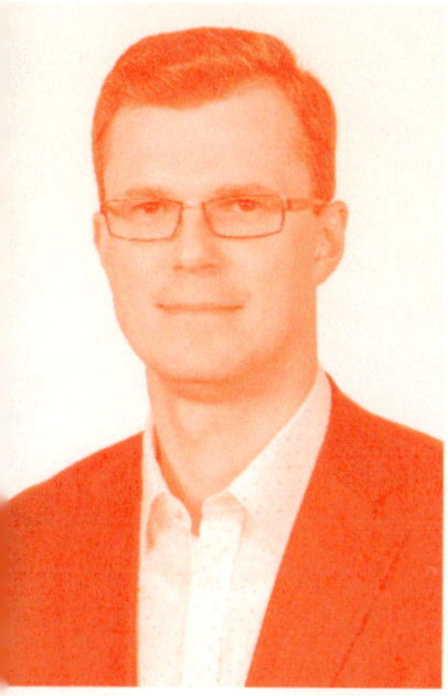
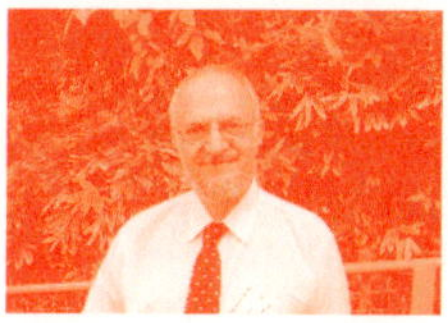
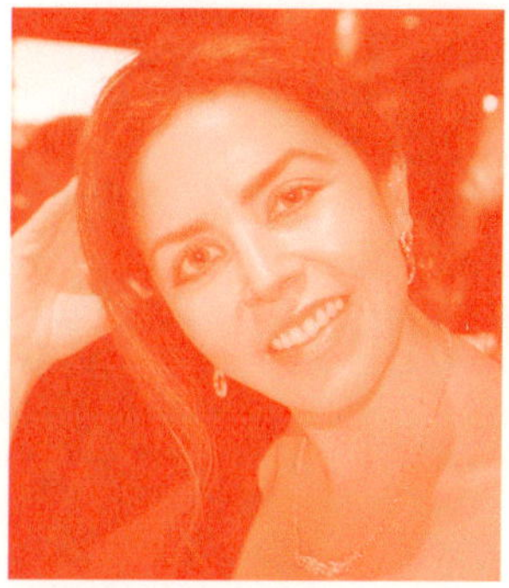

Supporting open minds since 2005

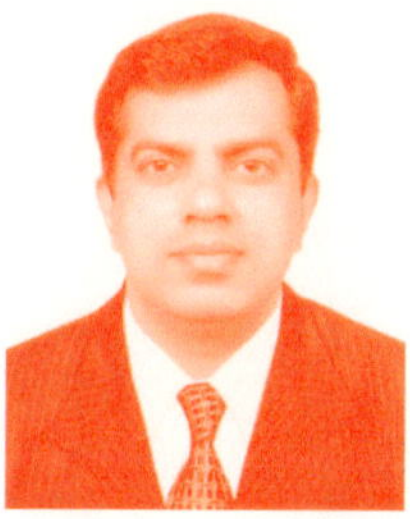
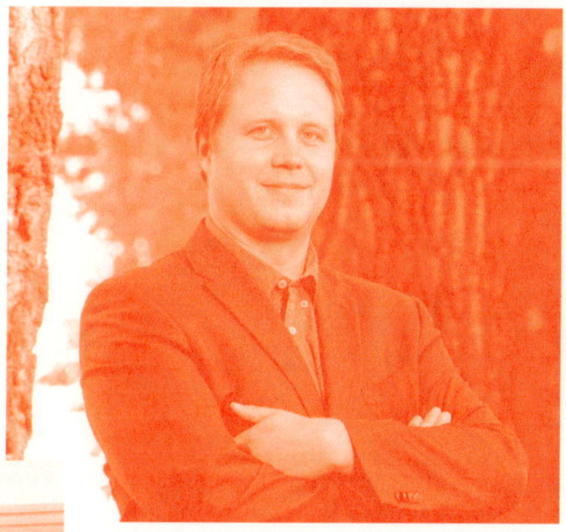
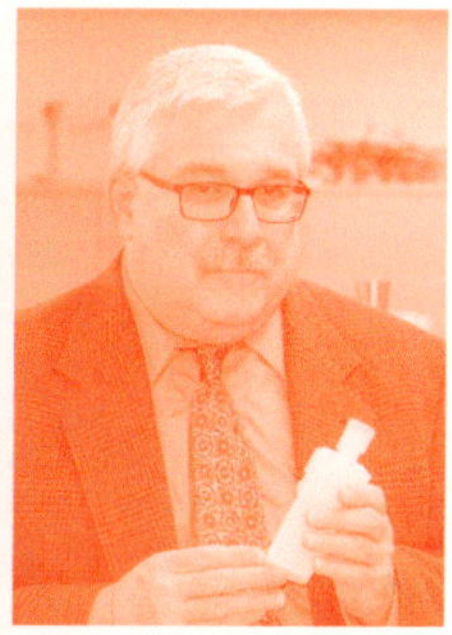
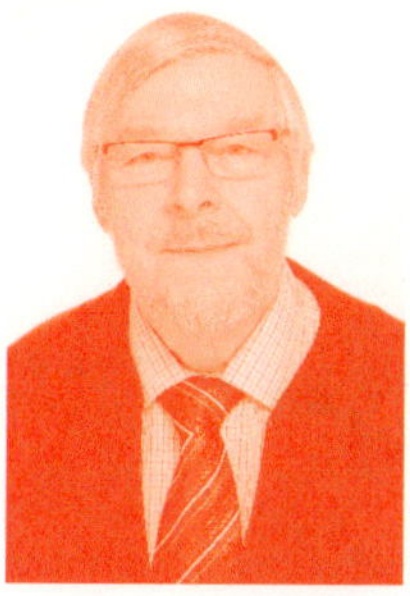
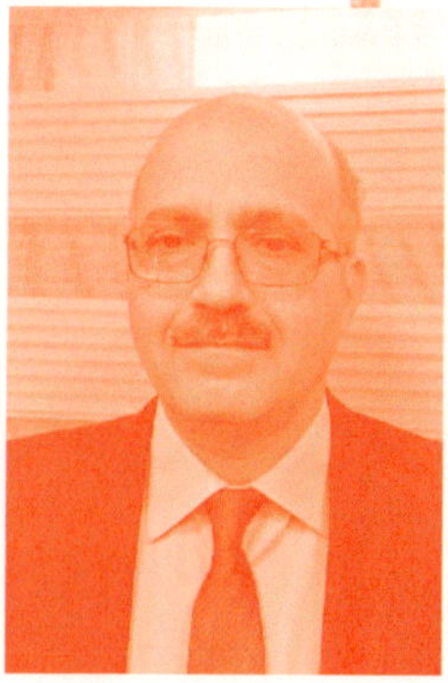
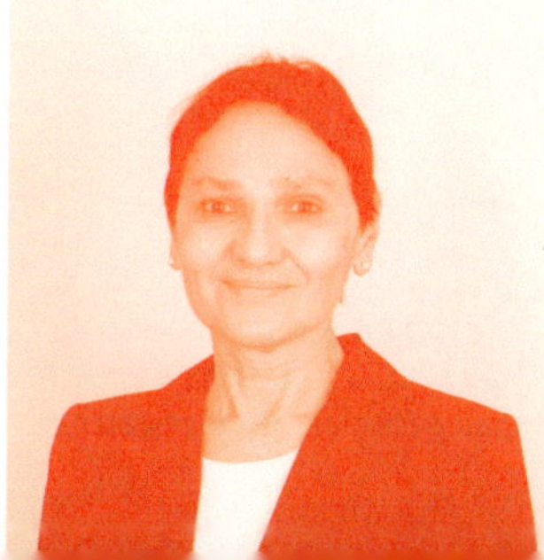
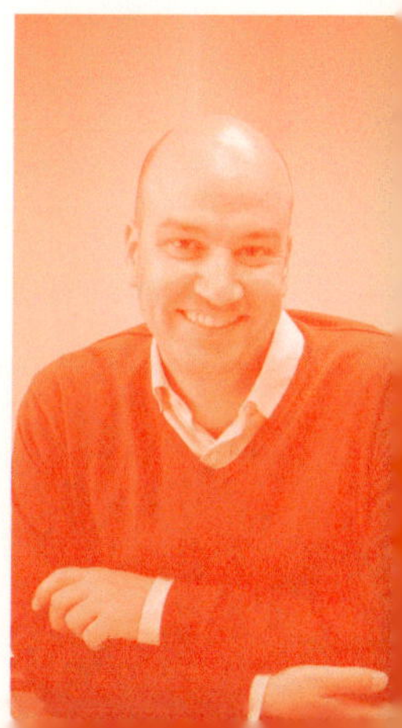

Weight Management
http://dx.doi.org/10.5772/intechopen.80199
Edited by Hubertus Himmerich

Contributors
Ermal Bojdani, Flavia De Souza, Aishwarya Rajagopalan, Troy R. Nold, Anderson Chen, Alesia A. Cloutier, Dil Tahera, Stefania Cella, Paolo Cotrufo, Mara Iannaccone, Annarosa Cipriano, Emilio Gutiérrez, Olaia Carrera, Martin Fischer, Arved Weimann, Nadine Oberänder, Hassan M. Heshmati, Abigail H. Natenshon, Fatima Elif Ergüney Okumuş, José Alonso Suclla-Velásquez, Connie Smedts, Charmode Sundip Hemant, Ximena Terra, Carlos González-Quilen, Esther Rodríguez-Gallego, Raúl Beltrán-Debón, Montserrat Pinent, Anna Ardévol, Maria Teresa Blay, Shahdevi Kurniawan, Hayder M. Alkuraishy, Ali I. Al-Gareeb, Naseer A. Al-Harchan, Kanagamani Krishnasamy, Upasana Upasana, Hubertus Himmerich, Valentina Cardi, Aishwarya Krishna Priya, Briana Applewhite, Anna Carr, Mary Cowan, Kate Tchanturia, Emmanuelle Dufour, Patrícia Colombo-Souza, Leonardo de Souza Piber, Jane de Eston Armond

© The Editor(s) and the Author(s) 2020
The rights of the editor(s) and the author(s) have been asserted in accordance with the Copyright, Designs and Patents Act 1988. All rights to the book as a whole are reserved by INTECHOPEN LIMITED. The book as a whole (compilation) cannot be reproduced, distributed or used for commercial or non-commercial purposes without INTECHOPEN LIMITED's written permission. Enquiries concerning the use of the book should be directed to INTECHOPEN LIMITED rights and permissions department (permissions@intechopen.com).
Violations are liable to prosecution under the governing Copyright Law.

cc BY

Individual chapters of this publication are distributed under the terms of the Creative Commons Attribution 3.0 Unported License which permits commercial use, distribution and reproduction of the individual chapters, provided the original author(s) and source publication are appropriately acknowledged. If so indicated, certain images may not be included under the Creative Commons license. In such cases users will need to obtain permission from the license holder to reproduce the material. More details and guidelines concerning content reuse and adaptation can be found at http://www.intechopen.com/copyright-policy.html.

Notice
Statements and opinions expressed in the chapters are these of the individual contributors and not necessarily those of the editors or publisher. No responsibility is accepted for the accuracy of information contained in the published chapters. The publisher assumes no responsibility for any damage or injury to persons or property arising out of the use of any materials, instructions, methods or ideas contained in the book.

First published in London, United Kingdom, 2020 by IntechOpen
IntechOpen is the global imprint of INTECHOPEN LIMITED, registered in England and Wales, registration number: 11086078, 7th floor, 10 Lower Thames Street, London, EC3R 6AF, United Kingdom
Printed in Croatia

British Library Cataloguing-in-Publication Data
A catalogue record for this book is available from the British Library

Additional hard and PDF copies can be obtained from orders@intechopen.com

Weight Management
Edited by Hubertus Himmerich
p. cm.
Print ISBN 978-1-83962-542-8
Online ISBN 978-1-83962-543-5
eBook (PDF) ISBN 978-1-83962-544-2

For EU product safety concerns:
IN TECH d.o.o., Prolaz Marije Krucifikse Kozulić 3, 51000 Rijeka, Croatia, info@intechopen.com or visit our website at intechopen.com.

We are IntechOpen, the world's leading publisher of Open Access books

Built by scientists, for scientists

5,000+
Open access books available

125,000+
International authors and editors

140M+
Downloads

151
Countries delivered to

Our authors are among the
Top 1%
most cited scientists

12.2%
Contributors from top 500 universities

CLARIVATE ANALYTICS BOOK CITATION INDEX INDEXED

WEB OF SCIENCE™

Selection of our books indexed in the Book Citation Index in Web of Science™ Core Collection (BKCI)

Interested in publishing with us?
Contact book.department@intechopen.com

Numbers displayed above are based on latest data collected.
For more information visit www.intechopen.com

Meet the editor

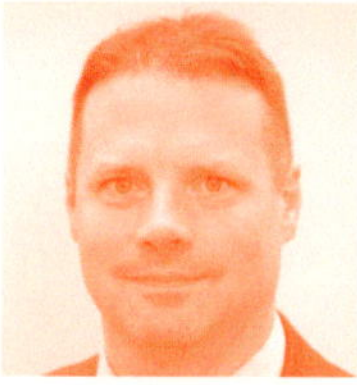

Since 2015, Professor Dr. Med. Hubertus Himmerich has been a Clinical Senior Lecturer in Eating Disorders at King's College London and a Consultant Psychiatrist on an inpatient ward for patients with eating disorders at the Bethlem Royal Hospital in London, UK. After studying medicine, he received his scientific and clinical training at the Max-Planck-Institute of Psychiatry in Munich and the Universities of Mainz and Marburg, Germany. In 2009 he was appointed Professor for Neurobiology of Affective Disorders at the University of Leipzig, Germany. His scientific focuses include appetite regulation, psychoimmunology and military mental health. He has led and performed national and international scientific projects with researchers from Europe, Australia and North America, and has published more than 150 articles in peer-reviewed scientific journals, books and book chapters.

Contents

Preface

Due to the increasing prevalence of eating disorders and obesity, weight management has become a crucial skill in current medical and psychotherapeutic practice. It requires knowledge of physical, psychological and social factors that influence body weight, clinical experience and the courage to try new therapeutic approaches such as novel diets and innovative psychological therapies, medications, anti-obesity devices or music therapy. This book covers the underpinnings and the pathophysiology of weight-related disorders, their far-reaching consequences and evidence-based as well as experimental therapies.

With great pleasure I have received in-depth, informative and exciting contributions from different disciplines by authors from Germany, India, Indonesia, Iraq, Italy, Perú, Spain, Turkey, the United Kingdom and the United States of America. Thus, I would like to thank all authors for their wonderful chapters and their hard work.

I would also like to thank IntechOpen and specifically Ms. Sandra Maljavac for making this scientific book project possible.

Hubertus Himmerich
Department of Psychological Medicine,
King's College London,
London, UK

Section 1

Etiological and Diagnostic Aspects of Weight-Related Disorders

Chapter 1

Risk and Maintenance Factors for Eating Disorders: An Exploration of Multivariate Models on Clinical and Non-Clinical Populations

Stefania Cella, Mara Iannaccone, Annarosa Cipriano and Paolo Cotrufo

Abstract

The recognition of factors involved in the development and maintenance of eating disorders (EDs) may support the choice of therapeutic strategies and improve the prevention/treatment of eating pathologies and their outcomes. Based on this consideration, the overall purpose of the chapter is to investigate how some psychological characteristics link to EDs. It is organized as follows. First, the epidemiological aspects, risk, and maintaining factors for ED are outlined. Next, we present the findings from our two studies. The purpose of the first study was to identify predictors associated with the severity of eating symptomatology. Then, the objective of the second study was to provide an understanding of the relationship among perceived parental bonding, self-esteem, perfectionism, body shame, body mass index, and ED risk and mainly to test a predictive ED risk model in a non-clinical sample. In conclusion, the major findings and practical implications are discussed.

Keywords: perceived parental bonding, self-esteem, perfectionism, body shame, body mass index, eating disorders, risk factors

1. Eating disorder risk and maintaining factors: an overview

Eating disorders (EDs) are highly prevalent psychological conditions characterized by abnormal eating behaviors that may lead to serious health problems and even cause death [1]. The existing diagnostic classifications of EDs include anorexia nervosa (AN), bulimia nervosa (BN), eating disorders not otherwise specified (EDNOS), avoidant/restrictive food intake disorder (ARFID), pica and rumination disorder. Additionally, the Diagnostic and Statistical Manual of Mental Disorders-5 (DSM-5) [2] supports binge eating disorder (BED) as a correct diagnosis on par with AN and BN.

In the framework of the European Study of the Epidemiology of Mental Disorders (ESEMeD) project, a lifetime prevalence rate of 0.93% for AN, 0.88% for BN, and 1.92% for BED have been found for females [3]. In a large population-based survey in the United States, Hudson and colleagues [4] have reported a lifetime prevalence of 0.9, 1.5, and 3.5% for AN, BN, and BED, respectively. More recently, a national survey has found a lifetime prevalence of DSM-5 defined AN, BN, and

BED of 0.80, 0.28, and 0.85%, respectively. Individuals with lifetime BED were found to have a later age of onset of ED and longer ED episodes duration [5].

Even though eating pathologies have been traditionally associated with females [6], males are also at risk for developing EDs [7, 8]. It was estimated that approximately 14% of AN [9], 10–15% of BN [10], and 40% of BED cases [11] were men. Prevalence rates of 0.3, 0.5, and 2.0% were found for AN, BN, and BED among men, who also accounted for approximately 25% of all EDs cases [4]. However, several studies have pointed out an upward trend in EDs prevalence rates among males [12–13]. Furthermore, empirical research shows that, in males, homosexual orientation is associated with higher body dissatisfaction and abnormal eating behaviors [14].

Adolescence to young adulthood is the peak risk period of onset for EDs symptomatology [15]. A recent longitudinal study, for instance, showed increases in weight preoccupation, body dissatisfaction, and bulimic behaviors from 11 to 25 years [16]. The Growing Up Today Study found that binge eating increased with age and peaked in late adolescence [17]. More generally, several authors have reported the presence of body dissatisfaction and drive for thinness even in children aged between 5 and 11 [18, 19] and have demonstrated that weight concerns, body dissatisfaction, and weight status increase with age [20, 21].

Some studies have found that the levels of EDs are highest in younger individuals [22]. Women with EDs with later age of onset (>25 years) might report less severe eating symptomatology compared with women with the typical age of onset (<25 years) [23].

In terms of the ED occurrence, several variables have been suggested as possible predisposing factors for these pathologies. In this section, we review some of the known risks and maintaining factors for the development of eating disturbances.

1.1 Parental bonding

It has long been recognized that family factors are essential features in the development, maintenance, and therapeutic outcome of EDs.

Selvini Palazzoli [24] was one of the first authors who observed some typical patterns in ED families functioning, such as an overprotective relationship with mother and a distant relationship with father.

Similarly, psychosomatic family model [25] suggested that a family environment characterized by enmeshment, overprotectiveness, and rigidity plays a key role in the etiology of AN. On the other hand, insecure attachment patterns were found to be prevalent in ED patients [26].

Overall, empirical evidence on parental bonding—generally assessed by the Parental Bonding Instrument [27]—highlights the importance of low paternal care and high maternal overprotection in the occurrence of ED symptomology in both clinical and non-clinical samples [28, 29]. Parental care refers to a continuum of behaviors ranging from affection and warmth to coldness and rejection. In contrast, parental protectiveness exists along a continuum that ranges from behaviors indicating encouragement of autonomy/independence as opposed to strict control with regulations and intrusiveness [27].

Yet, up till now, few studies have investigated whether parental bonding might be correlated with the severity of disordered eating symptoms. Among ED patients, high parental overprotection is associated with suicidal behavior [30]. Body image disturbances, considered as one of the major clinical features of eating pathology [31], resulted in being predicted by low parental care and high parental overprotection [29, 32].

In the study by Canetti and colleagues [33], anorexic participants reported perceiving both parents as less caring and fathers as more controlling than control group participants; moreover, maternal control and paternal care were associated with higher symptom severity. A recent cross-sectional study has shown that the quality of the father-daughter relationship (i.e., overprotective and avoidant) plays a critical role in understanding the ED onset and maintenance [29].

Similar findings were reported by Rienecke and colleagues [34], the presence of paternal criticism—and not maternal—showed a significant predictive power for less psychological improvement in ED psychopathology at the end of family-based treatment for adolescents AN.

Overall, the overprotective behavior of the parents might be a result of the ED and often starts as a consequence of the disorder [35]. Researchers suggest that eating pathology may influence family dynamics and environment, which in turn may unconsciously affect ED symptoms maintenance and evolution [36].

In terms of the psychological dynamics underlying the association between parental bonding and eating pathologies, several researchers have suggested the existence of potential mediating mechanisms involved in such association. Turner and colleagues [37], for instance, reported that paternal care and maternal overprotection had an indirect effect on ED symptoms through the mediating effect of maladaptive core beliefs (i.e., schemas related to defectiveness/shame and dependence/incompetence).

Likewise, maladaptive perfectionism was found to mediate the pathway from parental psychological control and ED patterns [38]. In our previous study [28], on a large sample of adolescents, the link between the parental bonding pattern typified by low paternal care/maternal overprotection and dysfunctional eating attitudes were found to be mediated by self-concept. Our data were consistent with the study of Perry and colleagues [39] in which a parental bonding pattern characterized by low care and over-protection affected self-concept formation, which, in turn, affected eating psychopathologies in adulthood.

1.2 Self-esteem

The literature on EDs shows that a patient's self-concept is fundamentally characterized by low self-esteem, which is considered a critical vulnerability factor in the development of these diseases [40]. In a review focusing on causes of EDs, low self-esteem is one of the prominent features strongly implicated in the onset of the pathology [41].

In a series of interesting papers exploring the self-esteem dimensions, Geller and colleagues found that shape- and weight-based self-esteem and intimate relationship-based self-esteem were related to higher ED symptoms [42, 43].

It seems that white women are most at risk for having low self-esteem and difficulty with eating problems [44]. Still, several studies have shown that an impoverished sense of self is an essential contributor to ED symptomatology [45], and it is correlated with a negative treatment outcome [46]. Similarly, in a study carried out by Brechan and Kvalem [47], the effect of body dissatisfaction on restrained eating, binge eating, and compensatory behavior was completely mediated by self-esteem.

However, some studies do not support the existence of a direct relationship between low self-esteem and eating pathology. In some studies, self-esteem did not emerge as a significant predictor of disordered eating [48, 49]. Moreover, some researchers suggest that future studies should focus on a more informative multifaceted construct of self-esteem [50] and investigate interactive effects with other predisposing factors for a better understanding of the link between self-esteem and eating problems [45]. In this regard, self-esteem has been suggested to predict disordered eating via body shame [51], also among obese youth [52]. A study by Goossens and colleagues [53] provided evidence for the hypothesis that an insecure relationship with parents may act as a mediating variable in the pathway from self-esteem and dysfunctional eating patterns.

1.3 Perfectionsim

Perfectionism is a personality trait that is characterized by setting excessively high personal standards of performance [54]. Frost and colleagues [54] viewed perfectionism as being constituted of adaptive (healthy) and maladaptive (dysfunctional) perfectionism.

In a cross-sectional research designed to explore perfectionism across different stages of EDs recovery, ED patients scored significantly higher than healthy controls on the maladaptive perfectionism factor [55]. Further studies have reported that elevated levels of both adaptive and maladaptive perfectionism are strongly associated with body dissatisfaction [56] and ED psychopathology [57–59], including BN [60]. A percentage of about 40% of AN patients (Mage = 15.3 years) have a very high score on self-oriented perfectionism and perfectionistic self-presentation. The authors concluded that in this subgroup of patients, it would be necessary to address these psychological characteristics to achieve a good outcome [61]. Several studies have highlighted that a higher level of perfectionism might be detrimental for disease duration and prognoses [62, 63], also among children and adolescents with EDs [64, 65]. Previous studies have shown that perfectionism predicts ED onset and maintaining [66]. Similarly, an experimental study has suggested that perfectionism represents a causal risk factor for ED pathology [67]. On the other hand, these findings are not systematically replicated in other studies: perfectionism—adaptive and maladaptive types—does not emerge as a risk factor for eating disturbances [68, 69], and the specific mechanism by which perfectionism uses its influence on eating psychopathology has, up till now, to be recognized.

In this regard, Bardone-Cone and colleagues [58] have reported that the investigation of mediating pathways from perfectionism to ED pathology was mostly absent from the literature. How perfectionism related to the EDs risk factors and potential mediating variables affecting the relationship between perfectionism and disordered eating remain mostly unknown.

Several studies support the association between low self-esteem, perfectionism, and varying degrees of ED patterns [70], "Indeed, the combination of low self-esteem and perfectionism is not unusual among those who binge, and especially those with BN, AN, or an atypical ED, and it may well contribute to the development of the problem" ([71], p. 65). Still, "as he was nearing the end of his life, Michelangelo began working on what many people believe to be his most important work, the Florentine Pietà. After working intensely for almost a decade, he entered his studio one day and took a sledgehammer to the sculpture. He broke away the hands and legs and nearly shattered the work before his assistants dragged him away. Why did Michelangelo attempt to destroy one of his greatest creations, a statue that has been described as among the finest works of the Renaissance? Disillusioned and isolated in the last decades of his life, Michelangelo had a heightened sense of perfectionism that was exarcebed by his failure to live up to the exceptions of his father, who viewed being a sculptor as akin to begin a manual laborer. Michelangelo, it seems, had self-esteem issues" ([72], p. 158).

Literature supports the hypothesis that a combination of low perception of control and low self-esteem moderates the effects of perfectionism on drive for thinness, BN, and body [73].

In conclusion, as previously suggested [74], the role of perfectionism in the etiology and maintenance of EDs remains unclear.

1.4 Body shame

Eating pathologies have been described as "disorders of shame" [75]. A positive relationship between shame and eating pathology has been found [76, 77].

However, several studies have concentrated upon shame explicitly associated with the body rather than to general shame.

Body shame is the shame one feels about one's body or any part of it [78]. Moreover, body shame can also relate to how one's body functions [79], and it represents a better concept than "body dissatisfaction" in work with EDs [80].

Body shame is a strong predictor of disordered eating [81, 82].

In a longitudinal study designed to explore the role of body shame and general shame in predicting increases in eating symptoms over 2.5 years in a sample of women with a past or current ED, body shame exclusively predicted an increase in AN symptoms [83]. Dorian and colleagues [84] have found that body shame is uniquely predictive of eating disturbance in a female clinical sample and in a male non-clinical sample. However, both body and characterological shame predicted eating psychopathology in a non-clinical female sample. In sum, body shame would seem to have a causal role in the ED onset.

In addition, the severity of ED symptomatology has been linked to feelings of bodily shame in the eating context [81, 85]. Troop and colleagues [83], for instance, found that shame was uniquely associated with the severity of both AN and BN symptoms. Goss and Gilbert [79] proposed a model based on the functional role of eating disordered beliefs and behaviors in the management of shame. The authors offered a model process based on risk factors (i.e., genetic factors, personality, early attachment history, abuse or rejection experiences, and cultural factors) that might predispose people to develop both shame proneness and ED proneness. These factors cause shame, and to defend themselves against adverse social outcomes, individuals may attempt to change their body shape and weight. Then, they may feel around in their ability to manage their weight, but when they are not able to do so, they feel further shame. This leads to a shame-pride circle that maintains the pathology.

Overall, shame can be described both as cause and consequence of symptoms in eating pathology [80]. Unfortunately, there are few findings about body shame, and much is unknown about how it operates in ED development. Literature supports the suggestion that body shame may act as a mediator in the relationship between self-esteem and disordered eating [51].

Regarding the determinants of body shame, some research has provided evidence associating poor perceived parenting and subsequent shame [86]. The perception of low parental care and high parental protectiveness in childhood was found to be related to shame in young adulthood [87]. Murray and colleagues [88] suggested that dysfunctional parenting practices may lead to individuals' feelings of inadequacy and worthlessness, so it might be clinically essential to examine the psychological consequences of such a family experience, such as shame. Specifically, the authors found that paternal overprotection was related to bulimic symptoms through the mediation effect of shame. On the other hand, it has been shown that parenting practices failed to predict the vulnerability to body image shame, directly or indirectly. In a study examining the determinants of body shame, Markham and colleagues [89] found that body-image esteem, global self-worth, appearance comparison, and internalization of the thin ideal accounted for 62% of the variance in body-image shame.

1.5 Body mass index

It would seem that the body mass index (BMI) plays a more critical role in promoting the risk factors for EDs than indirectly maintaining eating pathology [90].

Obese individuals are at higher risk for developing an eating pathology [91]. Indeed, a low BMI represents a protective factor against the development of disturbed eating in adolescent girls [92, 93]. Moreover, BMI in childhood is a significant predictor of restrained eating in early adolescence [94].

BMI at admission can be considered as a significant predictor of outcome in AN [95]. The link between BMI and mortality in BN has also been investigated. Severe BN patients may be at higher risk of death, especially if suicide has been attempted previously or in case of a low minimum BMI at admission [96].

In terms of the underlying mechanisms that linked BMI and eating psychopathology, in a study by Fan and colleagues [97], BMI was not found to have a direct influence on ED symptoms, and the authors concluded that weight control concerns and behaviors could mediate this relationship. To answer the question of what causes a high BMI, risk factors for obesity included parental fatness—although only a few longitudinal studies have investigated the parent-child fatness association—social factors, birth weight, timing or rate of maturation, physical activity, dietary factors, and other behavioral and psychological factors [98, 99].

Parental overweight is one of the main predictors for the development of childhood overweight and obesity [100], but parents can influence child body weight through specific feeding behaviors and practices, such as restriction, pressure to eat, and monitoring [101, 102], or more broadly through their general parental attitudes and style of interacting with children (for a review, see [103]). In a study about the influence of parental care in childhood on the risk of obesity in young adulthood, parental neglect was found to significantly affect the risk of adult obesity, independent of age and body mass index in childhood, sex, and social background. Instead, receiving overprotective parental support did not affect [104].

In terms of the psychological dynamics underlying parental-child relationship, possible mediating factors are considered. Overall, a growing body of research has focused on maternal sensitivity and emotion regulation. A poor quality of the early maternal-child relationship, characterized by low levels of maternal sensitivity, may be linked to childhood overweight and obesity through the development of potential difficulties in children's ability to regulate emotions [105]. In this regard, emotion dysregulation in early childhood is implicated in the development of obesity in early adolescence [106]. Similarly, empirical research suggested that authoritarian parenting (high control and low levels of emotionally responsiveness) may influence children's self-regulation skills [107] and, in turn, to be positively associated with child weight status [108, 109]. A longitudinal study showed that more inadequate maternal emotional regulation abilities during pregnancy were able to predict, at 7 months of age of the baby, the quality of the early mother-child feeding patterns [110], and the body mass index of the child at three years of age [111].

1.6 Multivariate etiologic models

Most of the studies about the ED onset have focused on the risk factors unconnectedly, precluding understanding about interactive effects.

In one of the few research in this area studies, Bardone-Cone and colleagues [112] found that perfectionism, body dissatisfaction, and self-esteem interact to predict bulimic symptoms. Specifically, women who perceived themselves to be overweight and who had elevated levels of perfectionism and lower levels of self-esteem were most at risk for bulimic symptoms. However, this interactive model has received mixed support [113–115], for example, it has been considered valid concerning maintenance and exacerbation, but not with the onset of bulimic symptoms [116]. Expanding the model to EDs patients under psychotherapy treatment, Watson and colleagues [74] found that binge eating and purging were not significantly predicted by the three-way interaction term neither in concurrent nor in prospective analyses (i.e., examined as a moderator of treatment outcome). The authors concluded raising concerns about the robustness of the three-way model. Otherwise, it could have been affected by an inadequate conceptualization of the perfectionism construct.

A study by Ghaderi [117] suggested that a combination of low self-esteem, high body concern, low perceived support from the family, and more relative use of escape avoidance coping constitute a risk profile that later would lead to the development of ED. However, the author did not investigate if and how the predictor variables interact with each other in explaining ED onset.

In terms of the mechanism that perpetuates EDs, according to the cognitive-behavioral theory of the maintenance of BN [118], a dysfunctional system for evaluating self-worth is central to the continuation of the pathology. People with eating disturbances judge themselves principally based on their eating behaviors, shape, or weight and their ability to control them. Most of the other clinical features can be considered as stemming directly from this overvaluation of eating, shape, and weight that represents the "core of psychopathology". This original theory of continuance on BN could embrace four additional maintaining mechanisms, which concern the influence of clinical perfectionism, low core self-esteem, mood intolerance, and interpersonal difficulties. However, a common mechanism is involved in the persistence of BN, AN, and the atypical EDs resulting in the transdiagnostic theory of the maintenance of the full range of eating disturbances [119]. Moving from this theory, Lampard and colleagues [120] concluded that a mixture of factors (i.e., transdiagnostic and disorder-specific) might be involved in the maintaining mechanism of ED disorder symptomatology. The transdiagnostic model of EDs might be applied to improve our understanding of muscle dysmorphia, additionally to eating psychopathology [121].

2. Identifying predictors associated with the severity of eating concerns in females with eating disorders

Investigating factors that contribute to the onset and development of EDs has been the focus of previous studies. Several variables have been suggested as possible predisposing and perpetuating factors for EDs pathologies: perceived parental bonding, self-esteem, perfectionism, and body shame are among the factors that have been investigated separately. However, studies explicitly evaluating different predictors associated with the risk and severity of eating symptoms are limited in the literature [122, 123].

Based on this consideration, we have conducted a study [124] to identify predictors associated with the severity of disordered eating symptomatology. Identifying which of the individual variables (self-esteem, perceived parental care and protectiveness, body shame, and perfectionism) significantly predicted the severity of eating symptomatology for ED patients was the main research question that has driven our work.

The study was approved by the ethics committee of the Faculty of Psychology (University of Campania "Luigi Vanvitelli").

We gathered data from inpatients and outpatients referred to specialized residential ED treatment units in Northern, Central, and Southern Italy. At intake, a clinical interview was administered by ED clinicians for the assessment of diagnosis. All participants had a primary ED diagnosis DSM-IV [125]. Participants were tested at early stages—in order to avoid strong treatment effects—and at variables points during the treatment.

We screened 80 female eating disordered patients aged 13–40 years old through the self-report measures of parental behavior, self-esteem, perfectionism, body shame, and ED risk.

It is worth noting that the comparisons between AN, BN, and BED patients on the study variables highlighted only a few statistically significant differences. Based on these findings, patients who fall below the different diagnostic categories for eating disturbances seem to share several psychological characteristics. However, results indicate that greater severity of the eating symptomatology could be related to the diagnosis of BN. In our opinion, these results seem to further support the hypothesis of a shared psychopathological core of EDs, and BN could be regarded as a "failed" AN [126, 127]. Future treatment research should broaden the clinical understanding of this suggestion.

In line with empirical research, maladaptive perfectionism was found to be strongly linked to eating concerns, followed by body shame and low self-esteem. On the other hand, differently from previous studies, parental care and protectiveness were not related to the level of eating symptomatology. Linear regression analysis, as displayed in **Table 1**, demonstrated that maladaptive perfectionism ($p < 0.001$), body shame ($p < 0.05$), and self-esteem ($p < 0.05$), significantly predicted ED symptom severity, and explained a significant proportion of variance in ED symptomatology (adjusted $R^2 = 0.450$).

While both adaptive and maladaptive perfectionism were found to be correlated to EDs symptomatology, only maladaptive perfectionism was significantly and positively associated with eating concerns. These findings seem to support recent studies pointing out the role of maladaptive perfectionism—but not adaptive—in the prediction of eating symptomatology [57]. However, this datum could be due to an inadequate assessment of the adaptive perfectionism. Future studies should look at perfectionism as a multidimensional construct and further investigate the specificity of both functional and dysfunctional perfectionism contribution and their interplay with ED maintenance.

In line with previous findings [84], shame about the body emerged as a significant predictor of the level of eating concerns. However, research is needed because few studies have investigated the role of shame in ED maintenance, and further investigation might examine other forms of shame (specific and generalized).

Interestingly, these results seem to contradict the findings of previous research [49], and suggest that low self-esteem is a strong predictor of ED symptomatology. In this sense, low self-esteem consistently emerges as one of the core features of ED pathology.

Model	B	Standard error	β	*T*	P	R^2	Adjusted R^2	*F*
1. Maladaptive Perfectionism (constant)	4.608 .615	9.884 .109	.538	4.666 5.642	.642 .000	.290	.281	31.838
2. Maladaptive Perfectionism (constant)	−19.382 .491	11.081 .106	.430	−1.749 4.651	.084 .000	.403	.387	25.961
Bodily Shame	2.629	.689	.353	3.815	.000			
3. Maladaptive Perfectionism (constant)	9.059 .389	13.892 .105	.341	.652 3.696	.516 .000	.471	.450	22.537
Bodily Shame	2.173	.669		3.248	.002			
Self-Esteem	-1.106	.354		-3.126	.003			

Table 1.
Stepwise regression model and statistics for dependent variable [124].

Unexpectedly, perceived parental care and protectiveness were not found being associated with the level of eating concerns. In contrast with ED literature, these findings might be due to cultural differences. Furthermore, it is possible that perceived parental bonding might participate in promoting the risk factors for eating pathology rather than indirectly maintaining the disturbance. It would be interesting to clarify this question.

In our opinion, it is helpful to recognize psychological variables significant for considerations in the treatment of these patients. Identifying potential predisposing and maintaining factors may enhance our understanding of ED symptomatology and support the choice of targeted therapeutic strategies to improve ED treatments and outcomes. Specific attention should be paid to helping ED patients to improve overall self-esteem. In addition, the treatment of maladaptive perfectionism and body shame might help in reducing ED symptomatology.

In conclusion, our findings stress the need to investigate these factors further as they might represent negative prognostic factors.

3. Structural equation modeling of possible risk factors for eating disorder onset in female and male adolescents

Given the limited number of studies evaluating multivariate models explaining ED risk, research intended to fill this empirical gap was undertaken. Specifically, we have conducted a study [128] to assess the relationships among perceived parental bonding, self-esteem, maladaptive and adaptive perfectionism, body shame, body mass index, and ED risk with structural equation modeling. Several predictions were advanced concerning these potentially contributing factors. We hypothesized that perceived parental bonding, self-esteem, perfectionism, and BMI do not have a direct effect on ED risk. In our opinion, one potential mean by which these variables are related to ED vulnerability is through their effects on body shame.

Obtaining a clearer picture of how ED relates to these variables could result in an enhanced understanding of the mechanism through which such factors may lead to eating pathology.

This research was conducted on a sample of 1156 high school students—males and females—who ranged in age from 13 to 20 years. Participants were screened through self-report measures of parental behavior, self-esteem, perfectionism, body shame, and ED risk. The height and weight of each individual were measured. This age group was chosen as this cohort is at the most significant risk for eating disturbances, with ED incidences peaking during adolescence to early adulthood [129].

The study received the institutional review board approval.

The results only partially supported the hypothesized model (**Figure 1**), and several interesting findings emerged.

Several studies have documented an association between a bonding behavior pattern characterized by low care and high protectiveness and eating symptomatology [130, 131]. In line with previous empirical research [36], the model tested showed that poor parental care does not have a direct effect on ED risk, but it has a significant indirect effect through low self-esteem. Parental care has also an indirect effect on ED risk through the mediational effect of the BMI. Thus, perceiving neglectful parents may put adolescents at risk of developing obesity and eating problems.

Bearing in mind this suggestion, it seems reasonable that a high BMI is predicted by low parental care, but not parental protectiveness.

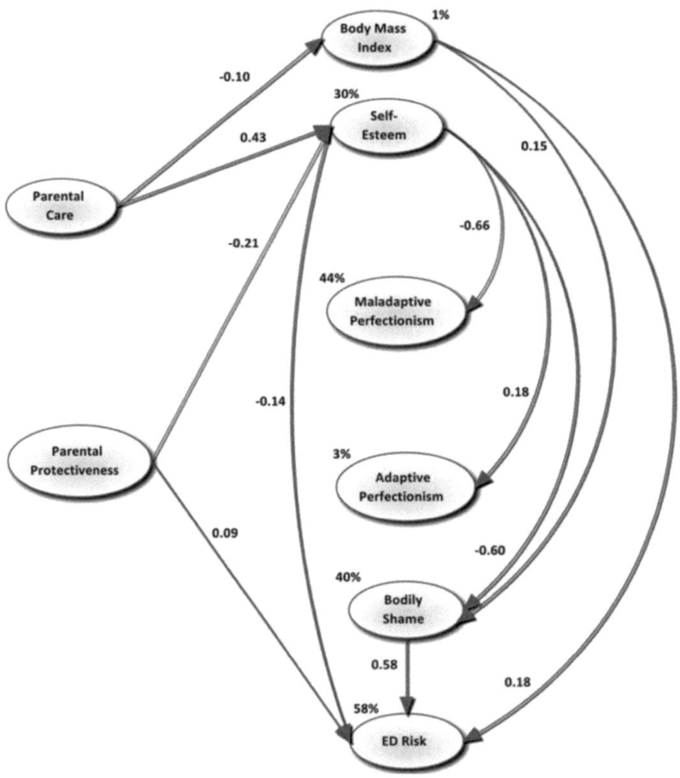

Figure 1.
Illustration of the final model with standardized path coefficients and percentage of variance explained [128].

Speculatively, it could be hypothesized that the relationship between parental overprotectiveness and ED risk might be mediated by the existence of other intervening variables, such as interoceptive awareness.

In this regard, parental protectiveness could not allow individuals to develop a sense of personal needs, altering their interoceptive awareness and, consequently, their eating behavior. Future empirical studies should investigate this suggestion.

Consistent with our hypothesis, parental protectiveness did have both direct and indirect effects—via low self-esteem—on ED risk, as previously suggested [39]. These findings are consistent with research that converges on the role of psychological control (i.e., parental protectiveness) in ED proneness. As such, this finding suggests that overprotectiveness may be more directly relevant to eating disturbance development. Research should further explore this datum and examine the unique contribution of each parent in the etiology of eating pathologies.

Results showed that self-esteem has a direct effect on both maladaptive and adaptive perfectionism. Specifically, the linkage between low self-esteem and maladaptive perfectionism was particularly strong. These findings offer further support to previous studies suggesting that striving to appear perfect is an attempt to compensate for low self-esteem [132]. Individuals with an ED may interpret their mistakes as evidence of personal deficiencies [133]. In this perspective, to be flawless represents an obligation.

Moreover, even if indirectly via self-esteem, a link between parental bonding and perfectionist orientation emerged. This datum partially supports the findings of Soenens and colleagues [38] who have evidenced a relationship between parental psychological control and maladaptive perfectionism.

Contrary to the initial hypothesis, parental care and protectiveness were not found as significant predictors of body shame. This agrees with findings from other researchers [89]. One potential explanation may be that parental bonding exerts an indirect influence on body shame via self-esteem and BMI. Indeed, as predicted, both low self-esteem and BMI emerged as significant predictors of increased vulnerability to body shame. In this regard, low self-esteem may be regarded as a source of body shame. People who perceive themselves as inadequate or unworthy may be at the most significant risk of experiencing body shame [89].

Model results showed that perfectionism did not predict body shame, contrary to our initial hypothesis. However, the non-significant pathway from both maladaptive and adaptive perfectionism to ED risk offers further support, alongside other studies [68], that these variables may not be vulnerability factors for eating disturbances.

Due to its association with self-esteem, perfectionism could be regarded as a psychological characteristic typically associated with eating disturbances, rather than a risk factor for EDs. However, future research is needed to investigate variables that may intervene in the pathway from perfectionism to ED risk.

In line with previous studies [51], body shame emerged as a mediator in the relationship between self-esteem and ED vulnerability—explaining 71% of the variance. Notwithstanding, self-esteem has also a direct influence on ED. These results further corroborate previous studies recognizing low self-esteem as a critical predictor of ED vulnerability [40, 41].

Although body shame partially mediated the relationship between BMI and eating disturbance vulnerability, BMI had also a positive effect on ED risk. Undeniably, a high BMI has long been considered as a strong ED risk factor [91]. Our results support findings of previous studies [82, 83] suggesting that the experience of shame related to one's body exerts a strong influence on eating disturbances vulnerability. Yet our results suggest that in addition to a direct effect, body shame also serves as a mediator between other risk factors and eating disturbance risk. In this regard, body shame may be a key variable in the pathway to eating disturbances risk and a core diagnostic feature of all eating disturbances. Notwithstanding, only a few studies have investigated the role of body shame in ED onset. Further studies on this construct would be beneficial.

Finally, the evaluation of measurement invariance allowed to conclude that the final model was invariant across gender: no gender differences emerged in the hypothesized pathway to ED risk. Therefore, our study suggests that adopting the same prevention and treatment programs for both males and females may be appropriate.

In conclusion, we extend the work of others who have separately examined the role of perceived parental bonding, self-esteem, body mass index, perfectionism, and shame in EDs, identifying the possible mechanisms through which these variables increase the likelihood of eating problem development.

This is the first study that conceptualizes how several risk factors may work together to create a pathway to eating pathologies. Collectively, perceived parental care and protectiveness, self-esteem, maladaptive and adaptive perfectionism, body shame, and BMI account for 58% of the variance in ED risk. Therefore, these initial findings suggest a promising model.

Provided that the present findings can be replicated longitudinally, they have noteworthy implications for EDs prevention and treatment. Identifying which interpersonal characteristics and personal factors are most relevant in the etiology of EDs may help mental health professionals designing targeted prevention and/or intervention programs during adolescence. Clinicians should consider the routine assessment and treatment of these factors. First and foremost, intervention programs ought to be addressed to reduce subjective feelings of ineffectiveness and shame. Particular attention should be paid to obese youth.

4. Conclusions

Among psychiatric illnesses, EDs have the highest rate of mortality [1], and early detection of cases is essential. Several researchers have investigated the factors that lead to these pathologies in the hope that this information would help in the design of more efficient programs of prevention and treatment. However, few studies have been devoted to understanding how these risk factors work in concert to promote eating disturbance development. A psychological model of risk factors for developing eating pathologies in female and male adolescents was validated in our study [128]. From this model, we can conclude that several ED risk factors are linked among them and occur together to cause the eating disturbance opening up the possibility of translating these findings into a form of intervention.

Notably, a potential mechanism for eating problem onset has been identified.

Overprotective parents often anticipate the physical needs of their children and compromise, albeit unconsciously, their ability to recognize their own need and their autonomy. The perception of parental hyper-involvement and lack of sufficient caring may produce a feeling of ineffectiveness and an impoverished self, which, in our opinion, maybe the root of eating psychopathologies. It would seem that the sense of ineffectiveness that these individuals feel toward themselves has been moved in their bodies through a defense mechanism that works by substituting the object of a painful or dangerous feeling with an acceptable object. Such a mechanism would produce body shame: "I am not inadequate, but my body is". In Freudian psychology, this unconscious mechanism of defense is called displacement [134]. From that perspective, EDs could be an attempt to modify and/or to punish the ashamed body, which has been considered responsible for an individual's ineffectiveness. The body becomes the stage of the illness. This potential mechanism of action (parental overprotectiveness/low care → low self-esteem → body shame → eating pathology) might work in both obese and normal-weight adolescents, but among obese people, this would occur more often because it comes more natural to consider a fat body responsible for the sense of ineffectiveness [52]. In that respect, a person with a high BMI would be at greater risk of developing an ED than others.

This investigation presents a unique contribution to the literature by illustrating a promise predictive ED risk model. However, it is not possible to use the present data to argue for specific casual links, and more research is needed to validate these hopeful results.

Understanding the potential causes of eating problems would permit us to formulate aids in planning prevention/treatment. This etiological model for eating pathology onset could be transformed into a model for early and preventive interventions. Prevention programs that specifically target risk factors may be of benefit. However, the practical utility and clinical significance of this model ought to be examined in prevention studies.

As well, understanding possible psychopathological maintenance mechanism present enormous potential for eating disturbance treatment. Another goal was to determine the relationship of well knows ED risk factors with the severity of eating symptomatology. More specifically, we carry out a study aimed at examining whether BMI, perceived parental care and protectiveness, self-esteem, body shame, and perfectionism (adaptive and maladaptive) provide more information about the level of eating concerns among ED patients [124]. The small size of the sample limited this study: consequently, the structural equation model test could not be used for the clinical population. Overall, our results suggest that maladaptive perfectionism, body shame, and low self-esteem may represent an obstruction for successful treatment, and consequently, it ought to be targeted in psychotherapy. Particular attention should be paid to people with high BMI because they may present more severe eating symptomatology. To sum up, the current results propose the necessity to consider these potential maintaining factors when designing treatment for this population.

The non-significant pathway from perfectionism to ED risk among non-clinical people seems to suggest that maladaptive perfectionism might represent a perpetuating factor in the ED maintenance exclusively. Perfectionism may correspond to a psychological correlate of the low self-esteem resulted from the need to compensate for a feeling of inadequacy as well as to a factor that makes the individuals more tenacious in achieving their own goal such as diet. In this perspective, perfectionism may be more substantially associated with AN.

On the other hand, parental bonding may play a key role in promoting the predisposing factors for eating pathologies rather than indirectly maintaining the pathology. As previously stated, parental bonding may create a vulnerability to eating disturbances principally through the development of a poor self-concept. The association between low self-esteem and eating disturbance development has been confirmed in our studies. By the potential mechanism of action described above, low self-esteem may represent the root of eating psychopathology and have a fundamental role in the onset as well as in the maintenance of the disorder.

The possible role of BMI in the beginning of EDs has also been established. It is known that obese people are more at risk of developing an ED. In our opinion, this might happen because obese individuals are more likely to move in their bodies the sense of ineffectiveness that they feel toward themselves, and this potential mechanism could also fuel the continuance of the pathology.

Finally, one of the strengths of these two studies includes the unique nature in investigating the role of body shame in EDs, a previously under-researched construct. Our data highlight the potential role of body shame as a critical variable in both ED onset and maintenance and as a core diagnostic feature of all eating disturbances. Further research is needed, but the preliminary results prove promising for application in a clinical setting.

Even though the current results contribute to valuable novel insights into EDs risk factors model, a large body of research proposes a biological model suggesting that genetic, immunological and metabolic aspects contribute to the development of EDs as well (for a review, see [135, 136]).

In conclusion, we focused on psychological risk factors that are important for the development and the maintenance of EDs. To differentiate between those predisposing, precipitating and perpetuating factors might help to develop more successful strategies for the prevention and treatment of these disorders.

Author details

Stefania Cella*, Mara Iannaccone, Annarosa Cipriano and Paolo Cotrufo
Observatory on Eating Disorders, Department of Psychology, University of Campania "Luigi Vanvitelli", Caserta, Italy

*Address all correspondence to: stefania.cella@unicampania.it

IntechOpen

© 2020 The Author(s). Licensee IntechOpen. This chapter is distributed under the terms of the Creative Commons Attribution License (http://creativecommons.org/licenses/by/3.0), which permits unrestricted use, distribution, and reproduction in any medium, provided the original work is properly cited.

References

[1] Arcelus J, Mitchell AJ, Wales J, Nielsen S. Mortality rates in patients with anorexia nervosa and other eating disorders: A meta-analysis of 36 studies. Archives of General Psychiatry. 2011;**68**(7):724-731. DOI: 10.1001/archgenpsychiatry.2011.74

[2] American Psychiatric Association. Diagnostic and Statistical Manual of Mental Disorders. 5th ed. Washington, DC: APA Press; 2013

[3] Preti A, de Girolamo G, Vilagut G, Alonso J, de Graaf R, Bruffaerts R, et al. The epidemiology of eating disorders in six European countries: Results of the ESEMeD-WMH project. Journal of Psychiatric Research. 2009;**43**(14):1125-1132. DOI: 10.1016/j.jpsychires.2009.04.003

[4] Hudson JI, Hiripi E, Pope HG, Kessler RC. The prevalence and correlates of eating disorders in the national comorbidity survey replication. Biological Psychiatry. 2007;**61**(3):348-358. DOI: 10.1016/j.biopsych.2006.03.040

[5] Udo T, Grilo CM. Prevalence and correlates of DSM-5-defined eating disorders in a nationally representative sample of U.S. adults. Biological Psychiatry. 2018;**84**(5):345-354. DOI: 10.1016/j.biopsych.2018.03.014

[6] Bruch H. Eating Disorders: Anorexia Nervosa, Obesity, and The Person Within. New York: Basic Books; 1973. p. 396

[7] Lipson SK, Sonneville KR. Eating disorder symptoms among undergraduate and graduate students at 12 U.S. colleges and universities. Eating Behaviors. 2017;**24**:81-88. DOI: 10.1016/j.eatbeh.2016.12.003

[8] Limbers CA, Cohen LA, Gray BA. Eating disorders in adolescent and young adult males: Prevalence, diagnosis, and treatment strategies. Adolescent Health, Medicine and Therapeutics. 2018;**9**:111-116. DOI: 10.2147/ahmt.s147480

[9] Hay P, Girosi F, Mond J. Prevalence and sociodemographic correlates of DSM-5 eating disorders in the Australian population. Journal of Eating Disorders. 2015;**3**(1):19. DOI: 10.1186/s40337-015-0056-0

[10] Carlat DJ, Camargo CA, Herzog DB. Eating disorders in males: A report on 135 patients. The American Journal of Psychiatry. 1997;**154**(8):1127-1132. DOI: 10.1176/ajp.154.8.1127

[11] Muise AM, Stein DG, Arbess G. Eating disorders in adolescent boys: A review of the adolescent and young adult literature. Journal of Adolescent Health. 2003;**33**:427-435. DOI: 10.1016/S1054-139X(03)00060-0

[12] Kjelsås E, Bjørnstrøm C, Götestam KG. Prevalence of eating disorders in female and male adolescents (14-15 years). Eating Behaviors. 2004;**5**(1):13-25. DOI: 10.1016/S1471-0153(03)00057-6

[13] Strother E, Lemberg R, Stanford SC, Turberville D. Eating disorders in men: Underdiagnosed, undertreated, and misunderstood. Eating Disorders. 2012;**20**(5):346-355. DOI: 10.1080/10640266.2012.715512

[14] Cella S, Iannaccone M, Ascione R, Cotrufo P. Body dissatisfaction, abnormal eating behaviours and eating disorder attitude in homo- and heterosexuals. Eating and Weight Disorders. 2010;**15**(3):e180-e185. DOI: 10.3275/6866

[15] Field AE, Sonneville KR, Micali N, Crosby RD, Swanson SA, Laird NM, et al. Prospective association of common

eating disorders and adverse outcomes. Pediatrics. 2012;**130**(2):e289-e295. DOI: 10.1542/peds.2011-3663

[16] Slane JD, Klump KL, McGue M, Iacono WG. Developmental trajectories of disordered eating from early adolescence to young adulthood: A longitudinal study. The International Journal of Eating Disorders. 2014;**47**(7):793-801. DOI: 10.1002/eat.22329

[17] Sonneville KR, Horton NJ, Micali N, Crosby RD, Swanson SA, Solmi F, et al. Longitudinal associations between binge eating and overeating and adverse outcomes among adolescents and young adults: Does loss of control matter? JAMA Pediatrics. 2013;**167**(2):149-155. DOI: 10.1001/2013.jamapediatrics.12

[18] Dion J, Hains J, Vachon P, Plouffe J, Laberge L, Perron M, et al. Correlates of body dissatisfaction in children. The Journal of Pediatrics. 2016;**171**:202-207. DOI: 10.1016/j.jpeds.2015.12.045

[19] Cotrufo P, Cella S. The possible link between puberty and the eating disorders onset. In: Fuchs JN, editor. Eating Disorders in Adult Women. New York: Nova Publishers; 2008. pp. 39-60

[20] Calzo JP, Sonneville KR, Haines J, Blood EA, Field AE, Austin SB. The development of associations among body mass index, body dissatisfaction, and weight and shape concern in adolescent boys and girls. Journal of Adolescent Health. 2012;**51**(5):517-523. DOI: 10.1016/j.jadohealth.2012.02.021

[21] Davison KK, Markey CN, Birch LL. A longitudinal examination of patterns in girls' weight concerns and body dissatisfaction from ages 5 to 9 years. The International Journal of Eating Disorders. 2003;**33**(3):320-332. DOI: 10.1002/eat.10142

[22] Seepersad R. The relation between eating disorders and self esteem in adolescents in Trinidad. Journal of the Department of Behavioural Sciences. 2012;**2**:102-127

[23] Bueno B, Krug I, Bulik CM, Jiménez-Murcia S, Granero R, Thornton L, et al. Late onset eating disorders in Spain: Clinical characteristics and therapeutic implications. Journal of Clinical Psychology. 2014;**70**(1):1-17. DOI: 10.1002/jclp.22006

[24] Selvini Palazzoli M. L'anoressia Mentale. Feltrinelli: Milano; 1963

[25] Minuchin S, Rosman BL, Baker L. Psychosomatic Families. Anorexia Nervosa in Context. Cambridge: Harvard University Press; 1978

[26] Dakanalis A, Timko CA, Zanetti MA, Rinaldi L, Prunas A, Carrà G, et al. Attachment insecurities, maladaptive perfectionism, and eating disorder symptoms: A latent mediated and moderated structural equation modeling analysis across diagnostic groups. Psychiatry Research. 2014;**215**(1):176-184. DOI: 10.1016/j.psychres.2013.10.039

[27] Parker G, Tupling H, Brown LB. A parental bonding instrument. The British Journal of Medical Psychology. 1979;**52**(1):1-10. DOI: 10.1111/j.2044-8341.1979.tb02487.x

[28] Cella S, Iannaccone M, Cotrufo P. How perceived parental bonding affects self-concept and drive for thinness: A community-based study. Eating Behaviors. 2014;**15**(1):110-115. DOI: 10.1007/s40519-019-00670-3

[29] Horesh N, Sommerfeld E, Wolf M, Zubery E, Zalsman G. Father-daughter relationship and the severity of eating disorders. European Psychiatry. 2015;**30**(1):114-120. DOI: 10.1016/j.eurpsy.2014.04.004

[30] Yamaguchi N, Kobayashi J, Tachikawa H, Sato S, Hori M,

Suzuki T, et al. Parental representation in eating disorder patients with suicide. Journal of Psychosomatic Research. 2000;**49**(2):131-136. DOI: 10.1016/S0022-3999(00)00146-X

[31] Glashouwer KA, Meulman C, de Jong PJ. Negative body image is not related to spontaneous body-scaled motoric behavior in undergraduate women. Frontiers in Psychology. 2019;**10**:580. DOI: 10.3389/fpsyg.2019.00580

[32] Grenon R, Tasca GA, Maxwell H, Balfour L, Proulx G, Bissada H. Parental bonds and body dissatisfaction in a clinical sample: The mediating roles of attachment anxiety and media internalization. Body Image. 2016;**19**:49-56. DOI: 10.1016/j.bodyim.2016.08.005

[33] Canetti L, Kanyas K, Lerer B, Latzer Y, Bachar E. Anorexia nervosa and parental bonding: The contribution of parent-grandparent relationships to eating disorder psychopathology. Journal of Clinical Psychology. 2008;**64**(6):703-716. DOI: 10.1002/jclp.20482

[34] Rienecke RD, Accurso EC, Lock J, Le Grange D. Expressed emotion, family functioning, and treatment outcome for adolescents with anorexia nervosa. European Eating Disorders Review. 2016;**24**(1):43-51. DOI: 10.1002/erv.2389

[35] Zabala MJ, Macdonald P, Treasure J. Appraisal of caregiving burden, expressed emotion and psychological distress in families of people with eating disorders: A systematic review. European Eating Disorders Review. 2009;**17**(5):338-349. DOI: 10.1002/erv.925

[36] Loeb KL, Lock J, Greif R, le Grange D. Transdiagnostic theory and application of family-based treatment for youth with eating disorders. Cognitive and Behavioral Practice. 2012;**19**(1):17-30. DOI: 10.1016/j.cbpra.2010.04.005

[37] Turner HM, Rose KS, Cooper MJ. Parental bonding and eating disorder symptoms in adolescents: The meditating role of core beliefs. Eating Behaviors. 2005;**6**(2):113-118. DOI: 10.1016/j.eatbeh.2004.08.010

[38] Soenens B, Vansteenkiste M, Vandereycken W, Luyten P, Sierens E, Goossens L. Perceived parental psychological control and eating-disordered symptoms: Maladaptive perfectionism as a possible intervening variable. The Journal of Nervous and Mental Disease. 2008;**196**(2):144-152. DOI: 10.1097/NMD.0b013e318162aabf

[39] Perry JA, Silvera DH, Neilands TB, Rosenvinge JH, Hanssen T. A study of the relationship between parental bonding, self-concept and eating disturbances in Norwegian and American college populations. Eating Behaviors. 2008;**9**(1):13-24. DOI: 10.1016/j.eatbeh.2007.01.007

[40] Courtney EA, Gamboz J, Johnson JG. Problematic eating behaviors in adolescents with low self-esteem and elevated depressive symptoms. Eating Behaviors. 2008;**9**(4):408-414. DOI: 10.1016/j.eatbeh.2008.06.001

[41] Polivy J, Herman CP. Causes of eating disorders. Annual Review of Psychology. 2002;**53**(1):187-213. DOI: 10.1146/annurev.psych.53.100901.135103

[42] Geller J, Zaitsoff SL, Srikameswaran S. Beyond shape and weight: Exploring the relationship between nonbody determinants of self-esteem and eating disorder symptoms in adolescent females. The International Journal of Eating Disorders. 2002;**32**(3):344-351. DOI: 10.1002/eat.10083

[43] Geller J, Srikameswaran S, Cockell SJ, Zaitsoff SL. Assessment of shape- and weight-based self-esteem in adolescents. The International Journal of Eating Disorders. 2000;**28**(3):339-345.

DOI: 10.1002/1098-108X(200011)28:3<339:AID-EAT12>3.0.CO;2-R

[44] Rhea DJ, Thatcher WG. Ethnicity, ethnic identity, self-esteem, and at-risk eating disordered behavior differences of urban adolescent females. Eating Disorders. 2013;**21**(3):223-237. DOI: 10.1080/10640266.2013.779177

[45] Shea ME, Pritchard ME. Is self-esteem the primary predictor of disordered eating? Personality and Individual Differences. 2007;**42**(8):1527-1537. DOI: 10.1016/j.paid.2006.10.026

[46] La Mela C, Maglietta M, Lucarelli S, Mori S, Sassaroli S. Pretreatment outcome indicators in an eating disorder outpatient group: The effects of self-esteem, personality disorders and dissociation. Comprehensive Psychiatry. 2013;**54**(7):933-942. DOI: 10.1016/j.comppsych.2013.03.024

[47] Brechan I, Kvalem IL. Relationship between body dissatisfaction and disordered eating: Mediating role of self-esteem and depression. Eating Behaviors. 2015;**17**:49-58. DOI: 10.1016/j.eatbeh.2014.12.008

[48] Jacobi C, Paul T, De Zwaan M, Nutzinger DO, Dahme B. Specificity of self-concept disturbances in eating disorders. The International Journal of Eating Disorders. 2004;**35**(2):204-210. DOI: 10.1002/eat.10240

[49] Young EA, Clopton JR, Bleckley MK.Perfectionism, low self-esteem, and family factors as predictors of bulimic behavior. Eating Behaviors. 2004;**5**(4):273-283. DOI: 10.1016/j.eatbeh.2003.12.001

[50] Collin P, Karatzias T, Power K, Howard R, Grierson D, Yellowlees A. Multi-dimensional self-esteem and magnitude of change in the treatment of anorexia nervosa. Psychiatry Research. 2016;**237**:175-181. DOI: 10.1016/j.psychres.2016.01.046

[51] Tylka TL, Sabik NJ. Integrating social comparison theory and self-esteem within objectification theory to predict women's disordered eating. Sex Roles. 2010;**63**(1):18-31. DOI: 10.1007/s11199-010-9785-3

[52] Iannaccone M, D'Olimpio F, Cella S, Cotrufo P. Self-esteem, body shame and eating disorder risk in obese and normal weight adolescents: A mediation model. Eating Behaviors. 2016;**21**:80-83. DOI: 10.1016/j.eatbeh.2015.12.010

[53] Goossens L, Braet C, Bosmans G, Decaluwé V. Loss of control over eating in pre-adolescent youth: The role of attachment and self-esteem. Eating Behaviors. 2011;**12**(4):289-295. DOI: 10.1016/j.eatbeh.2011.07.005

[54] Frost RO, Marten P, Lahart C, Rosenblate R. The dimensions of perfectionism. Cognitive Therapy and Research. 1990;**14**(5):449-468. DOI: 10.1007/BF01172967

[55] Bardone-Cone AM, Sturm K, Lawson MA, Robinson DP, Smith R. Perfectionism across stages of recovery from eating disorders. The International Journal of Eating Disorders. 2010;**43**(2):139-148. DOI: 10.1002/eat.20674

[56] Wade TD, Tiggemann M. The role of perfectionism in body dissatisfaction. Journal of Eating Disorders. 2013;**1**(1):2. DOI: 10.1186/2050-2974-1-2

[57] Boone L, Soenens B, Braet C, Goossens L. An empirical typology of perfectionism in early-to-mid adolescents and its relation with eating disorder symptoms. Behaviour Research and Therapy. 2010;**48**(7):686-691. DOI: 10.1016/j.brat.2010.03.022

[58] Bardone-Cone AM, Wonderlich SA, Frost RO, Bulik CM, Mitchell JE,

Uppala S, et al. Perfectionism and eating disorders: Current status and future directions. Clinical Psychology Review. 2007;**27**:384-405. DOI: 10.1016/j.cpr.2006.12.005

[59] Limburg K, Watson HJ, Hagger MS, Egan SJ. The relationship between perfectionism and psychopathology: A meta-analysis. Journal of Clinical Psychology. 2017;**73**:1301-1326. DOI: 10.1002/jclp.22435

[60] Kehayes ILL, Smith MM, Sherry SB, Vidovic V, Saklofske DH. Are perfectionism dimensions risk factors for bulimic symptoms? A meta-analysis of longitudinal studies. Personality and Individual Differences. 2019;**138**:117-125. DOI: 10.1016/j.paid.2018.09.022

[61] Castro-Fornieles J, Gual P, Lahortiga F, Gila A, Casulà V, Fuhrmann C, et al. Self-oriented perfectionism in eating disorders. The International Journal of Eating Disorders. 2007;**40**(6):562-568. DOI: 10.1002/eat.20393

[62] Egan SJ, Wade TD, Shafran R. Perfectionism as a transdiagnostic process: A clinical review. Clinical Psychology Review. 2011;**31**:203-212. DOI: 10.1016/j.cpr.2010.04.009

[63] Nilsson K, Sundbom E, Hägglöf B. A longitudinal study of perfectionism in adolescent onset anorexia nervosa-restricting type. European Eating Disorders Review. 2008;**16**(5):386-394. DOI: 10.1002/erv.850

[64] Vall E, Wade TD. Predictors of treatment outcome in individuals with eating disorders: A systematic review and meta-analysis. International Journal of Eating Disorders. 2015;**48**:946-971. DOI: 10.1002/eat.22411

[65] Johnston J, Shu CY, Hoiles KJ, Clarke PJF, Watson HJ, Dunlop PD, et al. Perfectionism is associated with higher eating disorder symptoms and lower remission in children and adolescents diagnosed with eating disorders. Eating Behaviors. 2018;**30**:55-60. DOI: 10.1016/j.eatbeh.2018.05.008

[66] Holland LA, Bodell LP, Keel PK. Psychological factors predict eating disorder onset and maintenance at 10-year follow-up. European Eating Disorders Review. 2013;**21**(5):405-410. DOI: 10.1002/erv.2241

[67] Boone L, Soenens B, Vansteenkiste M, Braet C. Is there a perfectionist in each of us? An experimental study on perfectionism and eating disorder symptoms. Appetite. 2012;**59**(2):531-540. DOI: 10.1016/j.appet.2012.06.015

[68] Levinson CA, Rodebaugh TL, White EK, Menatti AR, Weeks JW, Iacovino JM, et al. Social appearance anxiety, perfectionism, and fear of negative evaluation: Distinct or shared risk factors for social anxiety and eating disorders? Appetite. 2013;**67**:125-133. DOI: 10.1016/j.appet.2013.04.002

[69] Joyce F, Watson HJ, Egan SJ, Kane RT. Mediators between perfectionism and eating disorder psychopathology in a community sample. Eating Behaviors. 2012;**13**(4):361-365. DOI: 10.1016/j.eatbeh.2012.07.002

[70] Wade TD, Wilksch SM, Paxton SJ, Byrne SM, Austin SB. How perfectionism and ineffectiveness influence growth of eating disorder risk in young adolescent girls. Behaviour Research and Therapy. 2015;**66**:56-63. DOI: 10.1016/j.brat.2015.01.007

[71] Fairburn CG. Overcoming Binge Eating (Second Edition): The Proven Program to Learn Why You Binge and How You Can Stop. New York: Guilford Press; 2013. p. 243

[72] Robins RW, Trzesniewski KH. Self-esteem development across the lifespan.

Current Directions in Psychological Science. 2005;**14**(3):158-162. DOI: 10.1111/j.0963-7214.2005.00353.x

[73] Sassaroli S, Gallucci M, Ruggiero GM. Low perception of control as a cognitive factor of eating disorders. Its independent effects on measures of eating disorders and its interactive effects with perfectionism and self-esteem. Journal of Behavior Therapy and Experimental Psychiatry. 2008;**39**(4):467-488. DOI: 10.1016/j.jbtep.2007.11.005

[74] Watson HJ, Steele AL, Bergin JL, Fursland A, Wade TD. Bulimic symptomatology: The role of adaptive perfectionism, shape and weight concern, and self-esteem. Behaviour Research and Therapy. 2011;**49**(9):565-572. DOI: 10.1016/j.brat.2011.04.002

[75] Birtchnell J. The psychology of shame: Theory and treatment of shame-based syndromes. Personality and Individual Differences. 1997;**22**(5):781. DOI: 10.1016/s0191-8869(97)85593-6

[76] Goss K, Allan S. Shame, pride and eating disorders. Clinical Psychology and Psychotherapy. 2009;**16**:303-316. DOI: 10.1002/cpp.627

[77] Troop NA, Allan S, Serpell L, Treasure JL. Shame in women with a history of eating disorders. European Eating Disorders Review. 2008;**16**(6): 480-488. DOI: 10.1002/erv.858

[78] Andrews B, Qian M, Valentine JD. Predicting depressive symptoms with a new measure of shame: The Experience of Shame Scale. The British Journal of Clinical Psychology. 2002;**41**(1):29-42. DOI: 10.1348/014466502163778

[79] Goss K, Gilbert P. Eating disorders, shame and pride: A cognitive-behavioural functional analysis. In: Gilbert P, Miles J, editors. Body Shame: Conceptualisation, Research and Treatment. New York: Brunner Routledge; 2002. pp. 219-255

[80] Skårderud F. Shame and pride in anorexia nervosa: A qualitative descriptive study. European Eating Disorders Review. 2007;**15**(2):81-97. DOI: 10.1002/erv.774

[81] Swan S, Andrews B. The relationship between shame, eating disorders and disclosure in treatment. The British Journal of Clinical Psychology. 2003;**42**(4):367-378. DOI: 10.1348/014466503322528919

[82] Jankauskiene R, Pajaujiene S. Disordered eating attitudes and body shame among athletes, exercisers and sedentary female college students. The Journal of Sports Medicine and Physical Fitness. 2012;**52**(1):92-101

[83] Troop NA, Redshaw C. General shame and bodily shame in eating disorders: A 2.5-year longitudinal study. European Eating Disorders Review. 2012;**20**(5):373-378. DOI: 10.1002/erv.2160

[84] Doran J, Lewis CA. Components of shame and eating disturbance among clinical and non-clinical populations. European Eating Disorders Review. 2012;**20**:265-270. DOI: 10.1002/erv.1142

[85] Burney J, Irwin HJ. Shame and guilt in women with eating-disorder symptomatology. Journal of Clinical Psychology. 2000;**56**(1):51-61. DOI: 10.1002/(SICI)1097-4679(200001)56:1<51:AID-JCLP5>3.0.CO;2-W

[86] Keith L, Gillanders D, Simpson S. An exploration of the main sources of shame in an eating-disordered population. Clinical Psychology & Psychotherapy. 2009;**16**(4):317-327. DOI: 10.1002/cpp.629

[87] Lutwak N, Ferrari JR. Under–standing shame in adults: Retrospective perceptions of parental-bonding

during childhood. The Journal of Nervous and Mental Disease. 1997;**185**(10):595-598. DOI: 10.1097/00005053-199710000-00001

[88] Murray C, Waller G, Legg C. Family dysfunction and bulimic psychopathology: The mediating role of shame. The International Journal of Eating Disorders. 2000;**28**(1):84-89. DOI: 10.1002/(SICI)1098-108X(200007)28:1<84:AID-EAT10>3.0.CO;2-R

[89] Markham A, Thompson T, Bowling A. Determinants of body-image shame. Personality and Individual Differences. 2005;**38**(7):1529-1541. DOI: 10.1016/j.paid.2004.08.018

[90] Stice E. Risk and maintenance factors for eating pathology: A meta-analytic review. Psychological Bulletin. 2002;**128**:825-848. DOI: 10.1037/0033-2909.128.5.825

[91] Sim LA, Lebow J, Billings M. Eating disorders in adolescents with a history of obesity. Pediatrics. 2013;**132**(4):e1026-e1030. DOI: 10.1542/peds.2012-3940

[92] Westerberg-Jacobson J, Edlund B, Ghaderi A. A 5-year longitudinal study of the relationship between the wish to be thinner, lifestyle behaviours and disturbed eating in 9-20-year old girls. European Eating Disorders Review. 2010;**18**(3):207-219. DOI: 10.1002/erv.983

[93] Gustafsson SA, Edlund B, Kjellin L, Norring C. Risk and protective factors for disturbed eating in adolescent girls—Aspects of perfectionism and attitudes to eating and weight. European Eating Disorders Review. 2009;**17**(5):380-389. DOI: 10.1002/erv.930

[94] Forrester-Knauss C, Perren S, Alsaker FD. Does body mass index in childhood predict restraint eating in early adolescence? Appetite. 2012;**59**(3):921-926. DOI: 10.1016/j.appet.2012.08.026

[95] Bühren K, Von Ribbeck L, Schwarte R, Egberts K, Pfeiffer E, Fleischhaker C, et al. Body mass index in adolescent anorexia nervosa patients in relation to age, time point and site of admission. European Child & Adolescent Psychiatry. 2013;**22**(7):395-400. DOI: 10.1007/s00787-013-0376-z

[96] Huas C, Godart N, Caille A, Pham-Scottez A, Foulon C, Divac SM, et al. Mortality and its predictors in severe bulimia nervosa patients. European Eating Disorders Review. 2013;**21**(1):15-19. DOI: 10.1002/erv.2178

[97] Fan Y, Li Y, Liu A, Hu X, Ma G, Xu G. Associations between body mass index, weight control concerns and behaviors, and eating disorder symptoms among non-clinical Chinese adolescents. BMC Public Health. 2010;**10**:314. DOI: 10.1186/1471-2458-10-314

[98] Moon K, Krems C, Heuer T, Roth A, Hoffmann I. Predictors of BMI vary along the BMI range of german adults—Results of the german national nutrition survey II. Obesity Facts. 2017;**10**(1):38-49. DOI: 10.1159/000456665

[99] Francis LA, Ventura AK, Marini M, Birch LL. Parent overweight predicts daughters' increase in BMI and disinhibited overeating from 5 to 13 years. Obesity. 2007;**15**(6):1544-1553. DOI: 10.1038/oby.2007.183

[100] Moraeus L, Lissner L, Yngve A, Poortvliet E, Al-Ansari U, Sjöberg A. Multi-level influences on childhood obesity in Sweden: Societal factors, parental determinants and childs lifestyle. International Journal of Obesity. 2012;**36**(7):969-976. DOI: 10.1038/ijo.2012.79

[101] Yamborisut U, Visetchart P, Thasanasuwan W, Srichan W,

Unjana R. Parental feeding practice is associated with child's body mass index in Thai school-aged children: A case study in Don Tum district, Nakhon Pathom, Thailand. Journal of Health Research. 2018;**32**(1):82-94. DOI: 10.1108/JHR-11-2017-01

[102] Ventura AK, Birch LL. Does parenting affect children's eating and weight status? International Journal of Behavioral Nutrition and Physical Activity. 2008;**5**(1):15. DOI: 10.1186/1479-5868-5-15

[103] Vollmer RL, Mobley AR. Parenting styles, feeding styles, and their influence on child obesogenic behaviors and body weight. A review. Appetite. 2013;**17**:232-241. DOI: 10.1016/j.appet.2013.08.01

[104] Lissau I, Sørensen TIA, Lissau I. Parental neglect during childhood and increased risk of obesity in young adulthood. Lancet. 1994;**343**(8893):324-327. DOI: 10.1016/S0140-6736(94)91163-0

[105] Anderson SE, Gooze RA, Lemeshow S, Whitaker RC. Quality of early maternal-child relationship and risk of adolescent obesity. Pediatrics. 2012;**129**(1):132-140. DOI: 10.1542/peds.2011-0972

[106] Francis LA, Susman EJ. Self-regulation and rapid weight gain in children from age 3 to 12 years. Archives of Pediatrics & Adolescent Medicine. 2009;**163**(4):297-302. DOI: 10.1001/archpediatrics.2008.579

[107] Piotrowski JT, Lapierre MA, Linebarger DL. Investigating correlates of self-regulation in early childhood with a representative sample of English-speaking American families. Journal of Child and Family Studies. 2013;**22**(3):423-436. DOI: 10.1007/s10826-012-9595-z

[108] Kakinami L, Barnett TA, Séguin L, Paradis G. Parenting style and obesity risk in children. Preventive Medicine. 2015;**75**:18-22. DOI: 10.1016/j.ypmed.2015.03.005

[109] Melis Yavuz H, Selcuk B. Predictors of obesity and overweight in preschoolers: The role of parenting styles and feeding practices. Appetite. 2018;**120**:491-499. DOI: 10.1016/j.appet.2017.10.001

[110] De Campora G, Giromini L, Larciprete G, Li Volsi V, Zavattini GC. The impact of maternal overweight and emotion regulation on early eating behaviors. Eating Behaviors. 2014;**15**(3):403-409. DOI: 10.1016/j.eatbeh.2014.04.013

[111] De Campora G, Larciprete G, Delogu AM, Meldolesi C, Giromini L. A longitudinal study on emotional dysregulation and obesity risk: From pregnancy to 3 years of age of the baby. Appetite. 2016;**96**:95-101. DOI: 10.1016/j.appet.2015.09.012

[112] Bardone-Cone AM, Vohs KD, Abramson LY, Heatherton TF, Joiner TE. The confluence of perfectionism, body dissatisfaction, and low self-esteem predicts bulimic symptoms: Clinical implications. Behavior Therapy. 2000;**31**(2):265-280. DOI: 10.1016/S0005-7894(00)80015-5

[113] Steele A, Corsini N, Wade TD. The interaction of perfectionism, perceived weight status, and self-esteem to predict bulimic symptoms: The role of "benign" perfectionism. Behaviour Research and Therapy. 2007;**45**(7):1647-1655. DOI: 10.1016/j.brat.2006.08.007

[114] Shaw HE, Stice E, Springer DW. Perfectionism, body dissatisfaction, and self-esteem in predicting bulimic symptomatology: Lack of replication. International Journal of Eating Disorders. 2004;**36**(1):41-47. DOI: 10.1002/eat.20016

[115] La Mela C, Maglietta M, Caini S, Casu GP, Lucarelli S, Mori S, et al.

Perfectionism, weight and shape concerns, and low self-esteem: Testing a model to predict bulimic symptoms. Eating Behaviors. 2015;**19**:155-158. DOI: 10.1016/j.eatbeh.2015.09.002

[116] Holm-Denoma JM, Gordon KH, Bardone-Cone AM, Vohs KD, Abramson LY, Heatherton TF, et al. A test of an interactive model of bulimic symptomatology in adult women. Behavior Therapy. 2005;**36**(4):311-321. DOI: 10.1016/S0005-7894(05)80113-3

[117] Ghaderi A. Structural modeling analysis of prospective risk factors for eating disorder. Eating Behaviors. 2003;**3**(4):387-396. DOI: 10.1016/S1471-0153(02)00089-2

[118] Fairburn CG, Cooper PJ. The clinical features of bulimia nervosa. In: Brownwell KD, Foreyt JP, editors. British Journal of Psychiatry. New York: Basic Books; 1984. pp. 238-246. DOI: 10.1192/bjp.144.3.238

[119] Fairburn CG, Cooper Z, Shafran R. Cognitive behaviour therapy for eating disorders: A "transdiagnostic" theory and treatment. Behaviour Research and Therapy. 2003;**41**:509-528. DOI: 10.1192/bjp.144.3.238

[120] Lampard AM, Tasca GA, Balfour L, Bissada H. An evaluation of the transdiagnostic cognitive-behavioural model of eating disorders. European Eating Disorders Review. 2013;**21**(2):99-107. DOI: 10.1002/erv.2214

[121] Murray SB, Rieger E, Karlov L, Touyz SW. An investigation of the transdiagnostic model of eating disorders in the context of muscle dysmorphia. European Eating Disorders Review. 2013;**21**(2):160-164. DOI: 10.1002/erv.2194

[122] Hilbert A, Pike KM, Goldschmidt AB, Wilfley DE, Fairburn CG, Dohm FA, et al. Risk factors across the eating disorders. Psychiatry Research. 2014;**220**(1-2): 500-506. DOI: 10.1016/j.psychres.2014.05.054

[123] Stice E, Marti CN, Durant S. Risk factors for onset of eating disorders: Evidence of multiple risk pathways from an 8-year prospective study. Behaviour Research and Therapy. 2011;**49**(10):622-627. DOI: 10.1016/j.brat.2011.06.009

[124] Cella S, Cipriano A, Iannaccone M, Cotrufo P. Identifying predictors associated with the severity of eating concerns in females with eating disorders. Research in Psychotherapy: Psychopathology, Process and Outcome. 2017;**20**(1):91-99. DOI: 10.4081/ripppo.2017.199

[125] American Psychiatric Association. Diagnostic and Statistical Manual of Mental Disorders. 4th ed. Washington, DC: APA Press; 1994

[126] Cotrufo P. Anoressia del sessuale femminile. Dal caos alla costituzione del limite. Franco Angeli: Milano; 2005. p. 144

[127] Cotrufo P, Gnisci A, Caputo I. Brief report: Psychological characteristics of less severe forms of eating disorders: An epidemiological study among 259 female adolescents. Journal of Adolescence. 2005;**28**(1):147-154. DOI: 10.1016/j.adolescence.2004.07.006

[128] Cella S, Iannaccone M, Cotrufo P. Does body shame mediate the relationship between parental bonding, self-esteem, maladaptive perfectionism, body mass index and eating disorders? A structural equation model. Eating and Weight Disorders [journal on the Internet]. 2019 March 11. DOI: 10.1007/s40519-019-00670-3. [Epub ahead of print]

[129] Stice E, Shaw H, Marti CN. A meta-analytic review of eating disorder prevention programs: Encouraging

findings. Annual Review of Clinical Psychology. 2007;**3**(1):207-231. DOI: 10.1146/annurev.clinpsy.3.022806.091447

[130] Jáuregui Lobera I, Bolaños Ríos P, Garrido Casals O. Parenting styles and eating disorders. Journal of Psychiatric and Mental Health Nursing. 2011;**18**(8):728-735. DOI: 10.1111/j.1365-2850.2011.01723.x

[131] Fassino S, Amianto F, Rocca G, Abbate Daga G. Parental bonding and eating psychopathology in bulimia nervosa: Personality traits as possible mediators. Epidemiologia e Psichiatria Sociale. 2010;**19**(3):214-222. DOI: 10.1017/s1121189x00001147

[132] Hewitt PL, Flett GL. Dimensions of perfectionism, daily stress, and depression: A test of the specific vulnerability hypothesis. Journal of Abnormal Psychology. 1993;**102**(1): 58-65. DOI: 10.1037/0021-843X.102.1.58

[133] Hewitt PL, Flett GL, Ediger E. Perfectionism traits and perfectionistic self-presentation in eating disorder attitudes, characteristics, and symptoms. The International Journal of Eating Disorders. 1995;**18**(4):317-326. DOI: 10.1002/1098-108X(199512)18:4<317::AID-EAT2260180404>3.0.CO;2-2

[134] Freud A. Das Ich und die Abweh–rmechanismen./The Ego and the Defense Mechanisms. Vienna: Int. Psychoanal. Verlag; 1936. p. 208

[135] Bulik CM, Kleiman SC, Yilmaz Z. Genetic influences on eating disorders. Current Opinion in Psychiatry. 2016;**29**(6):383-388. DOI: 10.1097/YCO.0000000000000275

[136] Himmerich H, Bentley J, Kan C, Treasure J. Genetic risk factors for eating disorders: An update and insights into pathophysiology. Therapeutic Advances in Psychopharmacology. 2019;**9**:1-20. DOI: 10.1177/204512531881473

Chapter 2

Weight Management: Inflammation

Upasana

Abstract

Nowadays, obesity is considered as one of the fastest escalating nutritional disorders that reached pandemic throughout the world. Obesity is a condition in which overaccumulation of energy in the form of fat happens in an individual's subcutaneous and/or abdominal visceral tissue. It is described as an abnormal growth of adipose tissue due to the enlargement of fat cell size (hypertrophic obesity) or fat cell number (hyperplastic obesity) or a condition of both. Earlier, it was reported that the most common type of obesity that affects the general population is the polygenic form that results from a result of a positive energy balance between energy consumption and its expenditure – or a combination of both. The pandemic of obesity has enforced to analyze the link between the role of inflammation and complications of overweight and obesity. This led to crossroads of the field of nutrition, diet therapy, physiology, immunology, and epidemiology and makes the understanding that they are linked inexplicably. The remodeling of obesity as an inflammatory state has led a wide impression in our conceptualization of obesity-related diseases. In this chapter, we highlight the endocrine aspect of adipose tissue, the effect of dysregulated secretion of adipokines due to inflammation and dietary components that affect obesity related to inflammation.

Keywords: nutritional disorder, obesity, adipokines, inflammation, dietary components

1. Introduction

A famous ancient proverb states that "Eat breakfast like a king, lunch like a prince, and dinner like a pauper." In today's era, these words have long been discarded. The magnitude of obesity has reached in pandemic proportion due to new technology and modern life, which makes life easier and less active along with the intake of high energy dense food for better taste [1–3]. This is one of the biggest public health concerns of today's era, which affects the individual not only physically but also physiologically and psychologically.

The World Health Organization (WHO) has reported that obesity has been growing at an alarming rate worldwide and has nearly been tripled between 1975 and 2016. It was also reported by WHO in the year 2016 that more than 1.9 billion adults, 18 years and older, were overweight; of these over 650 million were obese (https://www.who.int/news-room/fact-sheets/detail/obesity-and-overweight) [4].

Nowadays, obesity is regarded as a complex dysfunctional neuroendocrine problem in which genetic makeup and environmental factors act in concert. The nongenetic risk factors encompass a wide range of social, physiological,

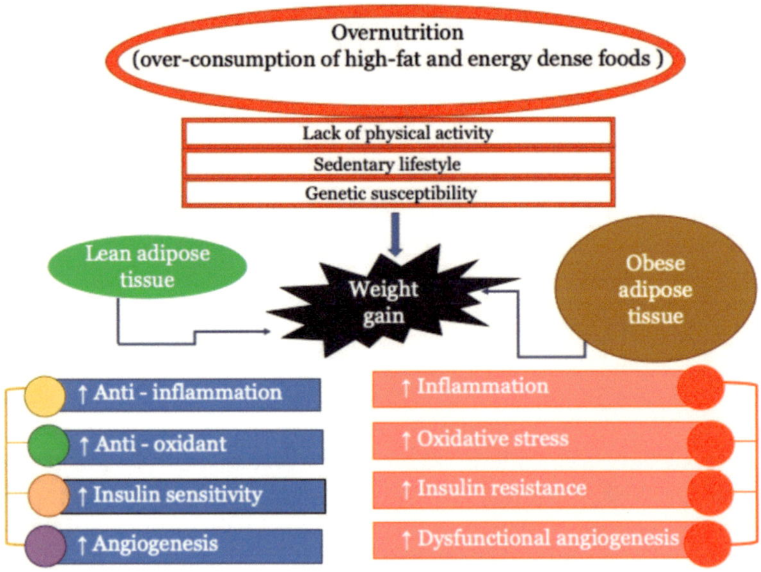

Figure 1.
Overnutrition (overconsumption of high-fat and energy dense foods), lack of physical activity, sedentary lifestyle, and genetic susceptibility are the leading factors associated with the development of obesity. In addition to dysfunctional angiogenesis, an obese state is characterized by an abnormal inflammatory response, low antioxidant capacity, and reduced insulin sensitivity that may eventually lead to the generation of inflammation, oxidative stress, and insulin resistance. The figure was modified from the following review paper by Dludla et al. [6].

environmental, and behavioral factors. Sedentary lifestyle and overconsumption of high-fat and energy dense foods are a major contributor to energy imbalance. The altered phenomenon of hunger and satiety, lack of physical activity, decreased thermogenesis, and resting metabolic rate over a long period of time may lead to the energy imbalance.

In addition, other external factors such as age, gender, food preference, breakfast skipping, medications, chemical toxicity, disorders of the endocrine system, socioeconomic status, and a psychological factor may give rise to weight gain problems. It is considered as a major contributor to the global burden of chronic diseases like hypertension, type 2 diabetes, hypercholesterolemia, heart diseases, insulin resistance, atherosclerosis, ischemic heart diseases, respiratory diseases, orthopedic disorders, several types of cancer, hormonal imbalance, disability, and many other diseases. Overweight and obesity also play a pivotal role in the development of low-grade inflammation, which contribute to the development of obesity-linked disorders, in particular to metabolic dysfunction [5]. However, a growing body of knowledge suggests that a possible convergence of an inflammatory state, which results in chronic inflammation and oxidative stress, is localized within adipose tissue [6] as shown in **Figure 1**. Adipose tissue inflammation plays a crucial role in promulgating obesity-related metabolic complications including the development of insulin resistance [6–8].

2. Adipose tissue: manager of inflammation

Over the past decades, it is well established that adipose tissue is not merely a fat storage depot but has been recognized as an endocrine organ capable of producing various bioactive substances. It then became evident that white adipose tissue (WAT) secretes ample of peptides. Few of them regulate the inflammatory processes such as leptin and adiponectin, whereas others are well-known cytokines such as interleukin (IL)-6, IL-1 and its receptor antagonist (IL-1Ra), and tumor necrosis factor (TNF)-α [9]. As we know, obesity is one of the major causes of atherosclerosis, which is recognized as a chronic vascular inflammatory process in which cytokines and chemokines play a dramatic role [9–10]. White adipose tissue plays an important role in metabolism and inflammation as illustrated in **Figure 2**.

Cytokines are categorized as interleukins, interferons, chemokines, hematopoietic factors, and growth factors. They are knotted in many biological processes such as growth, differentiation, cell division, apoptosis, immunity, and inflammation [9]. Cytokines are produced by numerous cell types of the hematopoietic lineage including T cells, B cells, mast cells, macrophages, dendritic cells, and natural killer cells. In spite of these, cytokines are also produced by nonhematopoietic cells such as epithelial cells, hepatocytes, and fibroblasts [9, 12]. Evidence revealed that IL-1, IL-6, and TNF-α are characterized as a proinflammatory cytokine that activates both acute and chronic inflammatory responses [9]. Inhibitors that control inflammation can be categorized as anti-inflammatory cytokines, soluble receptors to cytokines, and naturally occurring proteins. Types of anti-inflammatory cytokines are IL-10, IL-4, and TGF-β; soluble receptors to cytokines are IL-1 and TNF-α; and naturally occurring proteins are IL-1Ra receptors. The classification of cytokines is depicted in **Figure 3**.

Chemokines are a type of cytokine that is a part of family molecules that are indulged in the chemotaxis of inflammatory cells via the generation of local concentration gradients. Chemokines play an important role in various physiological and pathological processes such as cell recruitment process and development of lymphoid organs or metastases. In spite of these, chemokines also participate in metabolic and inflammatory disorders such as rheumatoid arthritis, glomerulonephritis,

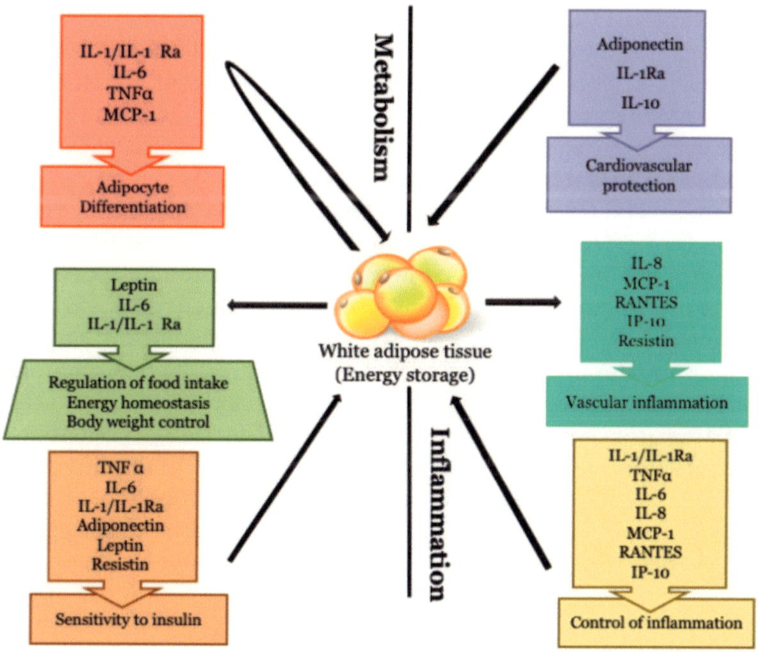

Figure 2.
Adipose tissue is a metabolically dynamic, highly active endocrine organ. White adipose tissue (WAT) produces a large variety of proteins regulating metabolism and inflammation, contributing to the maintenance of energy homeostasis and, probably, the pathogenesis of obesity-related metabolic and vascular complications. The figure was modified from the following research paper by Juge-Aubry et al. [9]. The following website was used for the extraction of image: https://scitechdaily.com/gc-1-turns-white-fat-brown-fat/ [11].

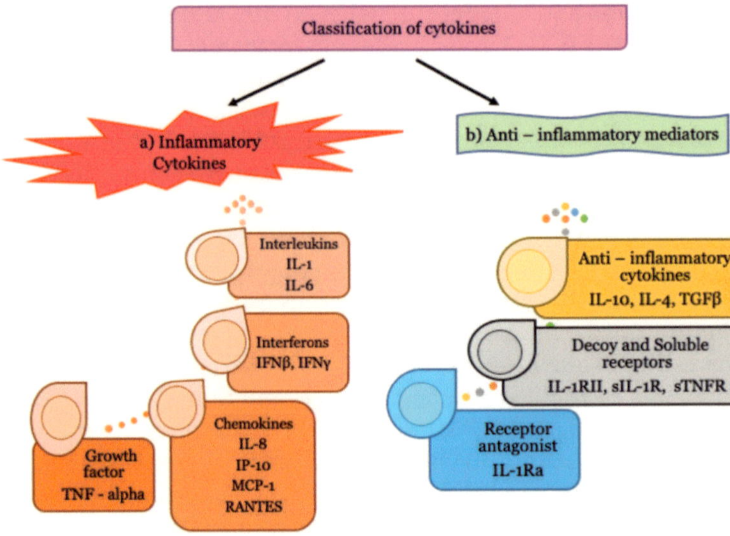

Figure 3.
Classification of cytokines. (a) Classes of inflammatory cytokines. (b) Anti-inflammatory mediators. The figure was modified from the following research paper by Juge-Aubry et al. [9].

and atherosclerosis via their innate ability to recruit and activate the inflammatory cells [9]. They are categorized into four subclasses according to the position of their cysteines (CXC, C, CX3C, and CC) [9, 13]. Chemokines that are produced from WAT are interferon-γ inducible protein 10 (IP-10 or CXCL10) and IL-8 (or CXCL8) belong to the CXC chemokines, while monocyte chemo-attractant protein-1 (MCP-1 or CCL2) and regulated upon activation normal T-cell express sequence (RANTES or CCL5) are CC chemokines [9, 13]. Previous studies showed that chemokines are paracrine rather than systemic factors, the significance of their secretion via adipose tissue may be seen in the context of fat depots found in close proximity to their target tissues, for example, subcutaneous fat in inflammatory skin diseases, perivascular adipose tissue in obesity-associated cardiovascular diseases, and perirenal fat in glomerulonephritis [9, 14].

In addition, several other metabolically important proteins with immunomodulatory actions are secreted by adipose tissue, including leptin, adiponectin, and resistin. The dysregulated expression of these factors, caused by excess adiposity and adipocyte dysfunction, has been linked to the pathogenesis of various disease processes through altered immune responses. As such, much attention has been paid to develop a better understanding of the immunoregulatory functions of adipose tissue. New factors secreted by adipose tissue have been identified that either promote inflammatory responses and metabolic dysfunction or contribute to the resolution of inflammation and have beneficial effects on obesity-linked metabolic disorders. These findings lend additional support to the notion that an imbalance of pro- and anti-inflammatory adipokines secreted by adipose tissue contributes to metabolic dysfunction [5].

3. Obesity: state of low-grade inflammation

Obesity is associated with alterations in immunity, a chronic low-grade inflammation, which is characterized by abnormal secretion of adipokines, that is, there is an increment in circulating proinflammatory cytokines and a decrement in anti-inflammatory cytokines. It is also linked with alteration in immunity. However, with the reduction in body weight, these parameters may reverse or come to the normal level. Although, it is still debatable how obesity triggers inflammation. Earlier, several hypotheses were proposed regarding the inflammation of obesity. The first one stated that overburden of nutrients in the adipocytes leads to intracellular stress that results in the stimulation of inflammatory cytokines [15–17].

The excessive nutrients may lead to aggregation of unfolded proteins in the endoplasmic reticulum (ER) via activation of the unfolded protein response (UPR) pathway [15, 17]. The pathway of UPR depends on basically three main sensors of ER, that is, PKR-like eukaryotic initiation factor 2α kinase (PERK), inositol-requiring enzyme 1 (IRE-1), and activating transcription factor 6 (ATF-6) [15, 18]. The activity of the C-Jun amino-terminal kinase (JNK) and inhibitor of IκB (IKK-β), serine-phosphorylation of insulin-receptor substrate protein 1 (IRS-1), and the nuclear factor-κB (NF-κB) pathway may increase by the activated sensors of ER that results in increased expression of proinflammatory cytokines [15–16, 19–21].

The second hypothesis enumerates that overburdened adipocytes with fat cells intensely increase the infiltration of macrophages, which may lead to subsequent differentiation and activation of cytotoxic T cells. As a result, initiation and propagation of inflammatory cytokines cascades occur [15, 22]. Third hypothesis proposes that as during obesity, enlargement of adipose tissue happens as a result tissue becomes relatively hypoxic. Hypoxia within the adipose tissues results in the activation of inflammatory pathways [15, 23–24]. Above all, the last hypothesis suggests that overburdened adipocytes themselves may directly activate immune pathogen sensors that result in chronic inflammation [15, 25].

4. Dietary components that affect obesity related to inflammation

The analysis of dietary intake is an approach to investigate a link between diet and overweight and obesity-related inflammation. Various studies reported that bioactive nutrients and dietary non-nutrients strongly influence health, metabolism, and progression of pathologic states that ultimately result in chronic degenerative diseases [26]. Many studies indicate that diet may affect body weight by controlling satiety and metabolic efficiency or by harmonizing insulin secretion and action [3, 27]. It is an essential key factor for immune response. Earlier, evidence revealed that undernutrition brings about immunosuppression due to susceptibility to infection. Whereas, overnutrition brings about immunoactivation due to susceptibility to inflammatory diseases. As a result, optimum nutrition is mandatory for a healthy immune balance of an individual [15] as shown in **Figure 4**.

Dietary components play an important role in obesity-related inflammation as enumerated below:

4.1 Carbohydrates

Carbohydrates are the main food source of a living organism and a major source of energy. Carbohydrates are also known as energy giving foods. The source of energy was estimated based on their glycemic index (GI) or glycemic load (GL) values. GI is the value given to the foods on how quickly they increase the glucose level postprandially and measures the quality of carbohydrate. GL calculates both the quality and quantity of carbohydrates [15, 28]. Earlier studies reported that, positive correlation exists between dietary GI and GL and biomarkers of inflammation because a low GI diet decreases the rate of glucose absorption in the body that subsequently reduces hyperglycemia and hyperinsulinemia that results in the reduction of systemic inflammation. Earlier, it was also reported that weight loss

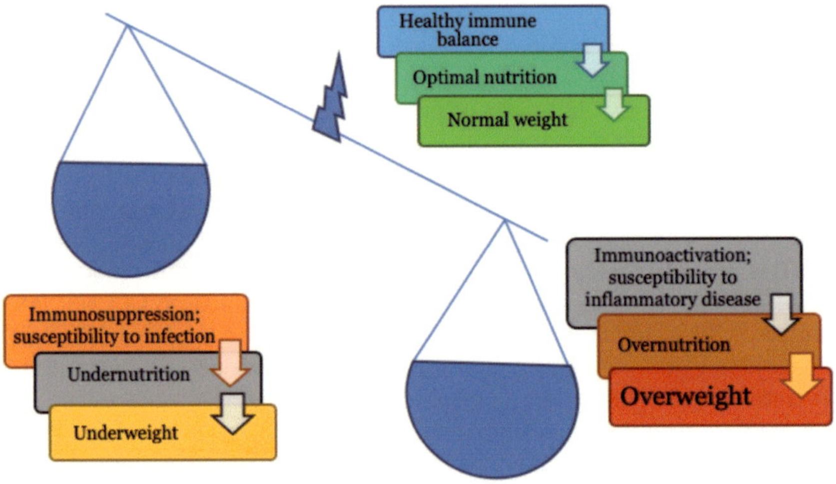

Figure 4.
Healthy immune balance between undernutrition and overnutrition. The figure was modified from the following research paper by Lee et al. [15].

leads to improvement in insulin sensitivity and a reduction in the level of proinflammatory cytokines. Various health organization also reported that low GI diets help in managing diabetes and coronary heart diseases and considered as a weapon against obesity [29–30].

Neuhouser et al. [31] revealed from randomized, crossover feeding study that respondents with high-fat mass (>32.0% for male and >25.0% for female) showed reduced CRP ($P = 0.02$) and marginally increased adiponectin ($P = 0.06$). Therefore, it was concluded that the quality of carbohydrates independent of energy was very important as low-GL foods improve the inflammatory and adipokine profiles of overweight and obese individuals [31]. Another study done by Levitan et al., among women ($n = 18{,}137$, >45 years of age), reported that diets characterized by lower GI and GL were associated with somewhat more favorable lipid profiles and lower CRP [32]. Interestingly, one of the epidemiological studies done by Vrolix and Mensick found that consumption of a diet with decreased GL does not decrease the metabolic risk parameters in overweight subjects [33]. Another study done by Kelly et al. also supports the above findings, that is, it does not found any additional benefit of including a low glycemic diet with exercise on insulin sensitivity and adipokine concentrations [34]. Above all, it may be stated that observational studies showed a positive association between intake of GI/GL diet and markers of inflammation. However, interventional studies do not found such an association.

4.2 Dietary fat

Fat is also one of the important sources of energy that serves both structural and metabolic functions of living organisms. The excessive accumulation of fat in the body leads to impairment of the immune system. A number of fatty acids have been studied including saturated, trans-fatty acids, and polyunsaturated fatty acids (PUFA) for their effect on inflammatory status [15].

4.2.1 Polyunsaturated fatty acids

The omega-3 (n-3) and omega-6 (n-6) PUFA families are precursors of eicosanoids, which play a vital role in the immune response [15]. Simpoulos [35] stated that high omega-6 fatty acids increase leptin and insulin resistance, whereas omega-3 fatty acids lead to homeostasis and weight loss. This is so because the high omega-6/omega-3 ratio is associated with overweight/obesity, whereas a balanced ratio decreases obesity and weight gain [35]. Another study showed that an increase in the intake of n-6:n-3 PUFA potentiates the inflammatory processes that ultimately lead to many inflammatory diseases such as nonalcoholic fatty liver disease (NAFLD), cardiovascular disease, diabetes, obesity, inflammatory bowel disease (IBD), rheumatoid arthritis, and Alzheimer's disease. This change in the ratio of consumption of n-3/n-6 fatty acids changes the production of important mediators and regulators of inflammation and immune response that leads toward the pro-inflammatory state. Hence, it was concluded in the study that increasing the ratio of (n-3)/(n-6) PUFA in the diet may lead to a reduction in the incidence of chronic inflammatory diseases [36].

A clinical trial and in-vitro experiment study reported that supplementation of fish oil delineates the expression of adipose inflammatory genes including inflammasome-associated IL-18 and IL-1b and circulating IL-18 levels. In spite of this, it was also stated that both eicosapentaenoic acid (EPA) and docosahexaenoic acid (DHA) decrease the inflammasome gene expression in obese human adipose and human adipocyte and macrophages [37]. Above all, various studies concluded that omega-3 fatty acids, namely EPA and DHA, have an anti-inflammatory effect.

4.2.2 Trans and saturated fatty acids

A review study was done by Rogero and Calder stated that saturated fatty acids induce inflammation by activating the TLR4 signaling pathway (TLR4 signaling pathway is recognized as the main pathway that triggers in obesity-induced inflammation) [38]. Another study revealed that the ingestion of excessive amounts of trans-fatty acids and saturated fatty acids is considered to be a risk factor for metabolic and degenerative diseases. It was also emphasized that saturated and trans-fatty acids favor a proinflammatory state leading to insulin resistance. These fatty acids can be indulged in several inflammatory pathways, contributing to disease progression in chronic inflammation, autoimmunity, allergy, cancer, atherosclerosis, hypertension, and heart hypertrophy as well as other metabolic and degenerative diseases. As a consequence, intake of dietary saturated and trans-fatty acids leads to lipotoxicity in several target organs by direct effects, represented by various inflammatory pathways, and through indirect effects, including an important alteration in the gut microbiota associated with endotoxemia process [39].

4.3 Fruits and vegetables

Fruits and vegetables comprise a myriad of nutrients, that is, vitamins, minerals, and many food compounds that have been inversely correlated with metabolic risk factors such as oxidative stress and inflammation. In a randomized controlled trial study, it was found that fruits and vegetables reduce the risk of metabolic disease that may be via modulation of gut microbiota. The study also revealed that fruits and vegetables decrease the secretion of interleukin-6 (IL-6) and lipopolysaccharide-binding protein (LBP) [40]. Another study done by Navarro et al. through factor analysis found that dietary patterns loaded with fruits and vegetables strongly negatively correlated with the secretion of hs-CRP among prepubertal girls [41]. An almost similar result was observed by Julia et al. that dietary pattern characterized by intake rich in vegetable and vegetable oil leads to the supply of essential fatty acids and antioxidant micronutrients showed a negative correlation with the risk of elevation of CRP [42]. Another cross-sectional study done on a group of 7574

Koreans found that an inverse correlation exists between vegetable pattern and CRP and the association appeared to be more predominant in men having hypertensive blood pressure [43]. Surprisingly, the study done by Salas-Salvado et al. (n = 772, 55–80 years of age) and Freese et al. (n = 77, 19–52 years of age) did not found any association between a diet rich in vegetables and fruits with inflammatory markers [adiponectin, CRP, IL-6, intercellular adhesion molecule-1 (ICAM-1), and vascular cell adhesion molecule-1 (VCAM-1)] [15, 44–45]. Another study done by Morand et al. (n = 24, mean age of 56 years) also showed a similar pattern of above finding that a single fruit supplementation (500 mL of orange juice/d for 4 weeks) did not change the levels of CRP, IL-6, ICAM-1, and VCAM-1 [15, 46].

4.4 Other nutrients

Oxidative stress and imbalance in immune responses play a crucial role in the development of obesity and its associated comorbidities. Various epidemiological shown that several vitamins and minerals have a favorable response on the level of inflammatory markers, that is, CRP, IL-6, and TNF-α.

4.4.1 Vitamin A

Various cross-sectional and intervention studies reported regarding overweight and obese respondents that they have lower circulating carotenoids in the plasma because of a high proportion of carotenoids, as lipid-soluble compounds, being stored in adipose tissue [15, 47]. The Women's Health Study (n = 2895, aged ≥45 years of age) reported that higher plasma concentrations of α- and β-carotene were associated with low levels of plasma CRP. In spite of this, plasma carotenoids were associated with obesity, HDL-cholesterol, LDL-cholesterol, HbA1c, and smoking [15, 48]. Another study done by Julia et al. suggested that the β-carotene status was inversely associated with low-grade inflammation [49]. Another cross-sectional meta-analysis study focusing on Syndrome X respondents showed an inverse association between total plasma carotenoids and metabolic syndrome. Respondents with the highest total circulating carotenoids had a 24% reduced risk for developing metabolic syndrome. Interestingly, when, individual carotenoids were included, and significant associations were found for β-carotene, lycopene, α-carotene, and β-cryptoxanthin [50–51].

4.4.2 Vitamin C

Vitamin C is effective in strengthening the immune system, capillary blood vessels, and protecting the dental health, as well as in the convenient use of iron, calcium, thiamine, riboflavin, folic acid, and vitamins A and E in the body. Vitamin C also acts as a cofactor for 15 different enzymes and shows the antioxidant activity as an electron donor reducing agent. It acts as a powerful free radical scavenger by protecting tissues against oxidative stress and reduces inflammation [52]. Totan et al. reported that vitamin C reduces the systemic inflammation by inhibiting CRP and TNF-α pathways. In spite of this, vitamin C inhibits hypoxia in adipose tissue that has the potential for protection against free radicals and decreasing lipid peroxidation. On the other hand, the study also revealed that vitamin C inhibits mature adipocyte formation and cell growth, inhibits lipolysis, and can be considered as a treatment model for obesity to offer solutions for abnormal fat accumulation [52]. Another study reported that vitamin C may improve inflammation by reducing the pro-inflammatory and inflammatory markers such as CRP, IL-6, and TNF-α [53]. Additionally, Fumeron et al. reported in the prospective, randomized, open-label trial study (n = 42, 18–80 years of age) that vitamin C supplementation (750 mg/d for 8 weeks) did not change blood levels of CRP [15, 54].

4.4.3 Magnesium

Magnesium is the second most abundant intracellular cation and is involved in about 300 biochemical reactions related to anabolic and catabolic actions in the body, such as glycolysis and protein and lipid metabolism [55–56]. The Women's Health Initiative Observational Study (n = 3713 postmenopausal women, aged 50–79 years) reported that intake of dietary magnesium was independently and inversely associated with plasma concentrations of hs-CRP, IL-6, and sVCAM-1 in postmenopausal women after an adjustment for multiple variables including dietary fiber, fruit, vegetables, folate, and saturated and trans-fatty intake [57]. Another study done by Guerrero-Romero and Rodriguez- Moran found that low serum Mg levels were independently related to elevated CRP concentration, in nondiabetic, nonhypertensive obese subjects (n = 371) [15, 58].

4.4.4 Flavonoids

Flavonoids, a group of natural substances with variable phenolic structures, are found in fruits, vegetables, grains, bark, roots, stems, flowers, tea, and wine. Nowadays, flavonoids are considered essential components in various applications such as nutraceutical, pharmaceutical, medicinal, and cosmetic. This is attributed to their anti-oxidative, anti-inflammatory, anti-mutagenic, and anti-carcinogenic properties coupled with their capacity to modulate key cellular enzyme function [59]. According to National Health and Nutrition Examination Survey (NHANES), a large, cross-sectional survey National Centre for Health Statistic (n = 9551 adults) showed that flavonoid consumption was inversely associated with obesity in both men and women in multivariate models. It was also observed that adults in the highest quartile of flavonoid intake had significantly lower body mass index and waist circumference than those in the lowest quartile of flavonoid intake ($P < 0.03$ and $P < 0.04$, respectively). The study also revealed that flavonoid intake was inversely related to C-reactive protein levels in women (p-trend, 0.01) [60]. The Nurses' Health Cohort Study (n = 2115 women, aged 43–70 years) reported that among flavonoid-rich foods, higher intake of grapefruit was significantly associated with lower concentrations of CRP and sTNF-R2. In spite of this, it was also reported in the study that flavonoids typically found in citrus fruits were modestly associated with lower plasma IL-18 concentrations [61]. Interestingly, a double-blind, placebo-controlled crossover study (n = 14, 35–53 years of age) reported that the supplementation of sea buckthorn flavonol extract for 4 weeks did not reduce CRP levels ($p < 0.05$) [15, 62].

4.4.5 Phytoestrogens

Phytoestrogens are plant-derived dietary compounds found in beans, seeds, and grains. The structure of phytoestrogens is similar to 17-β-oestradiol (E2), the primary female sex hormone. This structural similarity to E2 enables phytoestrogens to cause (anti) oestrogenic effects by binding to the oestrogen receptors [63]. Phytoestrogens had so many health benefits such as a lowered risk of menopausal symptoms such as hot flushes and osteoporosis, obesity, metabolic syndrome, and type 2 diabetes and lowered risks of cardiovascular disease, brain function disorders, breast cancer, prostate cancer, bowel cancer, and other cancers [63]. A randomized crossover clinical trial for 8 weeks (n = 42, postmenopausal women with metabolic syndrome) reported that soy nut consumption reduces interleukin-18 [64]. On the other hand, in a randomized, double-blind, controlled trial study (n = 50, post-menopausal women age = 58 ± 5 years), it was found that supplementation of soy isoflavone for 6 months had no effects on plasma CRP level [65].

4.4.6 Probiotics, prebiotics and synbiotics

According to the Food and Agriculture Organization of the United Nations (FAO) and WHO, probiotics are defined as "live microorganisms which, when administered in adequate amounts, confer a health benefit on the host" [66–67]. Earlier studies reported that probiotic bacteria, when administered orally, are able to modulate the immune system; however, differences exist in the immunomodulatory effects of different probiotic strains [15]. A randomized, double-blind, and placebo-controlled parallel-group intervention study compared *Lactobacillus rhamnosus* with *Bifidobacterium animalis* ssp. Lactis Bb12 and *Propionibacterium freudenreichii* ssp. Shermanii JS for 3 weeks in healthy respondents (n = 81, 23–58 years of age). The study showed no effect on serum levels of TNF-α, IL-6, IL-10, or IFN-γ but a decreased level of CRP in the *L. rhamnosus* supplementation group [15, 68].

According to FAO/WHO, prebiotics is defined as "non-digestible food ingredients that beneficially affect the host by selectively stimulating the growth and/or activity of one or a limited number of bacterial species already established in the colon, and thus improve the host health" [67, 69]. Russo et al. reported in the study that intake of 11% enriched inulin-enriched pasta for 5 weeks improved lipidic and glicidic metabolism as well as insulin resistance in healthy young subjects [70]. Another study reported that intake of oligofructose (type of prebiotics) supplementation (8 g/day for 3 weeks) in the elderly (n = 19, mean age = 85 years) showed a decrease in the expression of IL-6 mRNA in peripheral blood monocytes [71]. In contrary to the above study, the intervention study showed that supplementation of oligofructose (1.95–3.9 g/day for 12 weeks) did not affect plasma levels of IL-6 or TNF-α in poorly nourished elderly subjects (mean age of 70 years) [15, 72].

Synbiotics are defined as a combination of suitable probiotics and prebiotics that enhances survival and activity of the organism, for example, a fructooligosaccharide (FOS) in conjunction with a Bifidobacterium strain or lactitol in conjunction with *Lactobacillus* strains [73–74]. Ferrarese et al. reported in the study that diet supplementation with Synbiotics prepared using selected strains (such as *Lactobacillus gasseri* strains) showed to exert weight reduction and anti-inflammatory activity. In spite of this, it was also concluded that their administration, together with galactomannan and/or inulin fibers, may increase weight management effects due to synergistic effect on short-chain fatty acid production and microbiota "re-configuration" [75].

5. Discussion

The pandemic of obesity and its associated comorbidities derives our attention to the mechanism associated with a pathological condition. Earlier investigations revealed how cells and tissues respond to the stress of overnutrition and about the interplay between adipose tissue and other cell types that are critically involved in energy homeostasis. These findings also suggest the inflammatory response of obesity that might be beneficial or harmful, depending on the stage and degree of obesity, as well as other factors [76]. Previously, it was also reported that obesity and its associated comorbidities are due to intermingled interactions between genetic, metabolic, and environmental factors in which dietary pattern plays a central role [77].

The current review is a narrative review of the impact of inflammation on weight management. In this review, a model is outlined in which inflammation is closely associated with obesity. However, this is a simplified view. Earlier studies reveal that severely underweight people such as patients with anorexia nervosa (AN) also display an overproduction of inflammatory cytokines. Dalton et al. reported from an exploratory cross-sectional study that interleukin (IL)-6, IL-15, and vascular cell adhesion molecule (VCAM)-1 concentrations were significantly elevated, and concentrations of BDNF (brain-derived neurotrophic factor), tumor necrosis factor (TNF)-β, and vascular endothelial growth factor (VEGF)-A were significantly lower in anorexia nervosa (AN) participants [78]. An almost similar result was reported through meta-analysis by Solmi et al. that patients with anorexia nervosa (AN) have increased TNF-α, IL6, IL1-β, and TNF-R-II levels but decreased C-reactive protein and IL-6R [79]. Earlier studies also reported that immunosuppressive medications such as corticosteroids lead to visceral adiposity. Galitzky and Bouloumie reported that long-term exposure of glucocorticoids (GCs), either due to anti-inflammatory and immunosuppressive therapies or endocrine disturbances, accumulation of abdominal fat was observed in individuals with Cushing syndrome [80]. Lee et al. stated in the study that glucocorticoids (GCs) have profound effects on adipose tissue, adipogenesis, adipose tissue metabolic, and endocrine function. In the study, it was found that glucocorticoids (GCs) have multiple, depot-dependent effects on adipocyte gene expression and metabolism that enhances central fat deposition and lead to visceral obesity [81]. Further, contradicting study results are not included in the current study in order to provide a stringent model. Additionally, due to the limited space, important aspects of the topic such as physical activity and its influence on body weight regulation and cytokine production in detail are not included in the current study.

6. Conclusion

As we know that obesity is the condition of excessive accumulation of fat as a result of disequilibrium between energy intake and its expenditure. Several studies showed that adipose tissue acts as an endocrine organ that plays a critical role in maintaining the homeostasis of immunity. Studies also reported that obesity plays a pivotal role in the development of low-grade inflammation. As a result, optimal nutrition is required for maintaining a healthy immune balance. A healthy diet comprising of appropriate GI/GL, n-3 PUFAs, less amount of saturated and trans-fatty acids, vitamins, minerals, flavonoids, phytoestrogens, probiotics, prebiotics, and Synbiotics is beneficial in combating the obesity and its related complications.

Therefore, it is concluded that consuming different dietary components rather than a single component may prove beneficial in combating the burden of weight gain as its associated comorbidities.

Acknowledgements

I express my deep sense of gratitude to my beloved husband Mr. Nirmal Kumar for his untiring help, opinions, and valuable suggestions with overwhelming encouragement. I am also deeply regretted if I am not able to cite the papers of all those authors who have contributed to our understanding of this topic.

Conflict of interest

The author declares no conflict of interest.

Author details

Upasana
Mahila College Dalmianagar, Veer Kunwar Singh University, Arrah, Bihar, India

*Address all correspondence to: me.upasana87@gmail.com

IntechOpen

© 2020 The Author(s). Licensee IntechOpen. This chapter is distributed under the terms of the Creative Commons Attribution License (http://creativecommons.org/licenses/by/3.0), which permits unrestricted use, distribution, and reproduction in any medium, provided the original work is properly cited.

References

[1] Bray GA. Risks of obesity. Endocrinology and Metabolism Clinics of North America. 2003;**32**:787-804

[2] Formiguera X, Canton A. Obesity: Epidemiology and clinical aspects. Best Practice & Research. Clinical Gastroenterology. 2004;**18**(6):1125-1146

[3] Ali AT, Crowther NJ. Factors predisposing to obesity: A review of the literature. Journal of Endocrinology, Metabolism & Diabetes of South Africa. 2009;**14**(2):81-84

[4] WHO: Obesity and overweight. Available from: https://www.who.int/news-room/fact-sheets/detail/obesity-and-overweight [Accessed: 03 March 2020]

[5] Ouchi N, Parker JL, Lugus JJ, Walsh K. Adipokines in inflammation and metabolic disease. Nature Reviews. Immunology. 2011;**11**:85-97

[6] Dludla PV, Nkambule BB, Jack B, Mkandla Z, Mutize T, Silvestri S, et al. Inflammation and oxidative stress in an obese state and the protective effects of gallic acids. Nutrients. 2019;**11**:23-29

[7] Francisqueti FV, Chiaverini LC, Santos KC, Minatel IO, Ronchi CB, Ferron AJ, et al. The role of oxidative stress on the pathophysiology of metabolic syndrome. Revista da Associação Médica Brasileira. 2017;**63**:85-91

[8] Lumeng CN, Saltiel AR. Inflammatory links between obesity and metabolic disease. Journal of Clinical Investigation. 2011;**121**:2111-2117

[9] Juge Aubry CE, Henrichot E, Meier CA. Adipose tissue: A regulator of inflammation. Best Practice & Research. Clinical Endocrinology & Metabolism. 2005;**19**(4):547-566

[10] Hansson GK. Inflammation, atherosclerosis, and coronary artery disease. The New England Journal of Medicine. 2005;**352**:1685-1695

[11] GC-1 Turns White fat into Brown fat. The Endocrine Society; 2015 [Accessed: 25 March 2020]

[12] Oppenheim JJ, Feldmann M. Introduction to the role of cytokines in innate host defense and adaptative immunity. In: Oppenheim JJ, Feldmann M, editors. Cytokine Reference, Volume 1: Ligands. San Diego: Academic Press; 2001. pp. 3-20

[13] Laing KJ, Secombes CJ. Chemokines. Developmental and Comparative Immunology. 2004;**28**:443-460

[14] Montani JP, Carroll JF, Dwyer TM, Antic V, Yang Z, Dulloo AG. Ectopic fat storage in heart, blood vessels and kidneys in the pathogenesis of cardiovascular diseases. International Journal of Obesity and Related Metabolic Disorders. 2004;**28** (Suppl 4):S58-S65

[15] Lee H, Lee In S, Choue R. Obesity, inflammation and diet. Pediatric Gastroenterology, Hepatology & Nutrition. 2013;**16**(3):143-152

[16] Gregor MF, Hotamisligil GS. Inflammatory mechanisms in obesity. Annual Review of Immunology. 2011;**29**:415-445

[17] Hotamisligil GS. Inflammation and metabolic disorders. Nature. 2006;**444**:860-867

[18] Ron D, Walter P. Signal integration in the endoplasmic reticulum unfolded protein response. Nature Reviews. Molecular Cell Biology. 2007;**8**:519-529

[19] Urano F, Wang X, Bertolotti A, Zhang Y, Chung P, Harding HP, et al.

Coupling of stress in the ER to activation of JNK protein kinases by transmembrane protein kinase IRE1. Science. 2000;**287**:664-666

[20] Deng J, Lu PD, Zhang Y, Scheuner D, Kaufman RJ, Sonenberg N, et al. Translational repression mediates activation of nuclear factor kappa B by phosphorylated translation initiation factor 2. Molecular and Cellular Biology. 2004;**24**:10161-10168

[21] Gregor MF, Hotamisligil GS. Thematic review series: Adipocyte biology. Adipocyte stress: The endoplasmic reticulum and metabolic disease. Journal of Lipid Research. 2007;**48**:1905-1914

[22] Surmi BK, Hasty AH. Macrophage infiltration into adipose tissue: Initiation, propagation and remodeling. Future Lipidology. 2008;**3**:545-556

[23] Hosogai N, Fukuhara A, Oshima K, Miyata Y, Tanaka S, Segawa K, et al. Adipose tissue hypoxia in obesity and its impact on adipocytokine dysregulation. Diabetes. 2007;**56**:901-911

[24] Ye J, Gao Z, Yin J, He Q. Hypoxia is a potential risk factor for chronic inflammation and adiponectin reduction in adipose tissue of ob/ob and dietary obese mice. American Journal of Physiology. Endocrinology and Metabolism. 2007;**293**:E1118-E1128

[25] Shi H, Kokoeva MV, Inouye K, Tzameli I, Yin H, Flier JS. TLR4 links innate immunity and fatty acid-induced insulin resistance. The Journal of Clinical Investigation. 2006;**116**:3015-3025

[26] Vaidya R, Udipi S. Metabolic syndrome in menopausal women: Modulation of contributory inflammatory markers by dietary substrates. Journal of Obesity & Metabolic Syndrome. 2015;**160**(2):155-160

[27] Liu S, Willett WC, Manson JE, Hu FB, Rosner B, Colditz G. Relation between changes in intakes of dietary fiber and grain products and changes in weight and development of obesity among middle aged women. The American Journal of Clinical Nutrition. 2003;**78**:920-927

[28] Salmeron J, Manson JE, Stampfer MJ, Colditz GA, Wing AL, Willett WC. Dietary fiber, glycemic load, and risk of non-insulin-dependent diabetes mellitus in women. Journal of the American Medical Association. 1997;**277**:472-477

[29] Augustin LS, Kendall CW, Jenkins DJ, Willett WC, Astrup A, Barclay AW, et al. Glycemic index, glycemic load and glycemic response: An International Scientific Consensus Summit from the International Carbohydrate Quality Consortium (ICQC). Nutrition, Metabolism, and Cardiovascular Diseases. 2015;**25**:795-815

[30] American Diabetes Association. Standards of medical care in diabetes-2011. Diabetes Care. 2011;**34**(Suppl 1):S11-S61

[31] Neuhouser ML, Schwarz Y, Wang C, Breymeyer K, Coronado G, Wang CY, et al. A low-glycemic load diet reduces serum C-reactive protein and modestly increases adiponectin in overweight and obese adults. The Journal of Nutrition. 2012;**142**:369-374

[32] Levitan EB, Cook NR, Stampfer MJ, Ridker PM, Rexrode KM, Buring JE, et al. Dietary glycemic index, dietary glycemic load, blood lipids, and C-reactive protein. Metabolism. 2008;**57**:437-443

[33] Vrolix R, Mensink RP. Effects of glycemic load on metabolic risk markers in subjects at increased risk of developing metabolic syndrome. The

American Journal of Clinical Nutrition. 2010;**92**:366-374

[34] Kelly KR, Navaneethan SD, Solomon TPJ, Haus JM, Cook M, Barkoukis H, et al. Lifestyle - induced decrease in in fat mass adiponectin secretion in obese adults. Medicine and Science in Sports and Exercise. 2014;**46**(5):920-926

[35] Simpoulos AP. An increase in the omega –6/omega-3 fatty acid ratio increases the risk for obesity. Nutrients. 2016;**8**:128-144

[36] Patterson E, Wall R, Fitzgerald GF, Ross RP, Stanton C. Health Implications of high dietary omega - 6 polyunsaturated fatty acids. Journal of Nutrition and Metabolism. 2012;**2012**:539426. DOI: 10.1155/2012/539426

[37] Lee KR, Midgette Y, Shah R. Fish oil derived omega 3 fatty acids suppress adipose NLRP3 inflammasome signaling in human study. Journal of the Endocrine Society. 2019;**3**(3):504-515

[38] Rogero MM, Calder PC. Obesity, inflammation, toll - like receptor 4 and fatty acids. Nutrients. 2018;**10**:432-450

[39] Estadella D, da Penha Oller do Nascimento CM, Oyama LM, Ribeiro EB, Damaso AR, Piana A. Lipotoxicity: Effects of dietary saturated and trans fatty acids. Mediators of Inflammation. 2012. DOI: 10.1155/2013/137579

[40] Kopf JC, Suhr MJ, Clarke J, Eyun S, Riethoven JM, Ramer-Tait AE, et al. Role of whole grains versus fruits and vegetables in reducing subclinical inflammation and promoting gastrointestinal health in individuals affected by overweight and obesity: A randomised controlled trial. Nutrition Journal. 2018;**17**:72-85

[41] Navarro P, de Dios O, Gavela-Perez T, Gorgojo L, Martin-Moreno JM, Soriano-Guillen L, et al. Vegetable and fruit intakes are associated with hs - CRP levels in pre - pubertal girls. Nutrients. 2017;**9**:224-233

[42] Julia C, Meunier N, Touvier M, Ahluwalia N, Sapin V, Papet I, et al. Dietary patterns and risk of elevated C-reactive protein concentrations 12 years later. The British Journal of Nutrition. 2013;**110**:747-754

[43] Lee Y, Kang D, Lee SA. Effect of dietary patterns on serum C-reactive protein level. Nutrition, Metabolism, and Cardiovascular Diseases. 2014;**24**(9):1004-1011

[44] Salas-Salvado J, Garcia-Arellano A, Estruch R, Marquez-Sandoval F, Corella D, Fiol M, et al. Components of the mediterranean-type food pattern and serum inflammatory markers among patients at high risk for cardiovascular disease. European Journal of Clinical Nutrition. 2008;**62**:651-659

[45] Freese R, Vaarala O, Turpeinen AM, Mutanen M. No difference in platelet activation or inflammation markers after diets rich or poor in vegetables, berries and apple in healthy subjects. European Journal of Nutrition. 2004;**43**:175-182

[46] Morand C, Dubray C, Milenkovic D, Lioger D, Martin JF, Scalbert A, et al. Hesperidin contributes to the vascular protective effects of orange juice: A randomized crossover study in healthy volunteers. The American Journal of Clinical Nutrition. 2011;**93**:73-80

[47] Brady WE, Mares-Perlman JA, Bowen P, Stacewicz-Sapuntzakis M. Human serum carotenoid concentrations are related to physiologic and lifestyle factors. The Journal of Nutrition. 1996;**126**:129-137

[48] Wang L, Gaziano JM, Norkus EP, Buring JE, Sesso HD. Associations of

plasma carotenoids with risk factors and biomarkers related to cardiovascular disease in middle-aged and older women. The American Journal of Clinical Nutrition. 2008;**88**:747-754

[49] Julia C, Galan P, Touvier M, Meunier N, Papet I, Sapin V, et al. Antioxidant status and the risk of elevated C- reactive protein 12 years later. Annals of Nutrition & Metabolism. 2014;**65**:289-298. DOI: 10.1159/000363194

[50] Beydoun MA, Chen X, Jha K, Beydoun HA, Zonderman AB, Canas JA. Carotenoids, vitamin A, and their association with the metabolic syndrome: A systematic review and meta-analysis. Nutrition Reviews. 2019;**77**:32-45

[51] Bohn T. Carotenoids and markers of oxidative stress in human observational studies and intervention trials: Implications for chronic diseases. Antioxidant. 2019;**8**(6):179. DOI: 10.3390/antiox8060179

[52] Totan B, Baygut H, Karadag MG. Vitamin C physiology: The known and the unknown in obesity. Journal of Food and Nutrition Research. 2019;7(8):613-618

[53] Ellulu MS. Obesity, cardiovascular disease, and role of vitamin C on inflammation: A review of facts and underlying mechanisms. Inflammopharmacology. 2017;**25**(3):313-328. DOI: 10.1007/s10787-017-0314-7

[54] Fumeron C, Nguyen-Khoa T, Saltiel C, Kebede M, Buisson C, Drueke TB, et al. Effects of oral vitamin C supplementation on oxidative stress and inflammation status in haemodialysis patients. Nephrology, Dialysis, Transplantation. 2005;**20**:1874-1879

[55] Barbagallo M, Dominguez LJ. Magnesium and aging. Current Pharmaceutical Design. 2010;**16**(7): 832-839

[56] de Oliveira ARS, Cruz KJC, Severo JS, Morais JBS, De Freitas TEC, Araujo RS, et al. Hypomagnesemia and its relation with chronic low-grade inflammation in obesity. Revista da Associação Médica Brasileira. 2017;**63**(2):156-163

[57] Chacko SA, Song Y, Nathan L, Tinker L, de Boer IH, Tylavsky F, et al. Relations of dietary magnesium intake to biomarkers of inflammation and endothelial dysfunction in an ethnically diverse cohort of postmenopausal women. Diabetes Care. 2010;**33**:304-310

[58] Guerrero-Romero F, Rodriguez-Moran M. Relationship between serum magnesium levels and C-reactive protein concentration, in non-diabetic, non-hypertensive obese subjects. International Journal of Obesity and Related Metabolic Disorders. 2002;**26**:469-474

[59] Panche AN, Diwan AD, Chandra SR. Flavonoids: An overview. Journal of Nutritional Science. 2016;**5**(e47):1-15

[60] Vernarelli JA, Lambert JD. Flavonoid intake is inversely associated with obesity and C-reactive protein, a marker for inflammation, in US adults. Nutrition & Diabetes. 2017;**7**:e276. DOI: 10.1038/nutd.2017.22

[61] Landberg R, Sun Q, Rimm EB, Cassidy A, Scalbert A, Mantzoros CS, et al. Selected dietary flavonoids are associated with markers of inflammation and endothelial dysfunction in U.S. women. The Journal of Nutrition. 2011;**141**:618-625

[62] Soumela JP, Ahotupa M, Yang B, Vasankari T, Kallio H. Absorption of flavonols derived from sea buckthorn (*Hippophae rhamnoides* L.) and their effect on emerging risk factors for cardiovascular disease in humans.

Journal of Agricultural and Food Chemistry. 2006;**54**:7364-7369

[63] Rietjens IMCM, Louisse J, Beekmann K. The potential health effects of dietary phytoestrogens. British Journal of Pharmacology. 2017;**174**:1263-1280. DOI: 10.1111/bph.13622

[64] Azabakht L, Esmallzadeh A, Kimiagar M, Hu FB, Mehrabi Y, Willett WC. Soy consumption, markers of inflammation, and endothelial function. Diabetes Care. 2017;**30**(4):967-973

[65] Aubertin-Leheudre M, Lord C, Khalil A, Dionne IJ. Effect of 6 months of exercise and isoflavone supplementation on clinical cardiovascular risk factors in obese postmenopausal women: A randomized, double-blind study. Menopause. 2007;**14**:624-629

[66] Food and Agriculture Organization. Probiotics in Food: Health and Nutritional Properties and Guidelines for Evaluation. Rome, Italy: FAO; 2006

[67] Cerdo T, Garcia-Santos JA, Bermudez MG, Campoy C. The role of probiotics and prebiotics in the prevention and treatment of obesity. Nutrients. 2019;**11**:635. DOI: 10.3390/nu11030635

[68] Kekkonen RA, Lummela N, Karjalainen H, Latvala S, Tynkkynen S, Jarvenpaa S, et al. Probiotic intervention has strain-specific anti-inflammatory effects in healthy adults. World Journal of Gastroenterology. 2008;**14**:2029-2036

[69] Pineiro M, Asp NG, Reid G, Macfarlane S, Morelli L, Brunser O, et al. FAO technical meeting on prebiotics. Journal of Clinical Gastroenterology. 2008;**42**:S156-S159

[70] Russo F, Riezzo G, Chiloiro M, de Michele G, Chimienti G, Marconi E, et al. Metabolic effects of a diet with inulin-enriched pasta in healthy young volunteers. Current Pharmaceutical Design. 2010;**16**(7):825-831

[71] Guigoz Y, Rochat F, Perruisseau-Carrier G, Rochat I, Schiffrin EJ. Effects of oligosaccharide on the faecal flora and non-specific immune system in elderly people. Nutrition Research. 2002;**22**:13-25

[72] Schiffrin EJ, Thomas DR, Kumar VB, Brown C, Hager C, Van't Hof MA, et al. Systemic inflammatory markers in older persons: The effect of oral nutritional supplementation with prebiotics. The Journal of Nutrition, Health & Aging. 2007;**11**:475-479

[73] Gibson GR, Roberfroid MB. Dietary modulation of the human colonic microbiota: Introducing the concept of prebiotics. The Journal of Nutrition. 1995;**125**(6):1401-1412

[74] Anandharaj M, Sivasankari B, Rani RP. Effects of probiotics, prebiotics, and synbiotics on hypercholesterolemia: A review. Chinese Journal of Biology. 2014. DOI: 10.1155/2014/572754

[75] Ferrarese R, Ceresola ER, Preti A, Canducci F. Probiotics, prebiotics and synbiotics for weight loss and metabolic syndrome in the microbiome era. European Review for Medical and Pharmacological Sciences. 2018;**22**:7588-7605. DOI: 10.26355/eurrev_201811_16301

[76] Reilly SM, Saltiel AR. Adapting to obesity with adipose tissue inflammation. Nature Reviews. Endocrinology. 2017;**13**:633-643. DOI: 10.1038/nrendo.2017.90

[77] Monteiro R, Azevedo I. Chronic inflammation in obesity and the metabolic syndrome. Mediators of Inflammation. 2010. DOI: 10.1155/2010/289645

[78] Dalton B, Campbell IC, Chung R, Breen G, Schmidt U, Himmerich H. Inflammatory markers in anorexia nervosa: An exploratory study. Nutrients. 2018;**10**:1573-1588. DOI: 10.3390/nu10111573

[79] Solmi M, Veronese N, Favaro A, Paolo S, Manzato E, Sergi G, et al. Inflammatory cytokines and anorexia nervosa: A meta-analysis of cross-sectional and longitudinal studies. Psychoneuroendocrinology. 2015;**51**:237-252. DOI: 10.1016/j.psyneuen.2014.09.031

[80] Galitzky J, Bouloumie A. Human visceral - fat - specific glucocorticoid tuning of adipogenesis. Cell Metabolism. 2013;**18**(1):3-5. DOI: 10.1016/j.cmet.2013.06.008

[81] Lee M, Pramyothin P, Karastergiou K, Fried SK. Deconstructing the roles of glucocorticoids in adipose tissue biology and the development of central obesity. Biochimica et Biophysica Acta. 2014;**1842**(3):473-481

Chapter 3

Orexin and Psychoneurobiology: A Hidden Treasure

Hayder M. Alkuraishy, Ali I. Al-Gareeb and Naseer A. Al-Harchan

Abstract

Orexin is a neuropeptide secreted from the lateral hypothalamus and prefrontal cortex concerned in wakefulness and excitement. This study aimed to review the possible neurobiological effect of orexin. A diversity of search strategies was adopted and assumed which included electronic database searches of Medline and PubMed using MeSH terms, keywords, and title words. Orexin plays a vital role in activation of learning, memory acquisition, and consolidation through activation of the monoaminergic system, which affects cognitive flexibility and cognitive function. Orexin stimulates adrenocorticotrophin (ACTH) and corticosteroid secretions via activation of the central corticotropin-releasing hormone (CRH). Cerebrospinal (CSF) and serum orexin serum levels are reduced in depression, schizophrenia, and narcolepsy. However, high orexin serum levels are revealed in drug addictions. Regarding neurodegenerative brain diseases, CSF and serum orexin levels are reduced in Parkinson's disease (PD), Alzheimer's disease (AD), Huntington's disease (HD), amyotrophic lateral sclerosis (ALS), and multiple sclerosis (MS). Orexin antagonist leads to significant reduction of sympathetic overactivity during withdrawal syndrome. Also, orexin antagonist improves sleep pattern. The orexinergic system is involved in different psychiatric and neurological disorders; therefore targeting of this system could be a possible novel pathway in the management of these disorders. In addition measurement of CSF and serum orexin levels might predict the relapse and withdrawal of addict patients.

Keywords: orexin, sleep disorders, psychiatric disorders, neurodegenerative disorders

1. Introduction

Orexin, also known as hypocretin, is a neuropeptide that regulates arousal, wakefulness, and appetite. The most common form of narcolepsy, in which the sufferer experiences brief losses of muscle tone (cataplexy), is caused by a lack of orexin in the brain due to destruction of the cells that produce it. There are only 10,000–20,000 orexin-producing neurons in the human brain, located predominantly in the perifornical area and lateral hypothalamus. They project widely throughout the central nervous system, regulating wakefulness, feeding, and other behaviors. The orexin system was initially suggested to be primarily involved in the stimulation of food intake, based on the finding that central administration of orexin-A and orexin-B increased food intake. In addition, it stimulates wakefulness, regulates energy expenditure, and modulates visceral function [1, 2].

IntechOpen

Two distinct types of orexin, orexin-A and orexin-B, were identified; they act on specific receptors called orexin receptor type 1 (OX1R) and orexin receptor type 2 (OX2R). Orexin-A activates both of these receptors equally, while orexin-B has a five times higher affinity to OX2R than OX1R. Upon activation, prepro-orexin will split to orexin-A and orexin-B, which act on their G protein-coupled receptors (**Figure 1**) [3].

Orexin receptors are distributed mainly in the lateral hypothalamus and adjacent areas, and their nerve fibers project to multiple brain regions. Orexinergic neurons in the lateral hypothalamus group are closely associated with reward-related functions. These neurons preferentially innervate the ventral tegmental area and the ventromedial prefrontal cortex. In contrast, the perifornical-dorsal group of orexinergic neurons is involved in functions related to arousal and autonomic response. These neurons project inter-hypothalamically, as well as to the brainstem, where the release of orexin modulates various autonomic processes. Indeed, accumulating evidence shows that the orexin/receptor system is ectopically expressed in several neurological disorders, suggesting that it plays an important role in the incidence and pathogenesis of these diseases [4].

It has been verified that hypothalamic orexigenic neurons are involved in reward functions, while prefrontal orexigenic neurons are linked in the regulation of autonomic and arousal functions. Moreover, orexin provokes and stimulates food intake via inhibition of autonomic digestive feedbacks. Orexigenic neurons are inhibited by leptin and food intake, while hypoglycemia and ghrelin activate orexigenic neurons. Amino acid and high-protein diets paradoxically provoke the hyperpolarization of orexigenic neurons and block glucose-induced orexigenic neuron activations [5]. Animal model studies have shown that orexin is a very important link between sleep and body metabolism since sleep deprivation leads to higher food intake and induction of catabolism [6].

Additionally, orexin stimulates different neurotransmitters which are linked to the activation of the central nervous system, including acetylcholine, histamine, noradrenaline, and dopamine. Therefore, mutations of orexin receptors lead to sleep disorders. Mice with orexin knockout are subjected to narcolepsy and excessive daytime sleepiness [7]. Alizamini et al. study showed that central

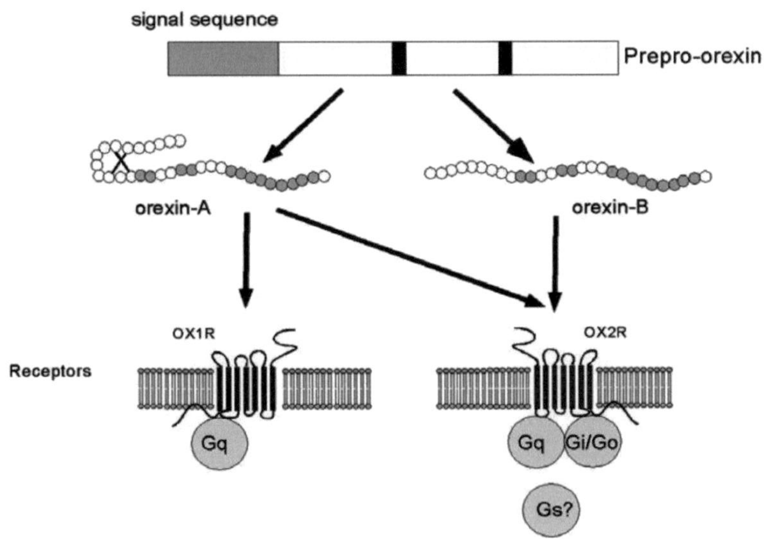

Figure 1.
Schematic representation of orexin system.

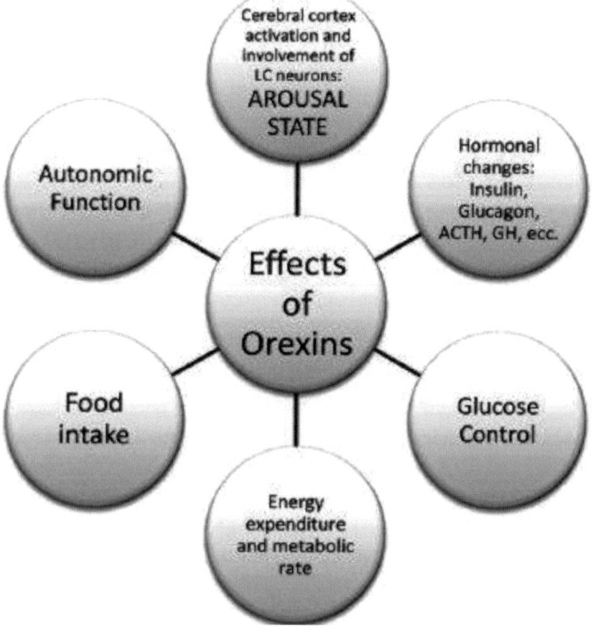

Figure 2.
Central and peripheral effects of orexin.

administration of orexin leads to stimulation of locomotion, psychomotor performance, body temperature, and energy expenditure. Furthermore, mice with orexin deficiency are subjected to obesity due to reduction of basal metabolic and energy expenditure rates. Beside, orexin knockout out mice is characterized by a reduction in brown adipose tissue thermogenesis with poor differentiation of pre-adipocyte into adipocytes in the adipose tissue [8]. Central and peripheral effects of orexin are illustrated in **Figure 2**.

The aim of this study was to provide a narrative review of the neurobiological effect of orexin system and to examine the association between orexin neurotransmission and different psychoneurological disorders, including depression, schizophrenia, addiction, Parkinson's disease, and dementia. Evidence from experimental, preclinical and clinical studies is evaluated for bidirectional relationships between orexin neurobiology and psychoneurological disorders. Given the nature of the subject area, it remains clear that this literature search cannot be regarded as a systemic review.

2. Method and search strategy

A diversity of search strategies was adopted and assumed which included electronic database searches of Medline and PubMed using MeSH terms, keywords, and title words. There is no limitation for publication year. The terms used for these searches were as follows: [orexin OR hypocretin] AND [cognitive function OR vigilance OR depression OR schizophrenia OR addiction OR Alzheimer dementia OR stroke OR sleep disorders]. [suvorexant OR orexin antagonists] AND [sleep disorders OR vigilance OR depression OR schizophrenia OR addiction]. Reference lists of identified and notorious articles were reviewed. Besides, only English articles were considered, and case reports were not involved in the review. The key features of recognized relevant search studies were considered, and the conclusions were summarized in a narrative review.

2.1 Orexin and cognitive function

Orexin regulates behavioral and neuroendocrine response during stressful conditions as these events lead to the impairment of cognitive flexibility and function. Also, patients with psychiatric disorders such as panic disorder are associated with significant reduction of hypothalamic orexin activations [9].

It has been shown that stress improves male cognitive flexibility, but it worsens female cognitive flexibility due to gender differences in stress-induced orexin neuropeptide activations. Women are twice as likely as men to suffer from stress-related psychiatric disorders, such as post-traumatic stress disorder (PTSD) and major depressive disorder (MDD); however, the biological basis of these sex differences is not fully understood. Interestingly, orexins are known to be dysregulated in these disorders. Both preclinical and clinical studies have reported higher orexin system expression in females, which contributes to exaggerated neuroendocrine and behavioral responses to stress. Therefore, orexins may be important in the etiology of stress-related psychiatric disorders that present differently in men and women [10]. Piantadosi et al. illustrated that stimulation of prefrontal cholinergic neurons leads to the release of orexin from hypothalamic neurons, which play an important role in cognitive activation since high orexin activates the arousal state and executive functions via activation of cortical cholinergic neurons [11]. Chieffi et al. study reported the beneficial effects of exercise in stimulation of orexin release due to enhancement of hippocampal activity as exercise attenuates hippocampal deterioration and depressive symptoms in elderly persons through regulation of orexin release [12].

Notably, cognitive impairment is the main feature of neurological and neuropsychiatric disorders as in dementia and narcolepsy, which are linked to orexin dysfunction. Therefore, intranasal orexin peptide may be an effective agent for cognitive dysfunction [13]. Astonishingly, orexin plays a crucial role in activation of learning and memory, as orexin-A provokes memory acquisition and consolidation through activation of monoaminergic system. Consequently, orexin antagonist leads to significant memory dysfunction in the experimental rats [14]. Kim et al. study revealed that orexin is an important key factor of hippocampal neurogenesis as orexin-A participates in the hippocampal neuronal proliferation and neuroprotection following stroke; thus orexin agonist participates in prevention of negative stroke outcomes [15]. On the other hand, Uslaner et al. exhibited that dual orexin receptor antagonists (DORA-22) is an effective sedative agent, with less cognitive disability than GABA allosteric modulators, which cause significant cognitive dysfunctions [16, 17]. Therefore, orexin improves cognitive functions as illustrated in different human and animal studies (**Table 1**).

2.2 Orexin and neuroendocrinology

Orexin is involved in the regulation of central and peripheral signals to regulate metabolic homeostasis. Alongside, orexin stimulates adrenocorticotrophin (ACTH) and corticosteroid secretions via activation of central corticotropin-releasing hormone (CRH) and vasopressin. Therefore, orexin through OX2R receptor controls the hypothalamic-pituitary-adrenal axis (HPA) [18]. Previously, Malendowicz et al. illustrated that chronic orexin administration led to dose-dependent increase in cortisol and aldosterone plasma levels independent of ACTH levels, indicating a

Species	Interventions	Results	References
Animals	Stimulation of prefrontal cholinergic neurons	↑ orexin	Piantadosi et al. [11]
Humans and animals	Exercise Orexin-A administration	↑ orexin Provokes memory acquisition and consolidation	Chieffi et al. [12]
Humans	Intranasal orexin-A administration	Improve cognition	Calva and Fadel [13]
Mice	Orexin-A administration	Stimulates angiogenesis and neuroprotection	Kim et al. [15]
Humans	Administration of orexin receptor antagonists	Stimulates angiogenesis and neuroprotection	Uslaner et al. [16]

Table 1.
Orexin and cognitive functions.

direct stimulating effect of orexin on the adrenal cortex [19]. But in spite of these findings, Patel et al. study confirmed insignificant effect of orexin antagonists on ACTH and cortisol serum levels as well as on the markers of the sympathetic nervous system [20].

It has been reported that orexin administration leads to significant suppression of the hypothalamic prolactin release, which is not upturned by dopamine receptor antagonists like metoclopramide suggesting a novel pathway in controlling of prolactin secretion. The mechanism of prolactin inhibition may be through inhibition of prolactin-releasing factor or stimulation of prolactin-inhibiting factor. But previous study illustrated insignificant effect of orexin antagonist on prolactin plasma levels [21, 22].

Many studies showed that the blood glucose is regulated by central orexin through regulation of hepatic glucose production, skeletal glucose consumption and thermogenesis. High orexin or dysrhythmic in orexin secretion is linked with the development of obesity and insulin resistance [23, 24]. Thus, suvorexant and other orexin antagonists are effective in the management of obesity and insulin resistance via amelioration of body adiposity and augmentation of energy expenditure that improve glucose metabolism. Moreover, orexin-A has important roles in the regulation of pancreatic islet biology through activation of insulin secretion and prolongation of pancreatic islets life span [25].

Tsuneki et al. study illustrated that suvorexant improves glucose tolerance through inhibition of hepatic gluconeogenic factors, when administrated at resting time. However, administration of suvorexant at awaking time illustrates insignificant effect on glucose tolerance due to differential effects on the orexin sleep/wake operating system [26].

In addition, Flores et al. study illustrated an interaction between endocannabinoid and orexigenic neurons as there is a similarity between OX1R and CB1 receptors with diffuse overlapping in the anatomical distribution of these neurons. Therefore, the pharmacological effect of cannabinoid may be through orexigenic receptors [27]. The neuroendocrine effects of orexin are summarized in **Table 2**.

2.3 Orexin and psychiatric disorders

2.3.1 Orexin and depression

Among important etiological factors involved in the pathophysiology of depression, disturbances of monoamines and HPA are the main mechanistic pathways

Species	Interventions	Results	References
Animals	Orexin administration	↑ ACTH, cortisol	Czerwinska et al. [18]
Animals	Orexin administration	↑ cortisol, aldosterone	Malendowicz et al. [19]
Humans	Orexin administration	No effect on ACTH and cortisol	Patel et al. [20]
Humans and animals	Orexin administration	Inhibits prolactin	Lyons et al. [21], Samson et al. [22]
Humans	High orexin levels	Insulin resistance and obesity	Gupta et al. [23], Cigdem et al. [24]
Humans and animals	Orexin administration	↑ insulin secretion	Mediavilla and Risco [25]
Animals	Administration of orexin antagonists	Improves glucose tolerance	Tsuneki et al. [26]

Table 2.
Neuroendocrine effects of orexin.

leading to functional disorders of neuroplasticity, which is regarded as a cardinal step in the onset of depression [28].

Diurnal variation in orexin serum levels revealed that high orexin levels are occurring at the middle of night. It has been reported that orexin level is significantly decreased in patients with depression in comparison with healthy subjects [29]. But paradoxical high orexin serum levels are seen in some depressed patients, which is normalized by selective serotonin reuptake inhibitors. Since, orexin-A CSF levels are negatively correlated with depressive symptoms [30].

Long-term antidepressant agents improve orexin serum levels regardless of the type of antidepressant medications [31]. Nevertheless, there are different findings concerning orexin levels in depression. Feng et al. reported that depression is linked to reduction of serotonergic neuronal activity which is responsible for modulation of orexinergic activity [32]. Thus reduction of serotonergic neuronal activity leads to activation of orexin neuroactivity leading to depression. However, orexin levels are significantly reduced in depression compared with healthy control [33].

The initial animal model study observed reduction in the orexinergic neurons by 18% with diminution in size of these neurons in comparison with normal rats. As well, prepro-orexin mRNA expression and orexin-A were reduced compared with control [34].

Previous preclinical study revealed a strong connection between low orexin and risk of depression which are inconsistent with previous studies that illustrated hypoactivity of orexinergic neurons in patients with depression since short-term antidepressant therapy improves sleep pattern through increasing and decreasing the expression of mRNA of orexin-A and orexin-B, respectively [35].

Ito et al. showed that administration of orexin-A leads to significant reduction of despair behavior in depression with important hippocampal neurogenesis via upregulation of neuropeptide Y (NPY). These changes are inhibited by co-administration of orexin-A antagonist [36].

Therefore, orexin levels are different according to the pathophysiology of depression. Low orexin in depressed patients is associated with hypersomnia, whereas high orexin in depressed patients is associated with insomnia and interrupted sleep [17]. Ji et al. illustrated that orexinergic neurons have direct connection to the ventral pallidum (VP) which is concerned with stress response and rewarding system. Orexin stimulates the VP and prevents depressive behavior. Therefore, high orexin in the VP is associated with elevated serum corticosterone serum levels during acute stress, which per se prevent a depressive reaction against stressful events through improvement of stress resilience [37].

2.3.2 Orexin and schizophrenia

The association between orexin and schizophrenia had not been previously explored precisely [38]. Clinical and preclinical findings proposed that orexin and orexin agonist are of great value and useful in treating cognitive deficit in schizophrenia [39]. There are widespread connection and interaction between orexin and dopaminergic neurons in midbrain, thalamocortical region, and amygdala suggesting the potential role of orexinergic neurons in schizophrenia [40].

Modafinil is an atypical dopamine reuptake inhibitor used in the treatment of narcolepsy and antipsychotic drug-induced sleep disorder (**Figure 3**) [41]. Modafinil has been revealed as a complement of drugs in therapy of schizophrenia, and it reduce negative symptoms with no effect on the positive symptoms. Modafinil improves locomotor and psychomotor performances through activation of orexinergic neurons [42].

Therefore, activations of orexinergic neurons by modafinil may be an imperative step for future antipsychotic medications. These findings document that dopaminergic agonists mainly at D1 and D2 receptors modify orexinergic neurotransmissions [43]. Also, dopamine antagonists that cause weight gain lead to activation of orexin pathway, but dopamine antagonists which do not cause weight gain do not activate orexin pathway [44]. Nevertheless, amphetamine which indirectly activates dopamine leads to activation of orexinergic neurotransmission despite induction of weight loss. Moreover, clozapine activates only orexinergic neurons in the prefrontal cortex [45]. Similarly, orexin antagonists abolish olanzapine and haloperidol effect on midbrain dopaminergic neurons, suggesting that orexin is an important neurotransmitter mediates the action of antipsychotic drugs [46]. As well, Chen et al. illustrated that orexin-A is stimulated and upregulated by non-obesegenic antipsychotic drugs [47]. Also, the high orexin level in patients with schizophrenia treated with antipsychotic drugs is regarded as a protective factor against the development and risk of drug-induced metabolic syndrome [48]. Furthermore, orexin agonist like modafinil ameliorates cognitive function, attention, and antipsychotic-induced sedation.

2.3.3 Orexin and addiction

The orexinergic system has broad projections and connections to different brain area which are concerned with drug-induced neuro-adaptation, including midbrain dopaminergic neurons, ventral tegmental area (VTA), nucleus accumbens (NA),

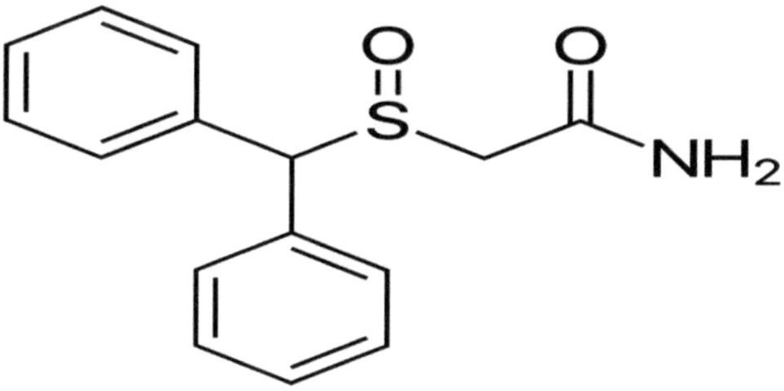

Figure 3.
Chemical structure of modafinil.

amygdala, and medial prefrontal cortex (mPFC). Drug abuse leads to augmentation of dopaminergic activity in NA through activation of orexinergic neurons at mesocorticolimbic pathway [49]. Correspondingly, experimental studies illustrated that OX1R and OX2R are highly expressed in the NA leading to inhibitory effect instead of excitatory effects seen on the VTA, amygdala, and mPFC. Therefore, a differential effect of orexin is receptor type dependent [50].

Acute administration of addicting drugs such as methamphetamine, nicotine, and amphetamine leads to activation of orexinergic neurons at the lateral hypothalamus. However, acute administration of cocaine and morphine does not affect orexinergic neurons. Besides, chronic administration of addict drugs causes activation of orexinergic neurons mainly at OX2R receptors, but chronic increasing dose of addict drugs leads to downregulation of orexinergic receptors [51]. Carr and Kalivas reported that orexin is an important mediator which enables cocaine to induce addiction-like behavior in rats due to dopaminergic neuronal changes [52]. Also, James et al. verified that orexinergic neurons at the lateral hypothalamus play a vital role in expression of addiction-like phenotype [53]. Thus, the orexinergic system is regarded as an important novel target for drug therapies to treat addiction.

Orexin serum level in chronic smoker subjects is related to craving in the phase of abstinence since it increased during addiction phase and reduced during withdrawal phase. This reduction leads to increase in craving and risk of relapse [54]. Therefore, orexin serum level is regarded as a potential biomarker predicts time and risk of smoking relapse.

Furthermore, Tsai and Huang reported that the orexin serum level is increased in heroin addicts who shifted to methadone maintenance therapy compared with controls suggesting that methadone increases orexin serum levels [55]. Similarly, orexin serum level is increased in chronic alcoholism, which is positively correlated with the severity of alcohol withdrawal. Alleviation of alcohol withdrawal syndrome is linked with reduction of the orexin serum level, which monitors the status of alcoholic patients during the abstinence period [56].

2.3.4 Orexin and sleep disorders

Narcolepsy is a sleep disorder that causes excessive daytime sleepiness or an intractable urge to sleep in, in which duration of rapid eye movement sleep (REM) is reduced. Cataplexy is a sudden reduction in muscle tones with preserved consciousness. Narcolepsy is commonly associated with cataplexy, which is triggered by emotional stimuli [57]. Methylphenidate, modafinil, and other psychostimulants are effective in the management of these sleep disorders [58]. Dysregulation of NREM sleep leads to narcolepsy only, whereas dysregulation of REM sleep leads to combined narcolepsy with cataplexy [59]. It has been reported that orexin increases vigilance through increasing awaking time and decreasing REM and NREM sleep periods. Both OX1R and OX2R are involved in the maintenance of arousal state directly or indirectly through the activation of monoaminergic neurons (noradrenalin, dopamine, histamine, and serotonin). Also, orexin activates cholinergic neurons in the basal forebrain, which is also important for arousal statues [60]. Yamanaka et al. study illustrated that activation of OX2R by orexin leads to wakefulness which is mediated by a histamine neurotransmitter since antihistamine blocks the excitatory effect of orexin, while activation of OX1R by orexin leads to wakefulness, through noradrenalin neurotransmitter [61]. Reduction of orexin level in the cerebrospinal fluid was documented in patients with narcolepsy and nowadays is regarded as one of the diagnostic criteria in the diagnosis of narcolepsy.

Likewise, human postmortem study found that orexin peptide and prepro-orexin mRNA are deficient in the pons and cerebral cortex [62]. Therefore, these findings unveil that orexin is an important neuropeptide in the regulation of sleep and consolidated wakefulness. **Table 3** summarized the potential role of orexin in common psychiatric disorders.

2.4 Orexin in neurodegenerative diseases

2.4.1 Parkinson's disease

Orexinergic neurons are severely affected in Parkinson's disease (PD); previously Fronczek et al. confirmed that orexinergic neuron density was reduced in the prefrontal cortex by 40% with significant reduction in CSF orexin levels in PD patients compared to the healthy control [63].

Furthermore, animal model study illustrated that 15% damage to the orexinergic neurons did not affect CSF orexin, while damage more than 70% leads to 50% decline in the CSF orexin [64]. These findings may explain the association of narcolepsy with PD since both dopamine and orexin interplay in the regulation of sleep pattern through activation of midbrain and thalamocortical pathway [65]. Feng et al. illustrated that in PD, there is a deficiency in hypoxia inducible factor 1 alpha (HIF1-α) due to mitochondrial dysfunction and the administration of orexin-A leads to significant neuroprotective effect on the dopaminergic neurons through the activation of HIF-α [66].

Moreover, orexin-A improves dopaminergic neurons in PD through the reduction of tyrosine hydroxylase (TH) and activation of brain-derived neurotrophic factor (BDNF) in the substantia nigra [43]. Therefore, orexin antagonist may increase risk of PD due to reduction of the neuroprotective and stimulating effects on the dopaminergic neurons at substantia nigra [67]. Sheng et al. found that orexin plays important roles in activation of the subthalamic nucleus which may give a new evidence for the participation of the subthalamic orexinergic system in PD. Importantly, orexin-A increased the protein level of brain-derived neurotrophic factor in dopaminergic neurons of the substantia nigra. The upregulation of BDNF is mainly via OX1R [68]. Long-term therapy with ropinirole in PD leads to significant reduction in the orexin activity which might explain the adverse effect of ropinirole-induced sleep disorder through inhibition of glutamatergic excitatory effect on the orexinergic neurons. Therefore, pharmacotherapy of PD should be re-evaluated in this context [69].

Psychiatric disorders	Species	Orexin levels	References
Depression	Human	Decreased	Kok et al. [29]
	Human	Increased	Grady et al. [30]
Schizophrenia	Human	Decreased	Mereu et al. [42]
			Patel et al. [20]
Chronic smoking	Animals	Increased	Al'Absi et al. [54]
Drug addictions	Human	Increased	James et al. [53]
Alcoholism	Human	Increased	Pan et al. [56]
Narcolepsy	Human	Decreased	Gabelle et al. [62]

Table 3.
Orexin and psychiatric disorders.

2.4.2 Alzheimer's disease

Alzheimer's disease (AD) is a neurodegenerative disease affecting different brain areas characterized by cognitive deficit and progressive memory loss [70]. AD also affects hypothalamic orexinergic neurons leading to excessive daytime sleepiness, which is correlated with low orexin CSF levels, as reduction 40% of the brain cell number is linked with a 14% reduction in orexin CSF levels [71]. Normally, orexin regulates cholinergic and monoaminergic neuron firing during sleep and wakefulness. In AD a reduction in the cholinergic pathway leads to disturbance in sleep patterns leading to daytime sleepiness and insomnia at night which are a hallmark of sleep rhythm in AD [72]. Besides, reduction of cholinergic activity causes overactivity of orexinergic neurons, which causes abnormal sleep and cognitive functions. These changes lead to an elevation of the orexin CSF level, which is linked with reduced REM sleep [73].

Dementia with Lewy bodies is characterized by an elevation in α-synuclein level, which is accumulated in orexin-containing neurons at the hypothalamus causing interference in orexin axonal transport. This effect leads to a reduction in the activity of the orexinergic system in dementia with Lewy bodies but not in AD [74]. Therefore, there are complexities in the orexinergic system according to the clinical presentation and sleep pattern in patients with AD.

2.4.3 Huntington's disease

Huntington's disease (HD) is a hereditary neurodegenerative disorder characterized by personality changes, motor disturbances, cognitive decline, and weight loss [75]. HD is caused by a defect in the gene encoding huntingtin, a protein with unclear function, which is essential for cell survival during development and in adult life [76]. In HD there is neurodegeneration involving the neostriatum and cerebral cortex, with the manifestation of intraneuronal aggregates of misfolded huntingtin. Moreover, in patients with end-stage HD, there is about 90% of neuronal loss in the tuber nucleus of the lateral hypothalamus. Orexin-A and orexin-B are synthesized from the same precursor gene and are expressed in the same neurons with their cell bodies concentrated to the lateral hypothalamus [77]. Preclinical and clinical studies observed that orexin serum and CSF levels are decreased by 72% in HD. In healthy subjects, orexin CSF level is >200pg/ml, but in HD and narcolepsy, this level is decreased below 110 pg/ml, due to degeneration of orexinergic neurons in the lateral hypothalamus. Therefore, CSF orexin level is regarded as a biomarker to evaluate the disease progression and usefulness of therapeutic intervention in patients with HD [78, 79]. However, Meier et al. illustrated that CSF and serum orexin levels are of no diagnostic value in prediction and follow-up of HD [80].

Recently, Cabanas et al. observed that orexin in HD has aberrant effects leading to abnormal sleep pattern, and thus orexin antagonist suvorexant may be of great value in restoring normal sleep and behavioral disturbance in HD [81] in addition, these neurons remain functional and illustrate paradoxical effect, it become more modifiable and affect by serotonine and noradrenaline, and less sensitive to the effect of suprachiasmatic nucleus (the master clock of the brain) causing abnormal biological circadian rhythm [81, 82].

Therefore, orexin level in HD is reduced, but the remaining functional orexinergic neurons lead to abnormal circadian biological rhythm causing behavioral, motor, and sleep disturbances.

2.4.4 Multiple sclerosis

Multiple sclerosis (MS) is a demyelinating disease in which the insulating covers of nerve cells in the brain and spinal cord are damaged. This damage disrupts the ability of parts of the nervous system to transmit signals, resulting in a range of signs and symptoms, including physical, mental, and sometimes psychiatric problems. Specific symptoms can include double vision, blindness in one eye, muscle weakness, and trouble with sensation or coordination. MS takes several forms, with new symptoms either occurring in isolated attacks (relapsing forms) or building up over time (progressive forms). Between attacks, symptoms may disappear completely; however, permanent neurological problems often remain, especially with the advancement of the disease [83, 84].

The three main characteristics of MS are the formation of lesions in the central nervous system, inflammation, and the destruction of myelin sheaths of neurons. These features interact in a complex and not yet fully understood manner to produce the breakdown of nerve tissue and in turn the signs and symptoms of the disease. Cholesterol crystals are believed to both impair myelin repair and aggravate inflammation. MS is believed to be an immune-mediated disorder that develops from an interaction of the individual's genetics and as yet unidentified environmental causes. Damage is believed to be caused, at least in part, by attack on the nervous system by a person's own immune system [85].

Considering the multiplicity of symptoms associated with multiple sclerosis (MS), there is possibility that hypocretin system function might be involved in the pathogenesis of the disease. Papuc et al. showed that high orexin CSF level in patients with MS as compared with healthy controls, but it positively correlated with fatigue level, suggesting a compensatory mechanism for the production of orexin in MS [86]. On the other hand, Nozaki et al. illustrated that orexin CSF level is reduced and correlated with symmetrical hypothalamic lesion and spinal cord damage in MS. Therefore, low orexin level was implicated in the pathogenesis of hypersomnia and cognitive deficit in patients with MS [87]. Recently, Pallais et al. confirmed that orexin has a neuroprotective effect in MS through inhibition of inflammatory and proinflammatory mediators mainly matrixmetaloproteinases (MMP-3, MMP-9) which are involved in damage of neuronal matrix proteins. Consequently, low CSF orexin level indicates underlying active disease [88].

Therefore, CSF orexin level is a valuable biomarker in the diagnosis and prediction of the severity of MS.

2.4.5 Amyotrophic lateral sclerosis

Amyotrophic lateral sclerosis (ALS), also known as motor neuron disease (MND), is a disease that leads the death of neurons controlling voluntary muscles. The underlying mechanism involves damage to both upper and lower motor neurons. ALS is characterized by stiff muscles, muscle twitching, and muscle weakness is still unknown. The cause of ALS is not known in 90% of cases but is believed to involve both genetic and environmental factors. The remaining 10% of cases is inherited [89]. Previously, Van Rooij et al. illustrated that CSF orexin level was normal in patients with ALS and not correlated with age and gender. However, a disturbance in the orexinergic system is involved in the pathogenesis of ALS [90]. Moreover, the pathogenesis of ALS is associated with lateral hypothalamic lesions, a site of the orexinergic system leading to sleep disturbances and hypersomnia [91].

Despite different and large body of literature survey, little is known about CSF orexin levels, in clinical and preclinical studies in ALS.

Therefore, orexin CSF level and orexinergic activity in different neurodegenerative diseases are summarized in **Table 4**.

2.5 Orexin antagonists and neurobiology

Regarding orexin antagonists, suvorexant is a dual orexin receptor antagonist was approved by the Food and Drug Administration (FDA) on 13 August 2014 [92]. Other orexin antagonists are almorexant, lemborexant, and filorexant are used in the management of insomnia and other sleep disorders. Also, these drugs may be of great value in the control of depressive disorders and peripheral diabetic neuropathy [93].

Suvorexant (**Figure 2**) is the first orexin antagonists approved in the United States for treatment of insomnia, which is effective in reduction of time to sleep onset and increase of total sleeping time [94]. Moreover, administration of SB-33867 which is an orexin antagonist leads to significant reduction of sympathetic tone causing a reduction in blood pressure, heart rate, and plasma noradrenalin. These findings suggest that orexin through OX1 receptor regulates sympathetic tone since intravenous administration of orexin leads to parallel increases in noradrenalin plasma levels [95].

Hatta et al. study confirmed the significant effect of suvorexant in the management of delirium in elderly patients in acute care units. The anti-delirium effect is due to the regulation of circadian biology [96]. Delirium is proposed to be related of suvorexant to disturbances and disorders in sleep pattern in critically ill patients in the intensive care unit. Also, attention disorders are caused by disturbances in the ascending reticular activating system (ARAS) which is responsible for maintenance of human arousal. Normally, the arousal state is regulated and stimulated by ARAS neurotransmitters and by hypothalamic orexin [97]. Therefore, orexin receptor antagonists may play important role in the regulation of hypothalamic and brain stem stress during acute injury. Moreover, a recent study by Kawada et al. illustrated that suvorexant add-on therapy to ramelteon in the management of sleep disorders in patients with acute stroke is more effective than when combined with benzodiazepines [98].

It has been verified that prolonged alcohol consumption is associated with sleep disturbance which is a powerful factor for relapse and setback to alcohol use. Suvorexant reduces the motivation properties of alcohol, so it plays a crucial role in the prevention of alcoholism [99].

Beside, Gentile et al. study revealed the possible role of suvorexant in reduction of motor impulsivity of cocaine-induced psychostimulant effects. Thus suvorexant may be effective in attenuation of cocaine withdrawal syndrome [100].

As well, suvorexant had placebo-like effect on EEG in comparison with zolpidem which has a significant reduction in the spectral density of rapid eye movement and non-rapid eye movement sleep (NREM) pattern [101].

Psychiatric disorders	Species	CSF orexin levels	References
Parkinson's disease	Human	Decreased	Fronczek et al. [63]
Alzheimer's disease	Human	Increased	Liguori et al. [73]
Huntington's disease	Human	Decreased	Mignot et al. [78]
	Animals	Normal	Papuc et al. [86]
Multiple sclerosis	Human	Decreased	Nozaki et al. [87]
ALS	Human	Normal	Van Rooij et al. [90]

Table 4.
Orexin and neurodegenerative diseases.

In spite of the wide uses of suvorexant in the management of sleep disorders and controlling insomnia, it did not reduce the psychomotor performances as documented by Vermeeren et al. study [102].

Orexin-A is involved in regulation of feeding; it stimulates nocturnal feeding through OX1 receptor. Therefore, OX1 receptor antagonist regulates feeding and reduced nocturnal feeding; thus, orexin antagonist could be useful in the treatment of obesity [103]. Orexin-A is implicated in the pathogenesis of obesity; it promotes hyperphagia through central activation of cannabinoid receptors and inhibition of melanocyte-stimulating hormone [104]. Both orexin-A and endocannabinoid increases glucose response of neuronal excitability in the arcuate nucleus leading to induction of feeding and obesity [104].

In summary, more research is required to reinforce the extant information on the importance of the limited number of factors studied to date and provide data on additional potentially relevant effects. Similarly, rubric for such research should shift from preclinical and animal model studies to clinical studies to illustrate disease progression and treatment effects in relation to orexin neurobiology. This study suggests that orexin system is a future target in the management of different psychoneurological disorders after delineating the specific role of orexin receptor agonists and antagonists. Moreover, measurement of orexin serum level which is an easy method may be of great value in evaluation and assessment of different neurological disorders. Also, ratio of orexin serum level/CSF orexin level may reflect the activity of endogenous orexinergic system.

3. Conclusion

Orexin system is regarded as a potential novel target in the management of schizophrenia, depression, addiction, and sleep disorders. Orexin serum level might predict relapse and withdrawal of addict patients.

Conflict of interest

None.

Funding and support

None.

Author details

Hayder M. Alkuraishy*, Ali I. Al-Gareeb and Naseer A. Al-Harchan
Department of Clinical Pharmacology, Medicine and Therapeutic, Medical Faculty, College of Medicine, Al-Mustansiriya University, Baghdad, Iraq

*Address all correspondence to: hayderm36@yahoo.com

IntechOpen

© 2020 The Author(s). Licensee IntechOpen. This chapter is distributed under the terms of the Creative Commons Attribution License (http://creativecommons.org/licenses/by/3.0), which permits unrestricted use, distribution, and reproduction in any medium, provided the original work is properly cited.

References

[1] Burdakov D. Reactive and predictive homeostasis: Roles of orexin/hypocretin neurons. Neuropharmacology. 2018:19. pii: S0028-3908(18)30811-6

[2] Airapetov MI, Sekste EA, Eresko SO, Bychkov ER, Lebedev AA, Shabanov PD. Chronic alcoholism influences the mRNA level of the orexin receptor type 1 (OX1R) in emotiogenic structures of the rat brain. Biomedit͡sinskai͡a Khimii͡a. 2018;**64**(5):451-454

[3] Lu GL, Lee MT, Chiou LC. Orexin-mediated restoration of hippocampal synaptic potentiation in mice with established cocaine-conditioned place preference. Addiction Biology. 2019;**24**(6):1153-1566

[4] Wei Q, Krolewski DM, Moore S, Kumar V, Li F, Martin B, et al. Uneven balance of power between hypothalamic peptidergic neurons in the control of feeding. Proceedings of the National Academy of Sciences of the United States of America. 2018;**115**(40):E9489-E9498

[5] Palomba L, Silvestri C, Imperatore R, Morello G, Piscitelli F, Martella A, et al. Negative regulation of leptin-induced reactive oxygen species (ROS) formation by cannabinoid CB1 receptor activation in hypothalamic neurons. Journal of Biological Chemistry. 2015;**290**(22):13669-13677

[6] Kaneko K, Yoshikawa M, Ohinata K. Novel orexigenic pathway prostaglandin D2-NPY system--involvement in orally active orexigenicδ opioid peptide. Neuropeptides. 2012;**46**(6):353-357

[7] Gozzi A, Turrini G, Piccoli L, Massagrande M, Amantini D, Antolini M, et al. Functional magnetic resonance imaging reveals different neural substrates for the effects of orexin-1 and orexin-2 receptor antagonists. PLoS One. 2011;**6**(1):e16406

[8] Alizamini MM, Kavianpour M, Karimi-Haghighi S, Fatahi Z, Haghparast A. Intra-hippocampal administration of orexin receptor antagonists dose-dependently attenuates reinstatement of morphine seeking behavior in extinguished rats. Peptides. 2018:31. pii: S0196-9781(18)30196-7

[9] Grafe LA, Cornfeld A, Luz S, Valentino R, Bhatnagar S. Orexins mediate sex differences in the stress response and in cognitive flexibility. Biological Psychiatry. 2017;**81**(8):683-692

[10] Lambe EK, Olausson P, Horst NK, Taylor JR, Aghajanian GK. Hypocretin and nicotine excite the same thalamocortical synapses in prefrontal cortex: Correlation with improved attention in rat. Journal of Neuroscience. 2005;**25**:5225-5229

[11] Piantadosi PT, Holmes A, Roberts BM, Bailey AM. Orexin receptor activity in the basal forebrain alters performance on an olfactory discrimination task. Brain Research. 2015;**1594**:215-222

[12] Chieffi S, Messina G, Villano I, Messina A, Esposito M, Monda V, et al. Exercise influence on hippocampal function: Possible involvement of orexin-A. Frontiers in Physiology. 2017;**8**:85

[13] Calva CB, Fadel JR. Intranasal administration of orexin peptides: Mechanisms and therapeutic potential for age-related cognitive dysfunction. Brain Research. 2018:24. pii: S0006-8993(18)30446-3

[14] Song J, Kim E, Kim CH, Song HT, Lee JE. The role of orexin in post-stroke

inflammation, cognitive decline, and depression. Molecular Brain. 2015;**8**:16

[15] Al-Kuraishy HM, Al-Gareeb AI, Naji MT, Al-Mamorry F. Role of vinpocetine in ischemic stroke and poststroke outcomes: A critical review. Brain Circulation. 2020;**6**(1):1-9

[16] Uslaner JM, Tye SJ, Eddins DM, Wang X, Fox SV, Savitz AT, et al. Orexin receptor antagonists differ from standard sleep drugs by promoting sleep at doses that do not disrupt cognition. Science Translational Medicine. 2013;**5**(179):179ra44

[17] Alijanpour S, Khakpai F, Ebrahimi-Ghiri M, Zarrindast MR. Co-administration of the low dose of orexin and nitrergic antagonists induces an antidepressant-like effect in mice. Biomedicine & Pharmacotherapy. 2018;**109**:589-594

[18] Czerwinska J, Chojnowska K, Kaminski T, Bogacka I, Smolinska N, Kaminska B. Orexin receptor expression in the hypothalamic-pituitary-adrenal and hypothalamic-pituitary-gonadal axes of free-living European beavers (*Castor fiber* L.) in different periods of the reproductive cycle. General and Comparative Endocrinology. 2017;**240**:103-113

[19] Malendowicz LK, Hochol A, Ziolkowska A, et al. Prolonged orexin administration stimulates steroid-hormone secretion, acting directly on the rat adrenal gland. International Journal of Molecular Medicine. 2001;**7**:401-404

[20] Patel AX, Miller SR, Nathan PJ, et al. Neuroendocrine and sympathetic responses to an orexin receptor antagonist, SB-649868, and alprazolam following insulin-induced hypoglycemia in humans. Psychopharmacology. 2014;**231**:3817-3828

[21] Al-Maiahy TJ, Al-Gareeb AI, Al-kuraishy HM. Prolactin and risk of preeclampsia: A single institution, cross-sectional study. Asian Pacific Journal of Reproduction. 2019;**8**(3):112-119

[22] Samson WK, Bagley SL, Ferguson AV, White MM. Hypocretin/orexin type 1 receptor in brain: Role in cardiovascular control and the neuroendocrine response to immobilization stress. American Journal of Physiology—Regulatory, Integrative and Comparative Physiology. 2007;**292**:R382-R387

[23] Al-Kuraishy HM, Al-Gareeb AI. Effect of orlistat alone or in combination with Garcinia cambogia on visceral adiposity index in obese patients. Journal of Intercultural Ethnopharmacology. 2016;**5**(4):408-418

[24] Cigdem Arica P, Kocael A, Tabak O, Taskin M, Zengin K, Uzun H. Plasma ghrelin, leptin, and orexin-A levels and insulin resistance after laparoscopic gastric band applications in morbidly obese patients. Minerva Medica. 2013;**104**(3):309-316

[25] Al-Kuraishy HM, Al-Gareeb AI. Effects of rosuvastatin alone or in combination with omega-3 fatty acid on adiponectin levels and cardiometabolic profile. Journal of Basic and Clinical Pharmacy. 2016;**8**(1):8-19

[26] Tsuneki H, Kon K, Ito H, Yamazaki M, Takahara S, Toyooka N, et al. Timed inhibition of orexin system by suvorexant improved sleep and glucose metabolism in type 2 diabetic db/db mice. Endocrinology. 2016;**157**(11):4146-4157

[27] Flores A, Maldonado R, Berrendero F. Cannabinoid–hypocretin cross-talk in the central nervous system: What we know so far. Frontiers in Neuroscience. 2013;**7**:256

[28] Al-kuraishy HM, Al-Gareeb AI. Eustress and malondialdehyde (MDA):

Role of *Panax ginseng*: Randomized placebo controlled study. Iranian Journal of Psychiatry. 2017;**12**(3):194-199

[29] Kok SW, Meinders AE, Overeem S, Lammers GJ, Roelfsema F, Frolich M, et al. Reduction of plasma leptin levels and loss of its circadian rhythmicity in hypocretin (orexin)-deficient narcoleptic humans. The Journal of Clinical Endocrinology & Metabolism. 2002;**87**(2):805-809

[30] Grady SP, Nishino S, Czeisler CA, Hepner D, Scammell TE. Diurnal variation in CSF orexin-A in healthy male subjects. Sleep. 2006;**29**(3):295-297

[31] Shariq AS, Rosenblat JD, Alageel A, Mansur RB, Rong C, Ho RC, et al. Evaluating the role of orexins in the pathophysiology and treatment of depression: A comprehensive review. Progress in Neuro-Psychopharmacology and Biological Psychiatry. 2019;**92**:1-7

[32] Feng P, Vurbic D, Wu Z, Hu Y, Strohl KP. Changes in brain orexin levels in a rat model of depression induced by neonatal administration of clomipramine. Journal of Psychopharmacology. 2008;**22**(7):784-791

[33] Ozsoy S, Olguner Eker O, Abdulrezzak U, Esel E. Relationship between orexin A and childhood maltreatment in female patients with depression and anxiety. Social Neuroscience. 2017;**12**(3):330-336

[34] Allard JS, Tizabi Y, Shaffery JP, Trouth CO, Manaye K. Stereological analysis of the hypothalamic hypocretin/orexin neurons in an animal model of depression. Neuropeptides. 2004;**38**(5):311-315

[35] Brundin L, Petersén Å, Björkqvist M, Träskman-Bendz L. Orexin and psychiatric symptoms in suicide attempters. Journal of Affective Disorders. 2007;**100**(1-3):259-263

[36] Ito N, Yabe T, Gamo Y, Nagai T, Oikawa T, Yamada H, et al. Icv administration of orexin-A induces an antidepressive-like effect through hippocampal cell proliferation. Neuroscience. 2008;**157**(4):720-732

[37] Ji MJ, Zhang XY, Chen Z, Wang JJ, Zhu JN. Orexin prevents depressive-like behavior by promoting stress resilience. Molecular Psychiatry. 2019;**24**(2):282

[38] Lambe EK, Liu RJ, Aghajanian GK. Schizophrenia, hypocretin (orexin), and the thalamocortical activating system. Schizophrenia Bulletin. 2007;**33**(6):1284-1290

[39] Borgland SL, Labouèbe G. Orexin/hypocretin in psychiatric disorders: Present state of knowledge and future potential. Neuropsychopharmacology. 2010;**35**(1):353

[40] Fadel J, Deutch AY. Anatomical substrates of orexin–dopamine interactions: Lateral hypothalamic projections to the ventral tegmental area. Neuroscience. 2002;**111**(2):379-387

[41] Andrade C, Kisely S, Monteiro I, Rao S. Antipsychotic augmentation with modafinil or armodafinil for negative symptoms of schizophrenia: Systematic review and meta-analysis of randomized controlled trials. Journal of Psychiatric Research. 2015;**60**:14-21

[42] Mereu M, Bonci A, Newman AH, Tanda G. The neurobiology of modafinil as an enhancer of cognitive performance and a potential treatment for substance use disorders. Psychopharmacology. 2013;**229**(3):415-434

[43] Bubser M, Fadel JR, Jackson LL, Meador-Woodruff JH, Jing D, Deutch AY. Dopaminergic regulation of orexin neurons. European Journal of Neuroscience. 2005;**21**(11):2993-3001

[44] Nakamura T, Uramura K, Nambu T, Yada T, Goto K, Yanagisawa M, et al.

Orexin-induced hyperlocomotion and stereotypy are mediated by the dopaminergic system. Brain Research. 2000;**873**(1):181-187

[45] Deutch AY, Bubser M. The orexins/hypocretins and schizophrenia. Schizophrenia Bulletin. 2007;**33**(6):1277-1283

[46] Rasmussen K, Hsu MA, Yang Y. The orexin-1 receptor antagonist SB-334867 blocks the effects of antipsychotics on the activity of A9 and A10 dopamine neurons: Implications for antipsychotic therapy. Neuropsychopharmacology. 2007;**32**(4):786

[47] Chen PY, Chen CH, Chang CK, Kao CF, Lu ML, Lin SK, et al. Orexin-A levels in relation to the risk of metabolic syndrome in patients with schizophrenia taking antipsychotics. International Journal of Neuropsychopharmacology. 2018;**22**(1):28-36

[48] Dalal MA, Schuld A, Pollmächer T. Lower CSF orexin A (hypocretin-1) levels in patients with schizophrenia treated with haloperidol compared to unmedicated subjects. Molecular Psychiatry. 2003;**8**(10):836

[49] Sharf R, Sarhan M, DiLeone RJ. Role of orexin/hypocretin in dependence and addiction. Brain Research. 2010;**1314**:130-138

[50] Marcus JN, Aschkenasi CJ, Lee CE, Chemelli RM, Saper CB, Yanagisawa M, et al. Differential expression of orexin receptors 1 and 2 in the rat brain. Journal of Comparative Neurology. 2001;**435**(1):6-25

[51] Zhang GC, Mao LM, Liu XY, Wang JQ. Long-lasting up-regulation of orexin receptor type 2 protein levels in the rat nucleus accumbens after chronic cocaine administration. Journal of Neurochemistry. 2007;**103**(1):400-407

[52] Carr D, Kalivas PW. Orexin: A gatekeeper of addiction. Nature Medicine. 2006;**12**(3):274

[53] James MH, Stopper CM, Zimmer BA, Koll NE, Bowrey HE, Aston-Jones G. Increased number and activity of a lateral subpopulation of hypothalamic orexin/hypocretin neurons underlies the expression of an addicted state in rats. Biological Psychiatry. 2019;**85**(11):925-935.

[54] Al'Absi M, Lemieux A, Hodges JS, Allen S. Circulating orexin changes during withdrawal are associated with nicotine craving and risk for smoking relapse. Addiction Biology. 2019;**24**(4):743-753

[55] Tsai MC, Huang TL. Orexin A in men with heroin use disorder undergoing methadone maintenance treatment. Psychiatry Research. 2018;**264**:412-415

[56] Pan JS, Zheng K, Liu JH, Gao ZY, Ye YG, et al. Orexin might predict status of alcohol dependence. Chinese Medical Journal. 2018;**131**(23):2866

[57] Dauvilliers Y, Arnulf I, Mignot E. Narcolepsy with cataplexy. The Lancet. 2007;**369**(9560):499-511

[58] Hollway JA, Mendoza-Burcham M, Andridge R, Aman MG, Handen B, Arnold LE, et al. Atomoxetine, parent training, and their effects on sleep in youth with autism spectrum disorder and attention-deficit/hyperactivity disorder. Journal of Child and Adolescent Psychopharmacology. 2018;**28**(2):130-135

[59] Sturzenegger C, Baumann CR, Lammers GJ, Kallweit U, van der Zande WL, Bassetti CL. Swiss Narcolepsy Scale: A simple screening tool for hypocretin-deficient narcolepsy with cataplexy. Clinical and Translational Neuroscience. 2018;**2**(2):2514183X18794175

[60] Almeneessier AS, Alzoghaibi M, BaHammam AA, Ibrahim MG, Olaish AH, Nashwan SZ, et al. The effects of diurnal intermittent fasting on the wake-promoting neurotransmitter orexin-A. Annals of Thoracic Medicine. 2018;**13**(1):48

[61] Yamanaka A, Tsujino N, Funahashi H, Honda K, Guan JL, Wang QP, et al. Orexins activate histaminergic neurons via the orexin 2 receptor. Biochemical and Biophysical Research Communications. 2002;**290**(4):1237-1245

[62] Gabelle A, Jaussent I, Hirtz C, Vialaret J, Navucet S, Grasselli C, et al. Cerebrospinal fluid levels of orexin-A and histamine, and sleep profile within the Alzheimer process. Neurobiology of Aging. 2017;**53**:59-66

[63] Fronczek R, Overeem S, Lee SY, Hegeman IM, Van Pelt J, Van Duinen SG, et al. Hypocretin (orexin) loss in Parkinson's disease. Brain. 2007;**130**(6):1577-1585

[64] Drouot X, Moutereau S, Nguyen JP, Lefaucheur JP, Creange A, Remy P, et al. Low levels of ventricular CSF orexin/hypocretin in advanced PD. Neurology. 2003;**61**(4):540-543

[65] Asai H, Hirano M, Furiya Y, Udaka F, Morikawa M, Kanbayashi T, et al. Cerebrospinal fluid-orexin levels and sleep attacks in four patients with Parkinson's disease. Clinical Neurology and Neurosurgery. 2009;**111**(4):341-344

[66] Feng Y, Liu T, Li XQ, Liu Y, Zhu XY, Jankovic J, et al. Neuroprotection by Orexin-A via HIF-1α induction in a cellular model of Parkinson's disease. Neuroscience Letters. 2014;**579**:35-40

[67] Liu MF, Xue Y, Liu C, Liu YH, Diao HL, Wang Y, et al. Orexin-A exerts neuroprotective effects via OX1R in Parkinson's disease. Frontiers in Neuroscience. 2018;**12**:835-845

[68] Sheng Q, Xue Y, Wang Y, Chen AQ, Liu C, Liu YH, et al. The subthalamic neurons are activated by both orexin-A and orexin-B. Neuroscience. 2018;**369**:97-108

[69] Michinaga S, Hisatsune A, Isohama Y, Katsuki H. An anti-Parkinson drug ropinirole depletes orexin from rat hypothalamic slice culture. Neuroscience Research. 2010;**68**(4):315-321

[70] Hyman BT. Heterogeneity and complexity in Alzheimer disease. In: Brain Pathology. Vol. 29. NJ, USA: Wiley; 2019. pp. 185-185

[71] Osorio RS, Ducca EL, Wohlleber ME, Tanzi EB, Gumb T, Twumasi A, et al. Orexin-A is associated with increases in cerebrospinal fluid phosphorylated-tau in cognitively normal elderly subjects. Sleep. 2016;**39**(6):1253-1260

[72] Triaca V, Calissano P. Impairment of the nerve growth factor pathway driving amyloid accumulation in cholinergic neurons: The incipit of the Alzheimer's disease story? Neural Regeneration Research. 2016;**11**(10):1553

[73] Liguori C, Romigi A, Nuccetelli M, Zannino S, Sancesario G, Martorana A, et al. Orexinergic system dysregulation, sleep impairment, and cognitive decline in Alzheimer disease. JAMA Neurology. 2014;**71**(12):1498-1505

[74] Lessig S, Ubhi K, Galasko D, Adame A, Pham E, Remidios K, et al. Reduced hypocretin (orexin) levels in dementia with Lewy bodies. Neuroreport. 2010;**21**(11):756

[75] Cheong RY, Gabery S, Petersén Å. The role of hypothalamic pathology for non-motor features of Huntington's disease. Journal of Huntington's Disease. 2019:1-7 (Preprint)

[76] Duarte AI, Sjögren M, Santos MS, Oliveira CR, Moreira PI, Björkqvist M.

Dual therapy with liraglutide and ghrelin promotes brain and peripheral energy metabolism in the R6/2 mouse model of Huntington's disease. Scientific Reports. 2018;**8**(1):1-4

[77] Petersén Å, Gil J, Maat-Schieman ML, Björkqvist M, Tanila H, Araujo IM, et al. Orexin loss in Huntington's disease. Human Molecular Genetics. 2005;**14**(1):39-47

[78] Mignot E, Lammers GJ, Ripley B, Okun M, Nevsimalova S, Overeem S, et al. The role of cerebrospinal fluid hypocretin measurement in the diagnosis of narcolepsy and other hypersomnias. Archives of Neurology. 2002;**59**(10):1553-1562

[79] Duffy CM, Hofmeister JJ, Nixon JP, Butterick TA. High fat diet increases cognitive decline and neuroinflammation in a model of orexin loss. Neurobiology of Learning and Memory. 2019;**157**:41-47

[80] Meier A, Mollenhauer B, Cohrs S, Rodenbeck A, Jordan W, Meller J, et al. Normal hypocretin-1 (orexin-A) levels in the cerebrospinal fluid of patients with Huntington's disease. Brain Research. 2005;**1063**(2):201-203

[81] Cabanas M, Pistono C, Puygrenier L, Rakesh D, Jeantet Y, Garret M, et al. Neurophysiological and behavioral effects of anti-orexinergic treatments in a mouse model of Huntington's disease. Neurotherapeutics. 2019;**16**(3):784-796

[82] Williams RH, Morton AJ, Burdakov D. Paradoxical function of orexin/hypocretin circuits in a mouse model of Huntington's disease. Neurobiology of Disease. 2011;**42**(3):438-445

[83] Thompson AJ, Banwell BL, Barkhof F, Carroll WM, Coetzee T, Comi G, et al. Diagnosis of multiple sclerosis: 2017 revisions of the McDonald criteria. The Lancet Neurology. 2018;**17**(2):162-173

[84] Montalban X, Hauser SL, Kappos L, Arnold DL, Bar-Or A, Comi G, et al. Ocrelizumab versus placebo in primary progressive multiple sclerosis. New England Journal of Medicine. 2017;**376**(3):209-220

[85] Fleischer V, Radetz A, Ciolac D, Muthuraman M, Gonzalez-Escamilla G, Zipp F, et al. Graph theoretical framework of brain networks in multiple sclerosis: A review of concepts. Neuroscience. 2019;**403**:35-53

[86] Papuć E, Zbigniew S, Paweł G, Konrad R. CSF hypocretin-1 concentrations correlate with the level of fatigue in multiple sclerosis patients. Neuroscience Letters. 2010;**474**(1):9-12

[87] Nozaki H, Shimohata T, Kanbayashi T, Sagawa Y, Katada SI, Satoh M, et al. A patient with anti-aquaporin 4 antibody who presented with recurrent hypersomnia, reduced orexin (hypocretin) level, and symmetrical hypothalamic lesions. Sleep Medicine. 2009;**10**(2):253-255

[88] Pallais JP, Kotz CM, Stanojlovic M. Orexin/hypocretinin in multiple sclerosis and experimental autoimmune encephalomyelitis. Neural Regeneration Research. 2020;**15**(6):1039

[89] Takata M, Tanaka H, Kimura M, Nagahara Y, Tanaka K, Kawasaki K, et al. Fasudil, a rho kinase inhibitor, limits motor neuron loss in experimental models of amyotrophic lateral sclerosis. British Journal of Pharmacology. 2013;**170**(2):341-351

[90] Van Rooij FG, Schelhaas HJ, Lammers GJ, Verbeek MM, Overeem S. CSF hypocretin-1 levels are normal in patients with amyotrophic lateral sclerosis. Amyotrophic Lateral Sclerosis. 2009;**10**(5-6):487-489

[91] Panda S, Gourie-Devi M, Sharma A. Sleep disorders in amyotrophic lateral sclerosis: A questionnaire-based study from India. Neurology India. 2018;**66**(3):700

[92] Herring WJ, Roth T, Krystal AD, Michelson D. Orexin receptor antagonists for the treatment of insomnia and potential treatment of other neuropsychiatric indications. Journal of Sleep Research. 2018;**18**:e12782

[93] Perrey DA, Zhang Y. Therapeutics development for addiction: Orexin-1 receptor antagonists. Brain Research. 2018:24. pii: S0006-8993(18)30447-5

[94] Herring WJ, Connor KM, Ivgy-May N, et al. Suvorexant in patients with insomnia: Results from two 3-month randomized controlled clinical trials. Biological Psychiatry. 2016;**79**:136-148. DOI: 10.1016/j.biopsych.2014.10.003

[95] Li A, Hindmarch CC, Nattie EE, Paton JF. Antagonism of orexin receptors significantly lowers blood pressure in spontaneously hypertensive rats. Journal of Physiology. 2013;**591**:4237-4248. DOI: 10.1113/jphysiol 2013.256271

[96] Hatta K, Kishi Y, Wada K, Takeuchi T, Ito S, Kurata A, et al. Preventive effects of suvorexant on delirium: A randomized placebo-controlled trial. Journal of Clinical Psychiatry. 2017;**78**(8):e970-e979

[97] Al-Kuraishy HM. Central additive effect of *Ginkgo biloba* and *Rhodiola rosea* on psychomotor vigilance task and short-term working memory accuracy. Journal of Intercultural Ethnopharmacology. 2016;**5**(1):7-19

[98] Kawada K, Ohta T, Tanaka K, Miyamura M, Tanaka S. Addition of suvorexant to ramelteon therapy for improved sleep quality with reduced delirium risk in acute stroke patients. Journal of Stroke & Cerebrovascular Diseases. 2018:12. pii: S1052-3057(18)30527-5

[99] Campbell EJ, Marchant NJ, Lawrence AJ. A sleeping giant: Suvorexant for the treatment of alcohol use disorder? Brain Research. 2018:3. pii: S0006-8993(18)30419-0

[100] Gentile TA, Simmons SJ, Watson MN, Connelly KL, Brailoiu E, Zhang Y, et al. Effects of suvorexant, a dual orexin/hypocretin receptor antagonist, on impulsive behavior associated with cocaine. Neuropsychopharmacology. 2018;**43**(5):1001-1009

[101] Struyk A, Gargano C, Drexel M, Stoch SA, Svetnik V, Ma J, et al. Pharmacodynamic effects of suvorexant and zolpidem on EEG during sleep in healthy subjects. European Neuropsychopharmacology. 2016;**26**(10):1649-1656

[102] Vermeeren A, Vets E, Vuurman EF, Van Oers AC, Jongen S, Laethem T, et al. On-the-road driving performance the morning after bedtime use of suvorexant 15 and 30 mg in healthy elderly. Psychopharmacology. 2016;**233**(18):3341-3351

[103] Nixon JP, Mavanji V, Butterick TA, Billington CJ, Kotz CM, Teske JA. Sleep disorders, obesity, and aging: The role of orexin. Ageing Research Reviews. 2015;**20**:63-73

[104] Morello G, Imperatore R, Palomba L, Finelli C, Labruna G, Pasanisi F, et al. Orexin-A represses satiety-inducing POMC neurons and contributes to obesity via stimulation of endocannabinoid signaling. Proceedings of the National Academy of Sciences. 2016;**113**(17):4759-4764

Chapter 4

Anorexia Nervosa

Fatima Elif Ergüney Okumuş

Abstract

Anorexia nervosa is characterized as having a significantly low body weight because of restricting energy intake or compensating to an excessive rate intentionally in order to attain or maintain an unrealistically thin ideal weight. Patients suffer multiple comorbid medical and psychiatric problems; moreover, deficits in treatment motivation are commonly seen, which causes a high rate of dropout from treatment programs. Thus, recent studies have focused on the etiology in order to develop efficient treatment options, as this can become a life-threatening problem. Prevention programs are also gaining attention, since full recovery can take a significant time and resources nevertheless may not be available for all cases. In this chapter, a brief history and basic diagnostic criteria of anorexia nervosa will be summarized. A review of comorbid psychiatric and medical conditions will be addressed. Prominent theories regarding its etiology and treatment options will be discussed in terms of a biopsychosocial approach. Finally, prevention studies will be highlighted.

Keywords: eating disorders, anorexia nervosa, body image, body dissatisfaction, compensatory behaviors, weight management strategies, dieting

1. Introduction

Weight management is essential for a healthy life, but in extreme cases, it can turn into a life-threatening condition. Eating behavior is an important dimension of weight management. For most of us, eating is an automatic response to hunger and can be as easy or normal as breathing. On the other hand, it may be a challenging area for people with eating disorders. Eating disorders (EDs) are serious psychiatric problems that have a multiple impact on health and well-being. The prominent types of EDs include anorexia nervosa (AN), bulimia nervosa (BN), and binge eating disorder (BED). This chapter will focus on anorexia nervosa and start with a brief history of AN. In the following sections, basic diagnostic criteria and a review of comorbid psychiatric and medical conditions will be addressed. Throughout the text, we will discuss prominent theories regarding its etiology and treatment options from a biopsychosocial perspective. Finally, prevention studies will be highlighted.

Anorexia nervosa is a complex disorder that includes physiological, behavioral, cognitive, and emotional components. Historical traces of anorexia can be found in ancient times. A group of women who starved themselves for religious reasons in Rome in 383 was reported [1]. Fasting is a common ritual in many religions and cultures, although starving triggered by psychological factors as a weight management strategy can lead to serious medical problems. Cases similar to AN have been reported since the fourteenth century, but as a psychological problem, preliminary cases were defined in 1873 and 1874 [2, 3]. The term anorexia nervosa means "nervous loss of appetite"; thus the early descriptions focused on food avoidance as the core problem. Then it was realized that people with AN do not suffer a loss of appetite; indeed their mind is extremely preoccupied with food. Hence, the psychological component became prominent, and the problem was conceptualized as a weight phobia and self-control. In fact, AN has been known about since the seventeenth century but was observed in the 1960s in western society and characterized as leading to a significantly low body weight because of restricting energy intake or compensating to an excessive rate intentionally, in order to attain or maintain an unrealistically thin ideal weight [4]. In the fifth edition of the *Diagnostic and Statistical Manual of Mental Disorders* (*DSM-5*), the title Feeding and Eating Disorders covers problems related to eating behaviors and unhealthy strategies for weight management [5]. Feeding disorders include pica, rumination disorder, and avoidant/restrictive food intake and can usually be seen in children, resulting in malnutrition or delay in growth due to unhealthy feeding behaviors. On the other hand, EDs are mostly seen in teenagers and adults. Their onset usually falls during puberty when body changes gain importance. DSM-5 defines three types of EDs, AN, BN, and BED. The underlying psychological mechanism is similar between these types as an intense fear of gaining weight and preoccupation with weight, body, and eating that leads to weight management strategies also known as compensatory behaviors like dieting, exercise, self-induced vomiting, misuse of laxatives, and diuretics [6]. The subtypes of EDs differ in body weight and weight management strategies. BN, BED, and other problems related to eating are beyond the scope of this chapter. Thus, we will first take a closer look at the clinical presentation of anorexia nervosa.

2. Clinical presentation

The current definition and clinical presentation of anorexia nervosa is determined by DSM-5 [5]. According to this diagnostic criterion, AN involves the following factors: The first criterion is a refusal to maintain a normal body weight despite being underweight. The factor of underweight or significantly low weight is usually determined by a body mass index (BMI) lower than 18.5 [7]. Nevertheless, not every underweight person is considered to have AN, though in this case being underweight is extremely important and in order to maintain this situation or to lose more weight, compensatory behaviors are evident. These unhealthy weight management strategies include excessive dieting or exercise, self-induced vomiting, and misuse of laxatives and diuretics, which leads to serious health problems including amenorrhea. The absence of at least three consecutive menstrual cycles was a diagnostic criterion for AN in the previous editions of the DSM [8]. Yet some women may have their periods even when they are underweight or there can be other metabolic problems resulting in amenorrhea. Moreover, it was making diagnoses difficult in men. In DSM-5, this original amenorrhea criterion was left out, in order to cover more cases.

Secondly, there is an intense fear of gaining weight or becoming fat, even though the body weight is less than normal. This fear is one of the most important factors that maintain compensatory behaviors and may not change despite weight loss. The third criterion is a disturbance in body image. Body image is a multidimensional framework that contains perceptions, attitudes, cognitions, emotions, and behaviors related to the body [9]. It can be defined as a representation of body in mind and is presumed to be the core psychological problem in AN [10]. People with AN have a body image distortion, resulting in a feeling of fatness independent of their weight; also negative attitudes towards the body, including body dissatisfaction, are prevalent [11]. Behaviors related with body such as excess weighing, body checking, and avoiding tight clothes might take up a lot of time on a daily basis. Negative body attitudes or body dissatisfaction has become almost a cultural norm in this age, especially for women, but for AN sufferers, these disturbances in body image are multifaceted and time-consuming, and this decreases functionality; also self-evaluation is mostly influenced by body shape and weight [12].

In AN diagnosis, two types were specified: restricting type and binge eating/purging type. Excessive dieting is prominent in the restricting type, whereas binge eating/purging type is characterized by recurrent binge eating episodes following by purging as a compensative behavior. A common definition for a binge eating episode is eating in a certain (e.g., at least 2 h) period of time an amount of food that is larger than most people would eat in a similar time period or condition accompanied by a sense of lack of control over eating (feeling that one cannot stop eating). Most commonly, self-induced vomiting or excessive dieting/exercise as purging behaviors follows this type of episode. The subtypes of AN are helpful in defining the clinical presentation of cases, but it should be noted that the predictive validity is weak, as transition between subtypes (both in AN and between AN and BN) is quite common [13]. The difference between the binge eating/purging type of AN and BN is that the AN cases are underweight. Also in AN, binge eating episodes might be subjective and may not always meet a clinical definition. However, there is also evidence that impulsivity, self-harming, social withdrawal, and comorbid psychiatric problems are more common in the binge eating/purging type, whereas perfectionism is more common in the restricting type [14]. Another problem in clinical presentation is that in most cases there is a lack of insight regarding their problem and deficits in treatment motivation are prevalent [15].

3. Comorbid medical and psychiatric conditions

Patients suffer multiple comorbid medical and psychiatric problems, as eating behavior affects health in multiple ways directly or indirectly [16].

Almost every system in the body is affected in AN, including gastrointestinal, cardiovascular, skeletal, nervous, endocrinological, and reproductive [17]. Physical examination results usually show low blood pressure, bradycardia, low body temperature, gastrointestinal problems, dehydration, hormonal deficits, amenorrhea or other menstrual problems, hair loss, and lanugo hair [18]. Cardiovascular problems include irregular heartbeats, heart attacks, and collapse of heart valves and may cause death [19]. Starvation affects menstrual functioning, resulting in poor reproductive health, with infertility problems. Even if anorexic women become pregnant, there is a high possibility of having small babies with complications or unhealthy children [20]. Self-induced vomiting may cause tooth erosion or calluses on hands [21]. AN usually begins at puberty, and this is an important time for the development of bones. Malnutrition can cause stunted growth and osteoporosis in the long term [22]. Anorexia is also associated with changes in the nervous system like loss of grey matter in the brain and reduction in pituitary size, resulting in deficits in attention, learning, memory, and visuospatial analyses [23, 24]. Above all, anorexia has the highest mortality rates among psychiatric disorders [25]. All of these medical problems can cause heart attacks or infections, but suicide is the most common cause of death [26].

In addition to physical problems, psychological complications are prevalent in AN. Almost half of the cases have a comorbid DSM diagnosis, especially depression being the most common among them [27]. Problems related to anxiety like social phobia and obsessive-compulsive disorders are highly associated with anorexia [28]. Trauma-related problems are more prevalent in the binge eating/purging type [29]. Comorbid psychological problems have a negative impact on prognosis and predicted suicide attempts [30]. As a result, AN is a chronic condition accompanied with a range of physical and psychological problems that interfere with daily functioning, and it has a high mortality rate.

4. Prognosis

Prognosis of anorexia is difficult, and full recovery is only possible in almost half of the cases [31]. Even when the physical symptoms are treated and the weight is maintained within the normal ranges, cognitive, emotional, and behavioral aspects of anorexia might continue. A complete recovery is only possible when all the symptoms are gone and especially when a positive body image is developed [10]. For this reason, recovery is considered as a long process that may take several years. Recurrent episodes of relapse are prevalent and accepted as within the nature of the disorder. Moreover, deficits in treatment motivation are quiet common, which causes a high rate of dropouts and chronicity of the problem [15]. Several factors may affect prognosis. For example, a very low BMI and a prolonged time before applying for treatment may worsen the process of prognosis [32]. Therefore, early detection and providing evidence-based treatment approaches are crucial to the course of anorexia.

5. Epidemiology

Estimating the prevalence of anorexia nervosa is problematic because it is a rare problem. The course of illness is variable, and sufferers are usually reluctant to report their situation or take part in studies [33]. Lifetime prevalence of DSM-5 diagnosis of AN in the West varies between 1 and 4% [27], but it has also been recently increasing in the non-Western world such as in Asia and the Middle East [34]. The problem is that most cases do not meet the full diagnostic criteria; resulting subthreshold EDs are more common in at-risk populations like high school and college samples [35]. Anorexia nervosa diagnosis is the most sexually based psychiatric problem, and the stereotypical patient is usually considered to be a young, white female from a higher socioeconomic class. This stereotype is not true all the time. However, the vast majority of the cases are women and the current male-female ratio is standing at 1:10 [5]. Nevertheless, recent studies show that between 3 and 20% of AN cases are male [36, 37]. Underdiagnoses of AN in men are a result of several factors that include sociocultural expectations towards women and the difference in symptom presentation in men. The mean age of onset is 17 in AN and the risk decreases with age [38]. However, onset of the disorder can be after age 40 or even later in some cases [39]. AN has been found to be less common among Black than White Americans [40], possibly due to underrepresentation in specialist eating disorder services and under detection in primary care [41]. Other than that, there is no systematic association between ethnicity/race or socioeconomic status and eating disorder occurrence [42]. Being in a sexual minority is a risk factor for EDs which is general for both women and men [43, 44]. In conclusion, it is noted that anorexia can affect people of all ages, genders, races, ethnic origins, socioeconomic status, and sexual orientations [45].

6. Etiology

Several theories have been proposed to understand the etiology of AN. Although these theories will be presented individually, it is recognized that a multidimensional approach is helpful to understand the causes of AN, even though such a comprehensive model has not yet been developed. Biological, psychological, and social factors interact with each other in the etiology. Prominent models include the genetic and neurobiological model, the psychodynamic model, the sociocultural model, and the cognitive behavioral model. Significant life events, personality, and a family system approach are also productive in understanding the causes of anorexia.

6.1 Genetic explanations

Genetic explanations focus on the biological mechanisms behind AN. Family, twin, and genetic studies found that AN runs in families [46]. A family history of AN puts people fourfold more at risk and relatives of women diagnosed with AN are 11 times more at risk of developing AN than controls [47, 48]. Moreover there is strong evidence that all types of EDs (AN, BN, and not otherwise specified EDs) track together in families without specificity [48]. Twin studies also show a genetic heredity for AN of between 28 and 74% but fail to identify specific genes [49]. In addition to these, anorexia interacts with other psychiatric problems. For example, people with a diagnosis of AN have a higher risk of developing OCD or vice versa [50]. Thus, genetic factors are considered responsible for 48–74% of the total variance in liability to AN [46]. Nevertheless, genetic factors cannot alone predict who will develop AN, as most of the cases do not have a familial history of EDs. Furthermore, methodological problems due to small sample size also reduce the likelihood of repetition of these studies.

It is evident that genes play an important role in the development of AN, although how these genetic predispositions interact with environmental factors has been a focus of research lately. Candidate gene and genome-wide studies are considered helpful in finding the answers. Research on candidate genes examined the serotonergic system (5-HT system), dopaminergic system, and opioidergic system that affect appetite, reward mechanism, mood, and weight; nevertheless, statistically significant results have not been presented so far [51]. Genome wide studies showed a relation between chromosomes 1, 11, and 12 and genes related to leptin regulation, lipid and glucose metabolism, serotonin receptor activities, and the immune system [52–55]. This genetic presentation is also consistent with the clinical presentation of anorexia. Further studies in these areas can be productive in order to explain the roles of genes in the AN etiology.

6.2 Neurobiological explanations

Neurobiological studies of AN focus on the brain areas, biological origins of symptoms, and neurochemical differences between people diagnosed with AN and healthy controls. Severe weight loss in anorexia causes a decrease in gray matter in several areas of the brain [56]. Moreover, a review of neuroimaging studies (PET, MRI, and fMRI) noted dysfunction in certain brain areas such as the amygdala, basal ganglia structures, and hippocampus [57]. On the other hand, research indicates dysfunctions in dopaminergic and serotonergic (5-HT) systems that are responsible for food, motivation, the reward system, executive function, emotion regulation, and impulse control [58]. Thus, food as a natural reward becomes a source of both threat and anxiety, which makes it easier to avoid or restrict [59]. Neuroimaging studies also support this explanation. In one fMRI study with AN patients, an increase in amygdala activity (threat perception) and a decrease in inferior parietal lobe activity (food-related pleasure and interest) were evident while patients were looking at food pictures [60]. Furthermore, AN patients give different responses to body-related words and pictures than controls. They pay more attention to these words and pictures, focusing on the parts of the body rather than focusing on the body as a whole; they experience cognitive, perceptual, and emotional changes when they look at their own body [61, 62]. These changes can be explained through the decrease in occipital and prefrontal cortex activity.

Lastly, the "insula hypothesis" is proposed as a neurological model of anorexia nervosa that states that a dysfunction of the neural circuitry integrated by the insula can be responsible for the clinical presentation of AN [63, 64]. Symptoms arise because of disability in the insula, which establish a homeostatic balance by linking the brain's perception, emotional response, and memory-related regions to each other. Thus, it is assumed that this dysfunction causes changes in reactions to foods, internal and external bodily sensations, and emotional processing.

6.3 Psychodynamic explanations

Psychodynamic explanations usually offer a unique way to understand patients' experiences of AN. These models emphasize the meanings and functions of symptoms and early childhood experiences that may cause fixation or unconscious conflicts related to individualization, separation, dependency, and control. From a psychoanalytic perspective, restriction of food symbolizes an area of control and a denial of growing up or becoming a woman [65]. Thus, the patient can stay as a child and can be looked after. Furthermore, family dynamics play an important role in these psychodynamic models. Excessive involvement, rigidity, inability to resolve conflict, and excessive protectionism are common dynamics in families of AN sufferers [66]. Bruch [67] also stated that this overinvolvement by "perfect" mothers may cause ineffectiveness in the child, resulting in these children may be not being able to identify and understand their needs or internal states. When food becomes a way of self-soothing, relaxing, and communicating, this pattern may result in eating related symptoms. Nevertheless, psychodynamic explanations are important to understand patients as individuals. However, generalization and causality is always a problem within these explanations. Moreover, these models fail to explain why childhood relationships are expressed through eating behaviors. In addition, it is always difficult to test or evaluate these explanations.

6.4 Cognitive behavioral explanations

Behavioral models of anorexia nervosa regard the disorder as a behavior that has been learned and is maintained through reinforcement. Individuals reduce their food intake as a means to lose weight due to the social pressure to be thin or other experiences, and this behavior is reinforced by sociocultural norms, feelings of being in control. These first explanations were criticized for not focusing on causal factors, and therefore cognitive explanations were proposed to be linked with these behaviors. Slade [68] pointed out that interpersonal problems and family conflicts underlie the perfectionistic tendency in anorexia, and this tendency is a triggering factor for dieting. Cognitive explanations focus on patients' thoughts about food, eating, weight, and shape which parallel Beck's model on depression [69]. Moreover, predisposing factors for self-starvation such as perfectionism, self-criticizing, and control were specified [70]. Thus, once the dieting and weight loss begin, they are reinforced and maintained easily as they become a way of gaining self-esteem. With the evidence-based studies, cognitive behavioral therapy (CBT) becomes the leading approach in both understanding and treating EDs in general [71]. CBT explains the etiology in AN as follows: dysfunctional thoughts of weight shape and body are influential in the development and persistence of symptoms, while weight control or compensatory methods (dieting, exercise, etc.) continue to reinforce the disorder. Symptoms are also conceptualized as a coping mechanism and a way of emotion regulation. Lately, Fairburn [6] has developed a transdiagnostic model of EDs that conceptualizes EDs beyond the diagnostic categories and targets the mechanism that is sustainable in all eating disorders. From Fairburn's transdiagnostic perspective, AN, BN, BED, and ED-NOS share the same core pathology that is cognitive in nature. For patients, the overvaluation of body shape and weight and their control is the most important part of life that defines and determines the worth of one's self. This pathology both causes and maintains eating and compensatory behaviors. In the case of anorexia, the consequences of malnutrition and hunger affect the cognitive ability of patients, which also causes rigidity in thoughts and behaviors.

6.5 Sociocultural explanations

Sociocultural models focus on the impact of culture and environment on body image and emphasize the importance of body image problems in the development of AN. Cultural expectations of thinness, usually termed "thin idealization," come from the media, family, friends, and peers [72]. Thinness is generalized within the scope of many positive meanings such as beauty, desirability, success, will, appreciation, charm, and control. Notably, exposure to images represented in the media that are often biologically unreachable for many women or even unreal (e.g., photoshopped) suggests thinness as a route to happiness, love, and success. Sociocultural models emphasize that the ideals of thinness are internalized through messages given by society, the media, peers, and family, resulting in eating and body problems and psychological symptoms in people who are dissatisfied with their body [73]. Lately, social media applications like Instagram and Tumblr and their impact on eating and body problems have become the focus of research in this area. Internalization of this thin ideal and an increase in body dissatisfaction are correlated with the prevalent pictures and the following of the accounts of thin people, celebrities, models, and actors [74]. Consequently, sociocultural factors play an important role in the thin idealization, but it is assumed that anorexia nervosa is developed through many factors including biological, cognitive, emotional, and social ones.

6.6 Risk factors in etiology

Several risk factors that include body dissatisfaction, dieting, being involved in body-related activities/sports/professions (dancing, ballet, athletics, modelling, acting, etc.), personality traits, family dynamics, and stress/trauma are stated as contributing to the etiology of anorexia [75]. Personality traits such as perfectionism, an obsessive-compulsive personality, and deficits in emotion regulation are prevalent in AN [76, 77]. These personality dimensions can be considered as both the predisposing and maintaining factors. Besides family dynamics, as we reviewed in the psychoanalytic model, are also important. Insecure attachment styles through stressful early childhood experiences and food-/body-related communications [78, 79] are the prominent factors related to the family. There is also some evidence of decreased family functioning in families of AN patients; however this might be a result of having an anorexic family member, as EDs affect families and caregivers [45]. Finally a wide range of traumatic experiences are prevalent in patients with AN. These include childhood neglect, every form of childhood abuse, witnessing violence, rape, loss of significant others, accidents, as well as interpersonal stress like bullying, humiliation, and body-related teasing [80]. The abovementioned factors may have neurodevelopmental effects on the HPA pathway and serotonergic system, which play a role in the brain's response to stress [81].

7. Treatment

Evidence-based research in this area suggests promising results in treatment. At the same time, the treatment processes are reported to be long and especially expensive, almost like schizophrenia, yet full recovery is only possible for half of the patients [82]. A multidimensional treatment with a multidisciplinary team is necessary in AN treatment, as the disorder contains biopsychosocial elements in nature. Medical nutritional therapy for weight gain and nutritional counseling is important, especially in the case of severe weight loss. Pharmacotherapy has a limited role in the treatment and however can be beneficial in some cases. Nevertheless, there is certain evidence that psychotherapy is essential in AN treatment, although a multidisciplinary approach is required that includes nutritional therapy and psychiatric and medical evaluation as well [83]. Inpatient treatment is suggested in cases with a low BMI (<13.5), rapid decrease in weight, risk of suicide, social isolation, failure of outpatient treatment, and medical risk factors (e.g., cardiac problems and lowered blood sugars) [84]. Specialized units and clinics are also required for AN treatment.

7.1 Medical nutritional therapy

Medical nutritional therapy is an essential part of treatment in AN, especially for inpatients. This form of therapy focuses on the evaluation of nutritional problems and risks, and after that nutritional counseling is provided to treat the nutritional disorder and to prepare the patient for the next stages of treatment. In medical nutritional therapy, the first choice is oral feeding (chewing and swallowing), but enteral/tube feeding (giving liquid food to the stomach or intestine) or, as a last resort, parenteral feeding (bypassing the digestive process) is also applicable [5, 83]. Refusals against weight gain are common in these treatments; the nutritional therapist also provides counseling to patients. In severely underweight patients, feeding may cause refeeding syndrome. Although weight gain is the first goal, weight maintenance is the ultimate goal in the long term. Hence, nutritional therapy has a value in the whole treatment process.

7.2 Pharmacotherapy

Research has focused on the impact of several pharmacological agents on anorexia, as neurobiological factors are important in the etiology. Even so, antipsychotics and antidepressants have only a limited role in treatment [85]. However, there is some evidence about olanzapine, an atypical antipsychotic, whose mechanism of action is unclear, which is thought to block serotonin and dopamine, which may be effective in weight gain [86]. In addition, appetite regulators (e.g., dronabinol) and hormone (e.g., estrogen) drugs may contribute to both weight gain and anxiety reduction [87]. In the treatment of AN, antidepressants do not provide the desired level of benefit, and it is suggested that this may be due to decreased 5-HT1A receptor activity, which is a consequence of starvation [88]. Nevertheless, almost half of the AN cases report using psychotropic medications despite lack of evidence supporting their efficacy, which is also concerning due to their severe side effects [89].

7.3 Psychotherapy

Psychotherapy is essential in anorexia treatment, and there is a range of psychotherapeutic approaches. The first psychological explanations of AN came from psychodynamic models, although psychodynamic treatments still have only limited effects [66]. Family therapy is the evidence-based psychotherapy type for younger AN patients, and some modifications are offered for adult patients [90]. CBT is the first step of treatment in BN and BED, and it also works for AN to some degree [91]. Other approaches include third wave behavioral therapies and eye movement desensitization and reprocessing (EMDR) therapy, which also show limited evidence of success in treatment.

7.3.1 Family-based approaches

Family dynamics are an important factor in the etiology of AN. The first studies in this area suggested family characteristics such as overinvolvement or inability to solve conflicts; however, family based approaches put families as part of the solution, not the source of the problem. These approaches originated from the Maudsley Hospital in London and focused on the family system as a whole. Several randomized control trials proved the efficacy of family-based treatments in adolescents with AN [92]. At a basic level, this kind of therapy analyzes predisposing and maintaining family dynamics of anorexia and then plans the treatment procedure accordingly. A three-step treatment plan is conducted that is almost a yearlong [93]. The first level focuses on families' parenting skills and whether decisions related to eating are under family control. They learn how to help their child to gain weight. The aim of the second level is to empower patients to gain control over their eating behaviors when they reach the normal weight range. Finally, the last level focuses on individualization and developing healthy social relations both between parent and child but also in peer relations too. Behavior change is central to this model. A family-based approach is also proposed for adult patients. The Maudsley Model of Anorexia Nervosa Treatment for Adults (MANTRA) involves caregivers in both formulation and administration during the treatment process [94]. This motivational and client-oriented cognitive interpersonal model is developed specifically for AN patients. It focuses on eating related problems and symptoms but also obsessive and anxious-avoidant personality traits that are central to the maintenance of AN.

7.3.2 Cognitive behavioral therapy

Cognitive behavioral therapy is the leading empirically supported treatment for BN and BED, but also there is evidence of its effectiveness in AN [83]. Enhanced CBT (CBT-E) is based on the transdiagnostic theory and is designed to treat eating psychopathology rather than being a DSM eating disorders diagnosis [6]. The word "enhanced" refers to new strategies and procedures to improve treatment outcomes and test the model in different groups (e.g., in patients, day-patients, adults, adolescents, etc.). CBT-E can also be conducted in a multistep approach (outpatient, intensive outpatient, and inpatient) by a multidisciplinary team according to the patient's needs. This intervention focuses on understanding the eating disorder mindset and its function. It is assumed that a change in the ED mindset will lead to symptom reduction. A standard CBT-E is a four-stage model. The first stage of treatment is aimed at creating a therapeutic alliance with assessment and case formulation. Regulation of eating behavior is the primary goal of this stage, through behavioral change. Patients are required to use self-monitoring sheets regarding their eating, and every session starts with a review of these records and in session weighing. The second stage (traditional CBT does not have this stage) is an overview and determination stage for possible barriers to change. Preoccupation with food and body is the main theme of the third stage. In addition, interpersonal problems, body checking behaviors, emotion regulation, ED mindset, and other individual factors related to the symptoms are central areas to work on. The last stage is focused on symptom prevention and possible future problems. Many cognitive and behavioral techniques including cognitive restructuring, exposure, and problem-solving training are used during this therapy.

Research indicates promising results regarding the efficacy of CBT-based interventions [95], especially on symptom prevention [91]. Thus, it is concluded that CBT-E is a cost-effective alternative to family-based treatments of anorexia [96].

7.3.3 Other psychotherapy approaches

Benefits of family-based interventions for adolescents are evident, and these approaches and CBT also work for adult cases to some degree although not for all. For these reasons the effect of different psychotherapies has gained attention. Research points to the effectiveness of psychodynamic therapy [97], third wave therapies (schema therapy, acceptance-commitment therapy, mindfulness-based interventions) [98], dialectical behavioral therapy [99], and EMDR [100], but no specific approach has shown clear superiority. Adding motivational techniques are also helpful [101], as deficits in treatment motivation are common among patients with AN. These findings suggest that a combination of nutritional therapy and anorexia nervosa-specific psychotherapy is an effective way to treat AN.

8. Prevention strategies

As mentioned above, AN is difficult to treat, as treatment might take a long time with high costs and may still not be possible in some cases. This has highlighted the importance of preventive studies. Prevention of EDs in general rather than AN-specific prevention is more common in research, since interchange between diagnoses and subthreshold EDs is more prevalent. Prevention strategies mainly work on two dimensions: first by reducing risk factors and second by targeting at-risk populations. Risk factors include thin idealization as a sociocultural element; dieting or excessive exercise as behavioral risk factors; and perfectionism, body dissatisfaction, and problems in emotion regulation as cognitive-emotional risk factors. These are more prevalent in high school and college samples as they constitute risky populations. Prevention programs can be school-based, computer-based, CBT-focused, media-literacy-focused, or on a sociopolitical level. A review of the details and effectiveness of these programs is beyond the scope of this chapter. However, longitudinal, structured programs have proven beneficial in reducing body dissatisfaction, disordered eating, and weight management behaviors [102]. Thus, adding preventive strategies to education and health systems can be a promising way of dealing with AN.

9. Conclusion

Anorexia nervosa is a complex psychiatric condition that is accompanied with a high morbidity and mortality risk. It is a rare problem and detection of cases with anorexia is hard as clinical presentation may vary; also voluntary admission to treatment facilities is low. Biological, psychological, and social factors intertwine in the etiology. Recent studies provide evidence of advances in understanding the psychobiological mechanisms that contribute to and maintain anorexia nervosa. Predisposing factors include genetic susceptibility and stressful early childhood experiences. On the other hand, psychological and social factors usually play a triggering role in the onset of symptoms. They also maintain the problem with changes in neural networks. Treatment of anorexia is a long and challenging process for patients, caregivers, and health professionals. Symptoms can become chronic when the necessary treatment is not provided. Even with the best treatment options, a full recovery is not possible in all cases. A multidimensional treatment provided by a multidisciplinary team in a specialized unit is fundamental for efficient treatment outcomes. Inpatient treatment can be required in severe cases. Nutritional therapy is an important part of treatment. Psychopharmacotherapy, on the other hand, has only a limited effect. Thus, psychotherapy is the leading factor in treatment. Evidence-based research indicates that adolescent patients with anorexia nervosa benefit from family-based interventions. Adults with anorexia nervosa have a good chance of achieving recovery or at least a substantial improvement in symptoms. CBT is an alternative to family-based interventions. Alongside these, a range of other anorexia-specific psychotherapy approaches is presented, although none of them has shown a clear superiority so far. This brings us to the importance of preventive studies regarding unhealthy eating and weight management behaviors. Future research will continue to focus on enhancing our understanding of the underlying biopsychosocial factors, in order to improve treatment and prevention.

Author details

Fatima Elif Ergüney Okumuş
Department of Psychology, Istanbul Sabahattin Zaim University, Istanbul, Turkey

*Address all correspondence to: elif.okumus@izu.edu.tr

IntechOpen

© 2020 The Author(s). Licensee IntechOpen. This chapter is distributed under the terms of the Creative Commons Attribution License (http://creativecommons.org/licenses/by/3.0), which permits unrestricted use, distribution, and reproduction in any medium, provided the original work is properly cited. CC BY

References

[1] Pearce JMS. Origins of anorexia nervosa. European Neurology. 2004;**52**(4):191-192. DOI: 10.1159/000082033

[2] Gull WW. Anorexia nervosa. Practical Comprehensive Treatment of Anorexia Nervosa. 1985;7:22-28

[3] Lasègue EC. De l'anorexie hystérique. Archives Générales de Médicines. 1873;**1**:385-403

[4] Bruch H. Anorexia nervosa: Therapy and theory. The American Journal of Psychiatry. 1982;**139**(12):1531-1538. DOI: 10.1176/ajp.139.12.1531

[5] American Psychiatric Association. Diagnostic and Statistical Manual of Mental Disorders (DSM-5®). Arlington: American Psychiatric Pub; 2013

[6] Fairburn CG. Cognitive Behavior Therapy and Eating Disorders. New York, USA: Guilford Press; 2008

[7] WHO. ICD-10: The ICD-10 Classification of Mental and Behavioural Disorders: Diagnostic Criteria for Research. Geneva, Switzerland: WHO; 1993

[8] American Psychiatric Association. Diagnostic and Statistical Manual of Mental Disorders. 4th ed., text rev. Washington, DC: Author; 2000

[9] Slade PD. What is body image? Behaviour Research and Therapy. 1994;**32**(5):497-502. DOI: 10.1016/0005-7967(94)90136-8

[10] Bruch H. Perceptual and conceptual disturbances in anorexia nervosa. Psychosomatic Medicine. 1962;**24**(2):187-194. DOI: 10.1.1.320.7064

[11] Cash TF, Deagle EA III. The nature and extent of body-image disturbances in anorexia nervosa and bulimia nervosa: A meta-analysis. International Journal of Eating Disorders. 1997;**22**(2):107-126. DOI: 10.1002/(SICI)1098-108X(199709)22:2<107::AID-EAT1>3.0.CO;2-J

[12] Smolak L, Levine MP. Adolescent transitions and the development of eating problems. In: Smolak L, Levine MP, Striegel-Moore R, editors. The Developmental Psychopathology of Eating Disorders: Implications for Research, Prevention, and Treatment. New Jersey: Erlbaum; 1996. pp. 207-233

[13] Eddy KT, Dorer DJ, Franko DL, Tahilani K, Thompson-Brenner H, Herzog DB. Diagnostic crossover in anorexia nervosa and bulimia nervosa: Implications for DSM-V. American Journal of Psychiatry. 2008;**165**(2):245-250. DOI: 10.1176/appi.ajp.2007.07060951

[14] Peat C, Mitchell JE, Hoek HW, Wonderlich SA. Validity and utility of subtyping anorexia nervosa. International Journal of Eating Disorders. 2009;**42**(7):590-594. DOI: 10.1002/eat.20717

[15] Abbate-Daga G, Amianto F, Delsedime N, De-Bacco C, Fassino S. Resistance to treatment and change in anorexia nervosa: A clinical overview. BMC Psychiatry. 2013;**13**(1):294. DOI: 10.1186/1471-244X-13-294

[16] Brambilla F, Monteleone P. Physical complications and physiological aberrations in eating disorders. Eating Disorders. 2003;**6**:139-222. DOI: 10.1002/0470867183.ch3

[17] Mehler PS, Blalock DV, Walden K, Kaur S, McBride J, Walsh K, et al. Medical findings in 1,026 consecutive adult inpatient–residential eating disordered patients. International Journal of Eating Disorders. 2018;**51**(4):305-313. DOI: 10.1002/eat.22830

[18] Brown C, Mehler PS. Medical complications of anorexia nervosa and their treatments: An update on some critical aspects. Eating and Weight Disorders-Studies on Anorexia, Bulimia and Obesity. 2015;**20**(4):419-425. DOI: 10.1007/s40519-015-0202-3

[19] Westmoreland P, Krantz MJ, Mehler PS. Medical complications of anorexia nervosa and bulimia. The American Journal of Medicine. 2016;**129**(1):30-37. DOI: 10.1016/j.amjmed.2015.06.031

[20] Linna MS, Raevuori A, Haukka J, Suvisaari JM, Suokas JT, Gissler M. Reproductive health outcomes in eating disorders. International Journal of Eating Disorders. 2013;**46**(8):826-833. DOI: 10.1002/eat.22179

[21] Romanos GE, Javcd F, Romanos EB, Williams RC. Oro-facial manifestations in patients with eating disorders. Appetite. 2012;**59**:499-504. DOI: 10.1016/j.appet.2012.06.016

[22] Ecklund K, Vajapeyam S, Feldman HA, Buzney CD, Mulkern RV, Kleinman PK, et al. Bone marrow changes in adolescent girls with anorexia nervosa. Journal of Bone and Mineral Research. 2010;**25**(2):298-304. DOI: 10.1359/jbmr.090805

[23] Plata-Salamán CR. Central nervous system mechanisms contributing to the cachexia–anorexia syndrome. Nutrition. 2000;**16**(10):1009-1012. DOI: 10.1016/S0899-9007(00)00413-5

[24] Szmukler GI, Andrewes D, Kingston K, Chen L, Stargatt R, Stanley R. Neuropsychological impairment in anorexia nervosa: Before and after refeeding. Journal of Clinical and Experimental Neuropsychology. 1992;**14**(2):347-352. DOI: 10.1080/01688639208402834

[25] Chesney E, Goodwin GM, Fazel S. Risks of all-cause and suicide mortality in mental disorders: A meta-review. World Psychiatry. 2014;**13**(2):153-160. DOI: 10.1002/wps.20128

[26] Pompili M, Mancinelli I, Girardi P, Ruberto A, Tatarelli R. Suicide in anorexia nervosa: A meta-analysis. International Journal of Eating Disorders. 2004;**36**(1):99-103. DOI: 10.1002/eat.20011

[27] Keski-Rahkonen A, Mustelin L. Epidemiology of eating disorders in Europe: Prevalence, incidence, comorbidity, course, consequences, and risk factors. Current Opinion in Psychiatry. 2016;**29**(6):340-345. DOI: 10.1097/YCO.0000000000000278

[28] Ulfvebrand S, Birgegård A, Norring C, Högdahl L, von Hausswolff-Juhlin Y. Psychiatric comorbidity in women and men with eating disorders results from a large clinical database. Psychiatry Research. 2015;**230**(2):294-299. DOI: 10.1016/j.psychres.2015.09.008

[29] Carter JC, Bewell C, Blackmore E, Woodside DB. The impact of childhood sexual abuse in anorexia nervosa. Child Abuse & Neglect. 2006;**30**(3):257-269. DOI: 10.1016/j.chiabu.2005.09.004

[30] Franko DL, Keel PK. Suicidality in eating disorders: Occurrence, correlates, and clinical implications. Clinical Psychology Review. 2006;**26**(6):769-782. DOI: 10.1016/j.cpr.2006.04.001

[31] Keski-Rahkonen A, Hoek HW, Susser ES, Linna MS, Sihvola E, Raevuori A, et al. Epidemiology and course of anorexia nervosa in the community. American Journal of Psychiatry. 2007;**164**(8):1259-1265. DOI: 10.1176/appi.ajp.2007.06081388

[32] Keel PK, Brown TA. Update on course and outcome in eating disorders. International Journal of Eating Disorders. 2010;**43**(3):195-204. DOI: 10.1002/eat.20810

[33] Ogden J. The Psychology of Eating: From Healthy to Disordered Behavior. West Sussex, UK: John Wiley & Sons; 2011

[34] Pike KM, Dunne PE. The rise of eating disorders in Asia: A review. Journal of Eating Disorders. 2015;**3**(1):33. DOI: 10.1186/s40337-015-0070-2

[35] Machado PP, Gonçalves S, Hoek HW. DSM-5 reduces the proportion of EDNOS cases: Evidence from community samples. International Journal of Eating Disorders. 2013;**46**(1):60-65. DOI: 10.1002/eat.22040

[36] Harada T, Yamauchi T, Kodama Y, Miyamoto S, Kiriike N, Inoue K. Clinical features of Japanese males with anorexia nervosa. Osaka City Medical Journal. 2016;**62**(2):85-93. DOI: 00306096-62-2-85

[37] Sweeting H, Walker L, MacLean A, Patterson C, Räisänen U, Hunt K. Prevalence of eating disorders in males: A review of rates reported in academic research and UK mass media. International Journal of Men's Health. 2015;**14**:2. DOI: 10.3149/jmh.1402.86

[38] Favaro A, Caregaro L, Tenconi E, Bosello R, Santonastaso P. Time trends in age at onset of anorexia nervosa and bulimia nervosa. The Journal of Clinical Psychiatry. 2009;**70**(12):1715-1721. DOI: 10.4088/jcp.09m05176blu

[39] Beck D, Casper R, Andersen A. Truly late onset of eating disorders: A study of 11 cases averaging 60 years of age at presentation. International Journal of Eating Disorders. 1996;**20**(4):389-395. DOI: 10.1002/(SICI)1098-108X(199612)20:4<389::AID-EAT6>3.0.CO;2-J

[40] Pike KM, Dunne PE, Addai E. Expanding the boundaries: Reconfiguring the demographics of the "typical" eating disordered patient. Current Psychiatry Reports. 2013;**15**(11):411. DOI: 10.1007/s11920-013-0411-2

[41] Striegel-Moore RH, Dohm FA, Kraemer HC, Taylor CB, Daniels S, Crawford PB, et al. Eating disorders in white and black women. American Journal of Psychiatry. 2003;**160**(7):1326-1331. DOI: 10.1176/appi.ajp.160.7.1326

[42] Mitchison D, Hay P, Slewa-Younan S, Mond J. The changing demographic profile of eating disorder behaviors in the community. BMC Public Health. 2014;**14**(1):943. DOI: 10.1186/1471-2458-14-943

[43] Frederick DA, Essayli JH. Male body image: The roles of sexual orientation and body mass index across five national US Studies. Psychology of Men & Masculinity. 2016;**17**(4):336. DOI: 10.1037/men0000031

[44] Matthews-Ewald MR, Zullig KJ, Ward RM. Sexual orientation and disordered eating behaviors among self-identified male and female college students. Eating Behaviors. 2014;**15**(3):441-444. DOI: 10.1016/j.eatbeh.2014.05.002

[45] Schaumberg K, Welch E, Breithaupt L, Hübel C, Baker JH, Munn-Chernoff MA, et al. The science behind the Academy for Eating Disorders' nine truths about eating disorders. European Eating Disorders Review. 2017;**25**(6):432-450. DOI: 10.1002/erv.2553

[46] Yilmaz Z, Hardaway JA, Bulik CM. Genetics and epigenetics of eating disorders. Advances in Genomics and Genetics. 2015;**5**:131-150. DOI: 10.2147/AGG.S55776

[47] Steinhausen HC, Jakobsen H, Helenius D, Munk-Jørgensen P, Strober M. A nation-wide study of the family aggregation and risk factors in anorexia nervosa over three generations.

International Journal of Eating Disorders. 2015;**48**(1):1-8. DOI: doi.org/10.1002/eat.22293

[48] Strober M, Freeman R, Lampert C, Diamond J, Kaye W. Controlled family study of anorexia nervosa and bulimia nervosa: Evidence of shared liability and transmission of partial syndromes. American Journal of Psychiatry. 2000;**157**(3):393-401. DOI: 10.1176/appi.ajp.157.3.393

[49] Hinney A, Volckmar AL. Genetics of eating disorders. Current Psychiatry Reports. 2013;**15**(12):423. DOI: 10.1007/s11920-013-0423-y

[50] Cederlöf M, Thornton LM, Baker J, Lichtenstein P, Larsson H, Rück C, et al. Etiological overlap between obsessive-compulsive disorder and anorexia nervosa: A longitudinal cohort, multigenerational family and twin study. World Psychiatry. 2015;**14**(3):333-338. DOI: 10.1002/wps.20251

[51] Bulik CM, Kleiman SC, Yilmaz Z. Genetic epidemiology of eating disorders. Current Opinion in Psychiatry. 2016;**29**(6):383. DOI: 10.1097/YCO.0000000000000275

[52] Nakabayashi K, Komaki G, Tajima A, Ando T, Ishikawa M, Nomoto J, et al. Identification of novel candidate loci for anorexia nervosa at 1q41 and 11q22 in Japanese by a genome-wide association analysis with microsatellite markers. Journal of Human Genetics. 2009;**54**(9):531. DOI: jhg200974

[53] Duncan L, Yilmaz Z, Walters R, Goldstein J, Anttila V, Bulik-Sullivan B, et al. Genome-wide association study reveals first locus for anorexia nervosa and metabolic correlations. The American Journal of Psychiatry. 2017;**174**(9):850-858. DOI: 10.1176/appi.ajp.2017.16121402

[54] Li D, Chang X, Connolly JJ, Tian L, Liu Y, Bhoj EJ, et al. A genome-wide association study of anorexia nervosa suggests a risk locus implicated in dysregulated leptin signaling. Scientific Reports. 2017;7(1):3847. DOI: s41598-017-01674-8

[55] Steiger H, Booij L, Kahan E, McGregor K, Thaler L, Fletcher E, et al. A longitudinal, epigenome-wide study of DNA methylation in anorexia nervosa: Results in actively ill, partially weight-restored, long-term remitted and non-eating-disordered women. Journal of Psychiatry & Neuroscience: JPN. 2019;**44**(3):205-213. DOI: 10.1503/jpn.170242

[56] Seitz J, Herpertz-Dahlmann B, Konrad K. Brain morphological changes in adolescent and adult patients with anorexia nervosa. Journal of Neural Transmission. 2016;**123**(8):949-959. DOI: 10.1007/s00702-016-1567-9

[57] Frank GK. Recent advances in neuroimaging to model eating disorder neurobiology. Current Psychiatry Reports. 2015;**17**(4):22. DOI: 10.1007/s11920-015-0559-z

[58] von Hausswolff-Juhlin Y, Brooks SJ, Larsson M. The neurobiology of eating disorders—A clinical perspective. Acta Psychiatrica Scandinavica. 2015;**131**(4):244-255. DOI: 10.1111/acps.12335

[59] Steinglass JE, Walsh BT. Neurobiological model of the persistence of anorexia nervosa. Journal of Eating Disorders. 2016;**4**(1):19. DOI: 10.1186/s40337-016-0106-2

[60] Santel S, Baving L, Krauel K, Münte TF, Rotte M. Hunger and satiety in anorexia nervosa: fMRI during cognitive processing of food pictures. Brain Research. 2006;**1114**(1):138-148. DOI: 10.1016/j.brainres.2006.07.045

[61] Miyake Y, Okamoto Y, Onoda K, Shirao N, Okamoto Y, Otagaki Y, et al. Neural processing of negative word

stimuli concerning body image in patients with eating disorders: An fMRI study. NeuroImage. 2010;**50**(3):1333-1339. DOI: 10.1016/j.neuroimage.2009.12.095

[62] Urgesi C, Fornasari L, Perini L, Canalaz F, Cremaschi S, Faleschini L, et al. Visual body perception in anorexia nervosa. International Journal of Eating Disorders. 2012;**45**(4):501-511. DOI: 10.1002/eat.20982

[63] Nunn K, Frampton I, Gordon I, Lask B. The fault is not in her parents but in her insula—A neurobiological hypothesis of anorexia nervosa. European Eating Disorders Review: The Professional Journal of the Eating Disorders Association. 2008;**16**(5):355-360. DOI: 10.1002/erv.890

[64] Nunn K, Frampton I, Fuglset TS, Törzsök-Sonnevend M, Lask B. Anorexia nervosa and the insula. Medical Hypotheses. 2011;**76**(3):353-357. DOI: 10.1016/j.mehy.2010.10.038

[65] Bruch H. The psychiatric differential diagnosis of anorexia nervosa. Anorexia Nervosa. The Journal of Nervous and Mental Disease. 1965;**141**:555-566

[66] Zerbe KJ. The crucial role of psychodynamic understanding in the treatment of eating disorders. Psychiatric Clinics of North America. 2001;**24**(2):305-313. DOI: 10.1016/S0193-953X(05)70226-4

[67] Bruch H. Four decades of eating disorders. Handbook of Psychotherapy for Anorexia Nervosa and Bulimia. New York: Guilford; 1985

[68] Slade P. Towards a functional analysis of anorexia nervosa and bulimia nervosa. British Journal of Clinical Psychology. 1982;**21**(3):167-179. DOI: 10.1111/j.2044-8260.1982.tb00549.x

[69] Beck AT. Cognitive Therapy and the Emotional Disorders. New York: International Universities Press; 1976

[70] Garner DM, Bermis KM. A cognitive-behavioral approach to anorexia nervosa. Cognitive Therapy and Research. 1982;**6**:123-150. DOI: 10.1007/BF01183887

[71] Fairburn C. A cognitive behavioural approach to the treatment of bulimia. Psychological Medicine. 1981;**11**(4):707-711. DOI: 10.1017/S0033291700041209

[72] Garner DM, Garfinkel PE. Socio-cultural factors in the development of anorexia nervosa. Psychological Medicine. 1980;**10**(4):647-656. DOI: 10.1017/S0033291700054945

[73] Stice E. Review of the evidence for a sociocultural model of bulimia nervosa and an exploration of the mechanisms of action. Clinical Psychology Review. 1994;**14**(7):633-661. DOI: 10.1016/0272-7358(94)90002-7

[74] Brown Z, Tiggemann M. Attractive celebrity and peer images on Instagram: Effect on women's mood and body image. Body Image. 2016;**19**:37-43. DOI: 10.1016/j.bodyim.2016.08.007

[75] Stice E, Gau JM, Rohde P, Shaw H. Risk factors that predict future onset of each DSM–5 eating disorder: Predictive specificity in high-risk adolescent females. Journal of Abnormal Psychology. 2017;**126**(1):38. DOI: 2016-47863-001

[76] Cassin SE, von Ranson KM. Personality and eating disorders: A decade in review. Clinical Psychology Review. 2005;**25**(7):895-916. DOI: 10.1016/j.cpr.2005.04.012

[77] Limburg K, Watson HJ, Hagger MS, Egan SJ. The relationship between perfectionism and psychopathology: A meta-analysis. Journal of Clinical Psychology. 2017;**73**(10):1301-1326. DOI: 10.1002/jclp.22435

[78] Tasca GA. Attachment and eating disorders: A research update. Current Opinion in Psychology. 2019;**25**:59-64. DOI: 10.1016/j.copsyc.2018.03.003

[79] Neumark-Sztainer D, Bauer KW, Friend S, Hannan PJ, Story M, Berge JM. Family weight talk and dieting: How much do they matter for body dissatisfaction and disordered eating behaviors in adolescent girls? Journal of Adolescent Health. 2010;**47**(3):270-276

[80] Mitchell KS, Mazzeo SE, Schlesinger MR, Brewerton TD, Smith BN. Comorbidity of partial and subthreshold PTSD among men and women with eating disorders in the national comorbidity survey-replication study. International Journal of Eating Disorders. 2012;**45**(3):307-315. DOI: 10.1002/eat.20965

[81] Steiger H, Gauvin L, Israël M, Koerner N, Kin NNY, Paris J, et al. Association of serotonin and cortisol indices with childhood abuse in bulimia nervosa. Archives of General Psychiatry. 2001;**58**(9):837-843. DOI: 10.1001/archpsyc.58.9.837

[82] Strober M, Freeman R, Morrell W. The long-term course of severe anorexia nervosa in adolescents: Survival analysis of recovery, relapse, and outcome predictors over 10-15 years in a prospective study. International Journal of Eating Disorders. 1997;**22**(4):339-360. DOI: 10.1002/(SICI)1098-108X(199712)22:4<339::AID-EAT1>3.0.CO;2-N

[83] NICE—National Institute for Health and Care Excellence. Eating Disorders: Recognition and Treatment. London, UK: National Institute for Health and Care Excellence; 2017

[84] Treasure TG, Szmukler G. The inpatient treatment of anorexia nervosa. In: Handbook of Eating Disorders: Theory, Treatment and Research. Chichester, England: Wiley; 1995

[85] Flament MF, Bissada H, Spettigue W. Evidence-based pharmacotherapy of eating disorders. International Journal of Neuropsychopharmacology. 2012;**15**(2):189-207. DOI: 10.1017/S1461145711000381

[86] McElroy SL, Guerdjikova AI, Mori N, Keck PE Jr. Psychopharmacologic treatment of eating disorders: Emerging findings. Current Psychiatry Reports. 2015;**17**:35. DOI: 10.1007/s11920-015-0573-1

[87] Miniati M, Marazziti D. Psychopharmacological options for adult patients with anorexia nervosa: The patients' and carers' perspectives integrated by the spectrum model. CNS Spectrums. 2019;**24**(2):225-226. DOI: 10.1017/S1092852917000700

[88] Kaye W. Neurobiology of anorexia and bulimia nervosa. Physiology & Behavior. 2008;**94**(1):121-135. DOI: 10.1016/j.physbeh.2007.11.037

[89] Fazeli PK, Calder GL, Miller KK, Misra M, Lawson EA, Meenaghan E, et al. Psychotropic medication use in anorexia nervosa between 1997 and 2009. International Journal of Eating Disorders. 2012;**45**(8):970-976. DOI: 10.1002/eat.22037

[90] Lock J, Gowers S. Effective interventions for adolescents with anorexia nervosa. Journal of Mental Health. 2005;**14**:599-610. DOI: 10.1080/09638230500400324

[91] Hay PJ, Touyz S, Sud R. Treatment for severe and enduring anorexia nervosa: A review. Australian & New Zealand Journal of Psychiatry. 2012;**46**(12):1136-1144. DOI: 10.1177/0004867412450469

[92] Le Grange D, Lock J, Agras WS, Bryson SW, Jo B. Randomized clinical

trial of family-based treatment and cognitive-behavioral therapy for adolescent bulimia nervosa. Journal of the American Academy of Child & Adolescent Psychiatry. 2015;**54**(11):886-894. DOI: 10.1016/j.jaac.2015.08.008

[93] Lock J. An update on evidence-based psychosocial treatments for eating disorders in children and adolescents. Journal of Clinical Child & Adolescent Psychology. 2015;**44**(5):707-721. DOI: 10.1080/15374416.2014.971458

[94] Schmidt U, Magill N, Renwick B, Keyes A, Kenyon M, Dejong H, et al. The Maudsley Outpatient Study of Treatments for Anorexia Nervosa and Related Conditions (MOSAIC): Comparison of the Maudsley Model of Anorexia Nervosa Treatment for Adults (MANTRA) with specialist supportive clinical management (SSCM) in outpatients with broadly defined anorexia nervosa: A randomized controlled trial. Journal of Consulting and Clinical Psychology. 2015;**83**(4):796. DOI: 10.1037/ccp0000019

[95] Fairburn CG, Cooper Z, Doll HA, O'Connor ME, Palmer RL, Dalle Grave R. Enhanced cognitive behaviour therapy for adults with anorexia nervosa: A UK–Italy study. Behaviour Research and Therapy. 2013;**51**(1):R2-R8. DOI: 10.1016/j.brat.2012.09.010

[96] Dalle Grave R, Calugi S, Doll HA, Fairburn CG. Enhanced cognitive behaviour therapy for adolescents with anorexia nervosa: An alternative to family therapy? Behaviour Research and Therapy. 2013;**51**(1):R9-R12. DOI: 10.1016/j.brat.2012.09.008

[97] Zipfel S, Wild B, Groß G, Friederich HC, Teufel M, Schellberg D, et al. Focal psychodynamic therapy, cognitive behaviour therapy, and optimised treatment as usual in outpatients with anorexia nervosa (ANTOP study): Randomised controlled trial. The Lancet. 2014;**383**(9912):127-137. DOI: 10.1016/S0140-6736(13)61746-8

[98] Linardon J, Fairburn CG, Fitzsimmons-Craft EE, Wilfley DE, Brennan L. The empirical status of the third-wave behaviour therapies for the treatment of eating disorders: A systematic review. Clinical Psychology Review. 2017;**58**:125-140. DOI: 10.1016/j.cpr.2017.10.005

[99] Chen EY, Segal K, Weissman J, Zeffiro TA, Gallop R, Linehan MM, et al. Adapting dialectical behavior therapy for outpatient adult anorexia nervosa—A pilot study. International Journal of Eating Disorders. 2015;**48**(1):123-132. DOI: 10.1002/eat.22360

[100] Zaccagnino M, Civilotti C, Cussino M, Callerame C, Fernandez I. EMDR in anorexia nervosa: From a theoretical framework to the treatment guidelines. In: Eating Disorders—A Paradigm of the Biopsychosocial Model of Illness. UK: IntechOpen; 2017. pp. 193-213. DOI: 10.5772/65695

[101] Geller J, Dunn EC. Integrating motivational interviewing and cognitive behavioral therapy in the treatment of eating disorders: Tailoring interventions to patient readiness for change. Cognitive and Behavioral Practice. 2011;**18**(1):5-15. DOI: 10.1016/j.cbpra.2009.05.005

[102] Rohde P, Stice E, Marti CN. Development and predictive effects of eating disorder risk factors during adolescence: Implications for prevention efforts. International Journal of Eating Disorders. 2015;**48**(2):187-198. DOI: 10.1002/eat.22270

Chapter 5

Diagnostic Methods in Childhood Obesity

Leonardo de Souza Piber, Patrícia Colombo-Souza and Jane de Eston Armond

Abstract

Childhood obesity, the most frequent pediatric disease, a worldwide public health problem, is considered a global epidemic and the main risk factor for obesity in adulthood. Among its consequences, cardiovascular and metabolic diseases stand out, which can be diagnosed during childhood, potentiate morbidity and mortality throughout life. Anthropometry, which includes the analysis of body mass index and the measurement of waist circumference, has proven efficacy in pediatric clinical evaluation. However, these diagnostic methods do not differentiate between subcutaneous and intra-abdominal or visceral fat. In this sense, diagnostic imaging methods complement the assessment of abdominal fat. In children, ultrasography appears as an innocuous, reproducible, and reliable diagnostic imaging method. The importance of knowing diagnostic methods for better monitoring of childhood obesity is emphasized.

Keywords: pediatric obesity, anthropometry, subcutaneous fat, intra-abdominal fat, ultrasonography, diagnostic methods, diagnostic imaging

1. Introduction

Obesity can be defined in a simplified way as a clinical condition in which there is an excessive accumulation of body fat, in the form of adipose tissue, and not just excess weight [1], as a consequence of a positive energy balance [2], capable of causing damage to the health of individuals [3], leading to reduced life expectancy [4]. It is known that the etiology of obesity is multifactorial, with both environmental and genetic aspects being involved in its genesis [3, 5].

It is believed that the determinants of excess weight make up a complex set of biological, behavioral, and environmental factors that interrelate and potentiate each other [2, 3].

Childhood is a phase of intense and rapid growth and physical, psychological, and social development, which causes an increase in nutritional needs. The advances in modern life have caused changes in the lifestyle of families around the world, causing these nutritional needs to be inadequately met, through the consumption of high-calorie diets, fats, voracious food, exchanging meals for quick snacks. These factors are linked to physical inactivity, the result of changes in children's games, which currently focus on video games and the excessive use of computers and television [6, 7].

The aforementioned aspects corroborate the increase in the prevalence of childhood obesity, a chronic disease characterized by increased body fat and influenced by genetic factors that, combined with environmental factors, make it difficult to maintain a healthy weight [6].

Childhood obesity, the most frequent pediatric disease [1] has also become a major public health problem in recent decades, being considered a global epidemic by the World Health Organization (WHO) [8–10], and the main risk factor for obesity in adulthood [1, 2, 10, 11].

Between 1980 and 1994, the proportion of children and adolescents considered obese increased 100% in the United States of America (USA). It is estimated that 15.3% of American children, aged between 6 and 11 years, suffer from obesity. The high prevalence of obesity has also been observed in populations in developing countries and with low socioeconomic status [12].

In Europe, in the last 10 years, this disease has grown around 10–40% in most countries [10, 12]. A study of 9-year-old Irish children found 19.3% to be overweight and 6.6% to be obese. Of children with parents of normal weight, 14.4% were overweight or obese, while 46.2% of children with obese parents were overweight or obese [9].

Parental obesity is well established as an important risk factor for childhood obesity [2]. Having an overweight father doubles the risk of childhood obesity, while obesity between the two parents further increases the risk. The relationship between the weight of the father and the son is complex, as it is a consequence of shared genetic and environmental factors [9].

Brazilian data on the prevalence of overweight and obesity in children aged 12–59 months; of these, 14.7% were overweight and 4.1% were obese [13, 14]. These results, both in relation to overweight and in relation to obesity, placed Brazil as the fourth most prevalent country when compared to 12 other countries in Latin America and with the data of Mexican children residing in the United States of North America [14].

In Brazil, there was an important increase in the number of overweight children in the country, mainly in the age group between 5 and 9 years. The number of overweight boys more than doubled between 1989 and 2009, from 15 to 34.8%, respectively. The number of obese people increased by more than 300% in this same age group, going from 4.1% in 1989 to 16.6% in 2008–2009. Among girls, this variation was even greater (from 2.4 to 11.8%) [15]. Obesity affects about 30% of children, mainly in middle- and high-income families [10].

Excess weight can cause serious health problems for children and adolescents due to the increased risk of cardiovascular diseases [16], dyslipidemia, glucose intolerance, diabetes, systemic arterial hypertension [17], respiratory diseases (obstructive airways, such as asthma and sleep apnea), orthopedic and postural disorders, dermatitis and some types of neoplasms; or even to become obese adults with a greater propensity to develop such pathologies [10, 12, 18, 19]. In addition to disorders in the emotional sphere [3] and non-alcoholic fatty liver disease (NAFLD) [7, 8, 10, 11, 20–22].

The growing trend in childhood obesity is related to the increase in the diagnosis of systemic arterial hypertension in children [6, 17, 23] and atherosclerosis in young people [24]. Metabolic changes resulting from obesity also increase the risk of developing hepatic steatosis [25], which has been proposed as one of the components or the hepatic manifestation of the metabolic syndrome [12]. Hepatic steatosis (HE) has an overall prevalence of 2.6% in children, ranging from 23 to 53% in obese children [10, 25].

NAFLD in childhood reduces life expectancy as it can progress to severe liver dysfunction [11, 22]. It is important to understand the natural history of HE not only because of the risk of progression of liver disease, but also because of the potential association with other pathologies such as type 2 diabetes mellitus and cardiovascular diseases [25].

Metabolic syndrome (MS), a group of disorders that includes obesity, insulin resistance, dyslipidemia, and hypertension, has been gaining importance due to its association with the subsequent development of cardiovascular disease and type 2 diabetes. The extent of coronary atherosclerosis in children and young adults increases considerably with the increasing number of multiple risk factors [17].

There is evidence that the atherosclerotic process starts in childhood [21], progresses with age and exhibits severity directly proportional to the number of risk factors presented by the individual. That is why it is believed that the primary prevention of cardiovascular diseases should begin in childhood, mainly through the process of education for the promotion of cardiovascular health with an emphasis on the importance of diet and the maintenance of a regular practice of physical activity for life [17, 26].

Pediatricians' attention to the consequences of obesity in childhood and adolescence probably started because of the significant increase in its prevalence in developed and developing countries [12]. In view of the increase in the frequency of overweight and obesity among children and adolescents, the diagnosis of nutritional status must be part of the routine medical evaluation [11, 15].

2. Visceral fat

Excess body fat (mainly visceral fat) has been associated with increased mortality, as there has been an increase in obesity prevalence rates [14]. It is assumed that visceral obesity is a risk factor for cardiovascular morbidity and mortality [27], regardless of the associated dyslipidemia, hypertension, and diabetes mellitus [28].

Since then, the relationship between subcutaneous, gluteal-femoral, and visceral fat with the action of insulin has been extensively studied and, today, it can be said that at least the association of visceral fat with the components of MS is well established [29].

It has been shown that the accumulation of visceral fat is related to the development of steatohepatitis and that this accumulation continuously influences the histological changes in NAFLD, from the beginning of the deposition of fat in the hepatocytes to the appearance of inflammatory changes [29, 30].

Both steatosis and abdominal visceral fat are independent correlates of cardiometabolic risk, but the associations are stronger between visceral fat and steatosis [29]. Currently, the type of fat distribution in the body, especially the accumulation of intra-abdominal fat (IAF), is considered the most important factor in the associations between these clinical entities [20].

Evidence suggests the importance of measuring abdominal obesity, in addition to general obesity, to assess health risks in the first decades of life [18].

Obesity, usually assessed by anthropometric measurements, has idiosyncrasies that are beyond common sense. For example, individuals with a low body mass index may have a high incidence of typical MS changes. Then, attention is drawn to the fact that it would not be the excess of total body fat but the distribution of that fat that would be related to insulin resistance and, consequently, to MS [29].

Over the years, research has shown that weight gain alone is less relevant than the distribution of body fat in determining metabolic changes [28]. Central obesity, characterized by the accumulation of fat in the trunk and abdomen, has visceral abdominal fat (VAF) as one of its components, whose thickness measurement is of great importance, as it is an indicator of cardiovascular risk due to metabolic changes resulting from this fat deposit [30, 31].

Visceral fat can be assessed by measuring waist circumference or by means of imaging tests, such as computed tomography (CT), magnetic resonance imaging (MRI), and ultrasonography (US).

3. Assessment of nutritional status

The assessment of nutritional status aims to verify growth and body proportions in an individual or in a community, with a view to establishing intervention attitudes. Thus, the standardization of the evaluation to be used for each age group is of fundamental importance, thus standardizing the criteria used by the health team [32].

With regard to the identification of cases of obesity in children, an important issue has been discussed, that is, which is the most accurate method to classify it [6].

When defining methods for assessing the nutritional status, those which best detect the nutritional problem that is intended to be corrected in the study population should be chosen. The costs for its use, the level of personal skill required to apply them properly, the time needed to perform them, the receptivity on the part of the population studied, and the possible health risks must be considered [32] .

Determining obesity is, establishing excess body fat [14]. This concern is justified by the increase in the prevalence of obesity worldwide and the potential risks of developing chronic diseases in adulthood [32].

Among the various methods, anthropometric diagnosis and imaging diagnosis stand out.

4. Assessment and diagnostic anthropometric

Anthropometry, which consists of assessing the physical dimensions and the global composition of the human body, has proved to be the single most used method for nutritional diagnosis at the population level, especially in childhood and adolescence, due to its ease of execution, low cost, and innocuity. Based on the publications of Jellife, edited by WHO, in the 1960s, based on studies that had started in the 1950s, anthropometry was systematized as a method of assessing nutritional status. It was from these studies that anthropometry developed rapidly in industrialized countries, which only occurred in the mid-1970s in developing countries. Since then, anthropometry has constantly evolved, being a useful method in population, clinical, and intervention studies, and its application has enabled advances in interpretations and in the search for mathematical formulations that improve the accuracy of body compartment estimation and its predictive power. Since 1978, WHO has adopted data from the National Center for Health Statistics (NCHS) as an international reference standard [32].

Anthropometric values represent, at the individual or population level, the degree of adjustment between the genetic potential for growth and the favorable and harmful environmental factors. The ideal anthropometric pattern, then, would be that obtained from populations or ethnic groups whose individuals had enjoyed the opportunity to fully develop their growth potential. In this sense, we use the statistical results obtained from populations in developed areas of the world, or in underdeveloped regions, from human groups of high socioeconomic standard, who probably had better opportunities to fulfill their genotypic growth possibilities [32].

Results from studies around the world have shown and show the possibility of using a single, international benchmark to assess growth and nutrition status in different regions. There is evidence that the growth in height and weight of healthy children of different ethnic origins, submitted to adequate living conditions, is similar up to 5 years of age [32].

Among the almost unlimited number of possible body measurements, the most frequently used measures are intended to determine body mass, expressed by weight; linear dimensions, especially height; body composition and energy and protein reserves, estimated by the main superficial soft tissues: subcutaneous fat and muscle mass [32].

4.1 Body mass index

Anthropometry, then, even considering its limitations, has been the most widely used method and also the one proposed by WHO [32].

It is recommended that the weight be measured in kilograms (kg), with an anthropometric scale, with the child barefoot, with light clothing and in an orthostatic position in the center of the scale, and that the height be measured in centimeters (cm), using a stadiometer, to the nearest 0.1 cm, with the child barefoot, with the back to the wall, feet together and parallel, in an upright position and looking forward in the horizon line.

The body mass index (BMI) is obtained by dividing body weight, in kilos, by height in square meters [2]; therefore, in kg/m2 [33–35], it is an anthropometric measure widely used to identify excess weight in children, adolescents, and adults [2, 6, 27, 36].

The stratification of nutritional status is obtained from the percentiles in the BMI/age ratio according to gender, from WHO, and allows children to be classified as eutrophic, overweight, or obese. Obesity is diagnosed in children with the percentile is equal to or greater than 97 and, overweight, in children with the percentiles between 85 (inclusive) and 97 [33–35].

The following BMI scores for age are considered, according to the WHO [33–35], illustrated in **Figure 1**.

The values of these anthropometric data should always be analyzed according to the child's age and sex, which are the main determinants of its evolution [2]. Although they are usual and simple procedures, they must be applied carefully, with standardization, and the instruments used must be calibrated frequently [32].

Obesity in children is not defined by an absolute number, but by a percentile [2, 37]. To establish a comparison of a set of anthropometric measurements with a reference standard, several scales can be used, the most common being the percentile and the Z score [32].

The percentiles are derived from the distribution in ascending order of the values of a parameter, observed for a given age or sex; the classification of a child

Value found for the child		Nutritional Diagnosis
percentile < 0.1	< Z score -3	Marked thinness
percentile ≥ 0.1 and ≤ 3	≥ Z score -3 and ≤ Score -2	Thinness
percentile > 3 and < 85	> Z score -2 and < Score +1	Eutrophy
percentile ≥ 85 and < 97	≥ Z score +1 and < Score +2	Overweight
percentile ≥ 97 and ≤ 99.9	≥ Z score +2 and ≤ score +3	Obesity
percentile > 99.9	> Z score +3	Severe obesity

Figure 1.
Reference values for diagnosing nutritional status using BMI curves for age. World Health Organization, Geneva (2000, 2006 and 2007).

in a given percentile allows to estimate how many children, of the same age and sex, are greater or lesser in relation to the evaluated parameter [2, 32]. The Z score means, in practical terms, the number of standard deviations that the data obtained are removed from their reference median [32].

The WHO Classification can be used for children regardless of age. Regarding the assessment of childhood obesity, the following criteria can be used: weight/height ratio equal to or greater than 120%; percentile equal to or greater than 97; or Z score equal to or greater than +2.0 [32].

To monitor growth, the curve (growth graph) is used in at least three successive measurements of weight and height, with intervals compatible with their growth rate according to age, allowing to assess the nutritional process. This instrument is extremely useful in establishing situations of nutritional risk [32].

Such curves are essential for both the diagnosis and the assessment of the patient's evolution during treatment. Only by viewing the child's graph can it be seen how small variations in weight and, consequently, in BMI can be significant [2].

The assessment of body composition becomes difficult in children due to its constant change during growth, in addition to not knowing what percentage of body fat increases the risks in relation to their health. It is mainly indicated to verify changes presented by children undergoing treatment for obesity [32]. When interpreting the data obtained in nutritional assessment, sexual maturation criteria should also be considered, given the great individual variability in the maturation process [2, 32].

BMI validity is based on the good correlation it presents with total body fat, especially with the amount of internal fat. However, it does not distinguish between fat mass and lean mass, making it difficult to differentiate between overweight with excess fat and that with hypertrophy of muscle mass [32, 36]. In addition, it does not determine the distribution of body fat [6] and does not reflect stunting, common among children of low socioeconomic status [32].

However, its ease of measurement must be considered since it uses anthropometric data of weight and height, which are easy to obtain and have good reproducibility [7, 32].

4.2 Waist circumference

The waist circumference (WC) defined by measuring the smallest circumference between the iliac crest and the costal margin is, in particular, a better predictor of visceral obesity, a condition that represents a high risk for the development of chronic noncommunicable diseases such as diabetes mellitus type 2, MS, HE, and cardiovascular diseases and, thus, it has been highlighted in national and international studies [6, 8, 38].

The use of this measure in screening and in primary health care helps in the early diagnosis and in the identification of those potential candidates to manifest such diseases in adulthood [1]. This measure is noninvasive, uses a minimum of equipment when compared to laboratory techniques, is fast to apply, easy to be used by trained evaluators, and is very affordable [38].

Waist circumference (WC) is measured in centimeters (cm), using a flexible and inelastic measuring tape, with the child in an orthostatic position, at the midpoint between the iliac crest and the costal rim, under clothing and at the end of a normal exhalation.

The authors stressed the importance of measuring waist circumference as a mandatory part of the pediatric semiological examination [22].

The classification of WC for each child is performed according to age, sex, and the percentiles of McCarthy et al. [39], considering the 90th and 95th percentiles to identify overweight and obesity, respectively (**Figure 2**).

Percentiles								
Genders	Ages*	5	10	25	50	75	90	95
Female	6+	46,3	47,3	49,2	51,5	54,2	57,0	58,9
	7+	47,4	48,4	50,3	52,7	55,6	58,7	60,8
	8+	48,5	49,6	51,5	54,1	57,1	60,4	62,7
	9+	49,5	50,6	52,7	55,3	58,5	62,0	64,5
	10+	50,7	51,8	53,9	56,7	60,0	63,6	66,2
Male	6+	47,2	48,2	50,7	52,2	54,6	57,1	58,7
	7+	47,9	48,9	50,9	53,3	56,1	58,8	60,7
	8+	48,7	49,9	52,1	54,7	57,8	60,9	62,9
	9+	49,7	51,0	53,4	56,4	59,7	63,2	65,4
	10+	50,8	52,3	55,0	58,2	61,9	65,6	67,9

Figure 2.
Parameters for classifying waist circumference between genders, adapted from McCarthy et al. [39].
** 6 + = group of children aged 6.00–6.99 years.*

4.3 Relationship between BMI and WC

Regarding the knowledge produced about the use of BMI or WC to assess the pattern of body fat, scholars of the subject in search of an answer demonstrated that there is a strong correlation coefficient between both measures, indicating that the waist circumference can determine, satisfactorily, children with high BMI [6, 7]. Investigations found important correlation values between BMI and WC, suggesting the joint use for the diagnosis of obesity, overweight, and central obesity [6], including in children and adolescents [7, 8].

BMI expresses changes that may occur in the distribution of fat, but does not verify the pattern of body fat. Thus, correlating this measure with other anthropometric measures is necessary, considering that the type of deposit of fat distribution is related to the health prognosis. However, WC is the measure that best represents the distribution of visceral fat and this, in turn, is more related to metabolic changes than subcutaneous fat, indicating the risk of children or adolescents to develop cardiovascular disease in future life. In addition, the relationship of this anthropometric measure with dyslipidemia, with arterial hypertension, and with the metabolic syndrome is evidenced in the literature and, therefore, should support professional practice [6].

McCarthy et al. stated that BMI may be a less sensitive indicator of fat among children and does not provide any indication of fat distribution. Information about WC in children can be as useful as BMI in population studies [39].

WC can be adopted as an alternative or additional measure to BMI in children. It is a direct measure that requires simple and inexpensive equipment, with the registration of a single value. BMI requires more complex equipment and mathematical calculations [39].

Researchers stressed the difference between ethnic groups and the importance of developing specific population patterns, as visceral adiposity is highly variable in children and is related to ethnicity [39]. The relative distribution of intra-abdominal tissue in relation to the subcutaneous abdominal region is significantly less in African American children than in whites [40].

For the same BMI, there may be individuals with more or less cardiovascular and metabolic risk, depending on the amount of intra-abdominal fat, which is also true for children [41]. It was shown that 23.4% of eutrophic children by BMI had high waist circumference [7].

4.4 Other anthropometric measurements

The waist-hip ratio and sagittal diameter are methods that indirectly determine visceral fat [28], predicting cardiovascular risk [38]. These anthropometric measures are methods used to assess body adiposity; however, they are unable to differentiate visceral from subcutaneous fat and have relatively high intra- and inter-examiner variability [29].

The assessment of adiposity through skinfold measurements is poorly reproducible and its usefulness in clinical practice is limited [15].

5. Diagnosis by imaging exams

Imaging exams are the methods of choice to assess and quantify visceral fat, since anthropometric measurements are unable to differentiate intra-abdominal from subcutaneous fat, as they are indirect measures [2, 29].

Dual-energy X-ray absorptiometry (DXA), a "scanning" technique considered to be reliable, whose mechanism occurs through two X-ray beams that cross the body, is used for the evaluation of the total and regional body composition of lean mass, fat mass, and bone mineral density. However, in the case of children, although it is a reference method, radiation exposure and high cost must be considered [6, 36].

Studies that concluded that anthropometric measurements have a strong correlation with the fat distribution indicated by DXA [6, 42] stand out. DXA estimates abdominal adiposity, but does not specifically quantify intra-abdominal fat [43].

Computed tomography (CT) is the gold standard method for the determination of visceral abdominal fat (VAF), due to its ability to differentiate between subcutaneous and visceral adiposity [44]. CT has the advantage of not depending on the operator's ability to identify structures during the examination and not be influenced by ultrasound transducer pressure on the abdomen during measurements. However, CT is an expensive method and submits patients to ionizing radiation, which limits its use mainly in epidemiological studies [31, 44].

Full-body CT measurements are accompanied by high radiation exposure and; therefore, they are not recommended for scientific purposes in healthy individuals. Thus, CT had to be restricted to some characteristic slices in most studies [36].

Magnetic resonance imaging (MRI) has also developed criteria for assessing visceral fat, with good accuracy [29, 44]; it is a method with which it is possible to assess the distribution of adipose tissue in children [10]. This test has the advantage of not emitting ionizing radiation [36] and the ability to quantify the fraction of fat [10]; however, it is more subject to artifacts than CT [29]. In addition, due to the high cost, greater need for sedation, and its limitation in claustrophobic patients, MRI has not been used routinely [10]. Among the limitations of the method for young children, there is the need to remain completely immobile during image capture [45].

Ultrasonography, in recent years, has been proposed as a noninvasive technique for the assessment of intra-abdominal fat [43], as it is a useful method for the determination of visceral adipose tissue [28, 44]. The possibility of measuring visceral fat attributes to US an important role in the assessment of MS [29].

In contrast to the disadvantages of CT, MRI, and anthropometric measurements, US has been establishing a simple, low-cost method, without radiation risk [29], free of side effects [10], with reproducibility and reliability already proven in the quantification of visceral fat [29], despite the need for specific equipment and well-trained observers, which can be repeated when necessary [28] and on a large scale, such as population screening [10].

Ultrasonography appears as one of the methods of diagnosis and characterization of abdominal fat, allowing the correlation of its findings with data from anthropometric physical examination in all age groups, being of great value in the evolutionary monitoring of obesity treatments.

In addition to measuring abdominal fat thickness, the method assesses the presence of liver fat. While some authors describe a sensitivity of ultrasonography in mode B for the detection of hepatic steatosis of just over 60%, other authors report a sensitivity of up to 90% [36].

Among its advantages, the ability to differentiate accumulation of intraperitoneal, pre-peritoneal, and subcutaneous fats, in addition to the safety of the examination, practicality, and speed, especially in the evaluation of the pediatric population, stands out.

US in children to measure pre-peritoneal fat and intra-peritoneal fat is a valid method for epidemiological and clinical studies [20, 46]. Statistical significance was observed between the thickness of intra-abdominal fat and subcutaneous tissue in relation to obesity in children [20]. US can be useful in measuring intraperitoneal fat in children and adolescents [20, 47]. The thickness of the subcutaneous fat showed no statistically significant difference between the sexes, between the age groups and in relation to the presence or not of steatosis. However, US can be used as a treatment control in individual cases [29].

The ultrasound technique consists of measuring the thickness of the subcutaneous and visceral abdominal fat, separately, using a transducer placed 1 cm (cm) above the umbilical scar. The thickness of the visceral adipose tissue obtained with this technique has a good correlation with the area of that same tissue quantified by computed tomography [29].

The knowledge acquired can be useful to employ a new method of assessing visceral fat and also to seek ultrasound parameters that change with the increase in BMI [20].

The techniques must be accurate and suitable for use both at the cross-sectional level (i.e., a single measure) and for monitoring the effects of interventions (behavioral, pharmacological, and surgical) aimed at promoting a healthy life [45].

6. Conclusions

Considering that the first signs and symptoms of obesity and its consequences can be determined in childhood, it becomes evident the importance of assessing subcutaneous and visceral fats in children, a population in which obesity may still be the only morbidity.

The pediatric detection and control of intra-abdominal obesity are important because it is associated with the metabolic syndrome in childhood, adolescence, and adulthood, and its progression can increase rates of morbidity and mortality due to cardiovascular disease among young adults.

Therefore, this population should be the target of prevention policies and programs, early diagnosis, and medical-nutritional monitoring, aiming to identify the risks of these pathologies and their health consequences.

Acknowledgements

The authors thank the professors and colleagues at the Santo Amaro University, especially Neil Ferreira Novo, Ph.D., Yara Juliano, Ph.D and Luciane Lucio Pereira, Ph.D.

The authors also thank their family and friends for constant encouragement.

Conflict of interest

The authors declare no conflict of interest.

Nomenclature

BMI	body mass index
CT	computed tomography
DXA	dual energy X-ray absorptiometry
Et al.	and others
HE	liver steatosis
IAF	intra-abdominal fat
NAFLD	non-alcoholic fatty liver disease
NCHS	National Center for Health Statistics
MRI	magnetic resonance imaging
MS	metabolic syndrome
US	ultrasonography
USA	United States of America
VAF	visceral abdominal fat
WC	waist circumference
WHO	World Health Organization
%	percent
$<$	less than
$\geq$	greater than or equal to
$\leq$	less than or equal to
$>$	greater than
cm	centimeter
kg	kilogram
kg/m^2	kilogram per square meter

Author details

Leonardo de Souza Piber*, Patrícia Colombo-Souza and Jane de Eston Armond
Santo Amaro University, São Paulo, Brazil

*Address all correspondence to: lpiber@prof.unisa.br

IntechOpen

© 2020 The Author(s). Licensee IntechOpen. This chapter is distributed under the terms of the Creative Commons Attribution License (http://creativecommons.org/licenses/by/3.0), which permits unrestricted use, distribution, and reproduction in any medium, provided the original work is properly cited.

References

[1] Pereira PF, Serrano HMS, Carvalho GQ, Lamounier JA, Peluzio MDCG, Franceschini SDCC, et al. Waist circumference as an indicator of body fat and metabolic changes in adolescents: Comparison between four references [Circunferência da cintura Como indicador de gordura corporal e alterações metabólicas em adolescentes: Comparação entre quatro referências]. Revista da Associação Médica Brasileira. 2010;**56**(6):665-669

[2] Troiano RP, Flegal KM. Overweight children and adolescents: Description, epidemiology, and demographics. Pediatrics. 1998;**101**(s2):497-504

[3] Enes CC, Slater B. Obesity in adolescence and its main determining factors [Obesidade na adolescência e seus principais fatores determinantes]. Revista Brasileira de Epidemiologia. 2010;**13**(1):163-171

[4] Haslam DW, James WP. Obesity. Lancet. 2005;**366**(9492):1197-1209 Review

[5] Brown CL, Halvorson EE, Cohen GM, Lazorick S, Skelton JA. Addressing childhood obesity: Opportunities for prevention. Pediatric Clinics of North America. 2015;**62**(5):1241-1261. DOI: 10.1016/j.pcl.2015.05.013

[6] Damasceno MMC, Fragoso LVC, Lima AKG, Lima ACS, Viana PCS. Correlation between body mass index and waist circumference in children [Correlação entre índice de Massa corporal e circunferência da cintura em crianças]. Acta Paulista de Enfermagem. 2010;**23**(5):652-657

[7] Dias LCGD, Gomes CB, Momentti AC, Furtado NR. Anthropometric characteristics and eating habits of schoolchildren: Indicative factors for nutritional education [Características antropométricas e hábitos alimentares de escolares: Fatores indicativos Para a educação nutricional]. Rev Ciênc Extens. 2014;**10**(3):56-68

[8] Duarte MAS, Silva GAPD. Hepatic steatosis in obese children and adolescents. Jornal de Pediatria. 2011;**87**(2):150-156

[9] Keane E, Layte R, Harrington J, Kearney PM, Perry IJ. Measured parental weight status and familial socio-economic status correlates with childhood overweight and obesity at age 9. PLoS One. 2012;**7**(8):e43503

[10] Soder RB, Baldisserotto M. Liver steatosis in childhood obesity: Imaging investigation [Esteatose hepática na obesidade infantil: Investigação por imagem]. Scientia Medica. 2009;**19**(4):202-208

[11] Padilha PC, Rocha HF, Alves N, Peres WAF. Prevalence of non-alcoholic liver disease in obese children and adolescents: A systematic review [Prevalência de doença hepática não-alcoólica em crianças e adolescentes obesos: Uma revisão sistemática]. Rev Paul Pediatr. 2010;**28**(4):387-393

[12] Lira AR, Oliveira FLC, Escrivão S, Meil MA, Colugnati FAB. Taddei JADAC. Liver steatosis in a school population of overweight and obese adolescents [Esteatose hepática em uma população escolar de adolescentes com sobrepeso e obesidade]. Jornal de Pediatria. 2010;**86**(1):45-52

[13] Martorell R, Khan LK, Hughes ML, Grummer-Strawn LM. Obesity in Latin American women and children. The Journal of Nutrition. 1998;**128**(9):1464-1473

[14] Behenck MS, Matheus SC, Silva JLT, Portela LOC. Methods of determining body fat. Métodos de determinação da gordura corporal. Revista Brasileira de Medicina. 2007;**61**(10):650-654

[15] Melo ME. Diagnosis of Childhood Obesity [Diagnóstico da Obesidade Infantil]. Brazilian Association for the Study of Obesity and Metabolic Syndrome-ABESO [Associação Brasileiro para o Estudo da Obesidade e da Síndrome Metabólica-ABESO]. Available from: http://wwwabesoorgbr/pagina/14/artigoss html [Internet]. 2009;**1**(1):2002-2003. Available from: https://abeso.org.br/wpcontent/uploads/2019/12/552fe98518b8a.pdf [Accessed: 30 May 2017]

[16] Umer A, Kelley GA, Cottrell LE, Giacobbi P Jr, Innes KE, Lilly CL. Childhood obesity and adult cardiovascular disease risk factors: A systematic review with meta-analysis. BMC Public Health. 2017;**17**(1):683. DOI: 10.1186/s12889-017-4691-z. Review

[17] Brandão AA, Magalhães ME, Pozzan R, França MDF, Pozzan R, Freitas EV, et al. Arterial hypertension in young people as a marker for primary cardiovascular prevention [Hipertensão arterial no jovem como marcador para a prevenção cardiovascular primária]. Revista da SOCERJ. 2002;**15**(4):247-255

[18] Burgos MS, Burgos LT, Camargo MD, Franke SIR, Prá D, Silva AMVD, et al. Association between anthropometric measurements and cardiovascular risk factors in children and adolescents [Associação entre medidas antropométricas e fatores de Risco cardiovascular em crianças e adolescentes]. Arquivos Brasileiros de Cardiologia. 2013;**101**(4):288-296

[19] Simmonds M, Llewellyn A, Owen CG, Woolacott N. Predicting adult obesity from childhood obesity: A systematic review and meta-analysis. Obesity Reviews. 2016;**17**(2):95-107. DOI: 10.1111/obr.12334

[20] Sakuno T, Tomita LM, Tomita CM, Giuliano IDCB, Ibagy A, Perin NMM, et al. Ultrasonographic evaluation of visceral and subcutaneous fat in obese children [Avaliação ultrassonográfica da gordura visceral e subcutânea em crianças obesas]. Rev Radio Bras. 2014;**47**(3):149-153

[21] Almeida CA, Pinho AP, Ricco RG, Elias CP. Abdominal circumference as an indicator of clinical and laboratory parameters associated with obesity in children and adolescents: Comparison between two reference tables. Jornal de Pediatria. 2007;**83**(2):181-185

[22] FeldsteinAE,CharatcharoenwitthayaP, Treeprasertsuk S, Benson JT, Enders FB, Angulo P. The natural history of non-alcoholic fatty liver disease in children: A follow-up study for up to 20 years. Gut. 2009;**58**(11):1538-1544

[23] Burgos MS, Reuter CP, Burgos LT, Pohl HH, Pauli LTS, Horta JA, et al. An analysis of blood pressure, obesity and cardiorespiratory fitness in schoolchildren [Uma análise entre índices pressóricos, obesidade e capacidade cardiorrespiratória em escolares]. Arquivos Brasileiros de Cardiologia. 2010;**94**(6):788-793

[24] McGill HC, McMahan CA, Malcom GT, Oalmann MC, Strong JP. Relation of glycohemoglobin and adiposity to atherosclerosis in youth. Arteriosclerosis, Thrombosis, and Vascular Biology. 1995;**15**(4):431-440

[25] Schwimmer JB, Deutsch R, Kahen T, Lavine JE, Stanley C, Behling C. Prevalence of fatty liver in children and adolescents. Pediatrics. 2006;**118**(4):1388-1393

[26] Silva MD, Rivera IR, Ferraz MRMT, Pinheiro AJT, Alves SWDS, Moura AA, et al. Prevalence of cardiovascular risk factors in children and adolescents from the education network in the city of Maceió [Prevalência de fatores de Risco cardiovascular em crianças e adolescentes da rede de ensino da cidade de Maceió]. Arquivos Brasileiros de Cardiologia. 2005;**84**(5):387-392

[27] Bastien M, Poirier P, Lemieux I, Després JP. Overview of epidemiology and contribution of obesity to cardiovascular disease. Progress in Cardiovascular Diseases. 2014;**56**(4): 369-381. DOI: 10.1016/j.pcad.2013.10.016

[28] Radominski RB, Vezozzo DP, Cerri GG, Halpern A. The use of ultrasound to assess abdominal fat distribution [O uso da ultra-sonografia na avaliação da distribuição de gordura abdominal]. Arquivos Brasileiros de Endocrinologia & Metabologia. 2000;**44**(1):5-12

[29] Eifler RV. The role of ultrasound in the measurement of subcutaneous and visceral fat and its correlation with hepatic steatosis [O papel da ultrassonografia na medida da gordura subcutânea e visceral e sua correlação com a esteatose hepática]. Radio Bras. 2013;**46**(5):273-278

[30] Leon LB, Becker SCC, Petry RC, Wink EF, Lantz F, Tovo CV. Non-alcoholic fatty liver disease in patients with normal body mass index: Etiology and associated risk factors in a tertiary hospital [Doença hepática gordurosa não alcoólica em pacientes com índice de Massa corporal normal: Etiologia e fatores de Risco associados em um hospital terciário]. Revista da AMRIGS. 2014;**58**(1):44-48

[31] Gouvêa HRD, Faria SL, Faria OP, Cardeal MDA, Bezerra A, Ito MK. Validation of ultrasound for the assessment of visceral abdominal fat in clinically severe obese patients [Validação da ultrassonografia para a avaliação da gordura abdominal visceral em obesos clinicamente graves]. Arquivos Brasileiros de Cirurgia Digestiva. 2013;**26**(Suplemento):43-46

[32] Sigulem DM, Devincenzi MU, Lessa AC. Diagnosis of the nutritional status of children and adolescents [Diagnóstico do estado nutricional da criança e do adolescente]. Journal of Pediatrics. 2000;**76**(3):275-284

[33] World Health Organization. Obesity: Preventing and managing the global epidemic. In: Technical Report Series 894. Genebra: WHO; 2000. pp. 268

[34] World Health Organization. Child Growth Standards: Length/Height-for-Age, Weight-for-Age, Weight-for-Length, Weight-for-Height and Body Mass Index-for-Age: Methods and Development. Geneva: WHO; 2006. pp. 312

[35] de Onis M, Onyango AW, Borghi E, Siyam A, Nishida C, Siekmann J. Development of a WHO growth reference for school-aged children and adolescents. Bulletin of the World Health Organization. 2007;**85**(9):660-667

[36] Machann J, Horstmann A, Born M, Hesse S, Hirsch FW. Diagnostic imaging in obesity. Best Practice & Research Clinical Endocrinology & Metabolism. 2013;**27**(2):261-277. DOI: 10.1016/j.beem.2013.02.003

[37] Sérgio A. National Program to Combat Obesity [Programa Nacional de Combate à Obesidade]. Lisbon: Directorate-General for Health; 2005. pp. 24

[38] Lima CGD, Basile LG, Silveira JQD, Vieira PM, Oliveira MRMD. Waist or abdominal circumference? A critical review of the methodological references [Circunferência da cintura ou abdominal? Uma revisão crítica dos referenciais metodológicos]. Rev Simbio-Logias. 2011;**4**(6):108-131

[39] McCarthy HD, Jarrett KV, Crawley HF. The development of waist circumference percentiles in British children aged 5.0-16.9 y. European Journal of Clinical Nutrition. 2001;**55**(10):902-907

[40] Goran MI, Nagy TR, Treuth MS, Trowbridge C, Dezenberg C, McGloin A, et al. Visceral fat in white

and African American prepubertal children. The American Journal of Clinical Nutrition. 1997;**65**(6):1703-1708

[41] Bustelo MM, Joga MM, Colomina IC, Buceta XS, Fernández MF. Waist circumference as an indicator of risk of morbidity in children [Circunferencia de cintura Como indicador de riesgo de morbilidad en niños]. Cadernos de Atención Primaria. 2007;**13**(4):242-247

[42] Martin-CalvoN,Moreno-GalarragaL, Martinez-Gonzalez MA. Association between body mass index, waist-to-height ratio and adiposity in children: A systematic review and meta-analysis. Nutrients. 2016;**8**(8). pii: E512. DOI: 10.3390/nu8080512 Review

[43] Ribeiro-Filho FF, Faria AN, Azjen S, Zanella MT, Ferreira SR. Methods of estimation of visceral fat: Advantages of ultrasonography. Obesity Research. 2003;**11**(12):1488-1494

[44] Cieśluk K, Dobroch J, Sawicka-Żukowska M, Krawczuk-Rybak M. Body composition measurements in paediatrics—A review. Part 2. Pediatric Endocrinology Diabetes and Metabolism. 2018;**24**(4):191-196. DOI: 10.5114/pedm.2018.83366 Review

[45] Lemos T, Gallagher D. Current body composition measurement techniques. Current Opinion in Endocrinology, Diabetes and Obesity. 2017;**24**(5):310-314. DOI: 10.1097/MED.0000000000000360 Review

[46] Mook-Kanamori DO, Holzhauer S, Hollestein LM, Durmus B, Manniesing R, Koek M, et al. Abdominal fat in children measured by ultrasound and computed tomography. Ultrasound in Medicine and Biology. 2009;**35**(12):1938-1946. DOI: 10.1016/j.ultrasmedbio.2009.07.002

[47] Jung JH, Jung MK, Kim KE, Kwon AR, Chae HW, Yoon CS, et al. Ultrasound measurement of pediatric visceral fat thickness: Correlations with metabolic and liver profiles. Annals of Pediatric Endocrinology & Metabolism. 2016;**21**(2):75-80. DOI: 10.6065/apem.2016.21.2.75

Section 2

Health Consequences of Weight-Related Disorders

Chapter 6

Obesity: A Risk Factor for Infection after Surgery

José Alonso Suclla-Velásquez and Connie Smedts

Abstract

Obesity is a prevalent health problem all over the world. It is associated with several diseases including infections. It impairs the immune system function by plenty of mechanisms. For instance, leptin and adiponectin are cytokines produced by the adipose tissue, both participating in immunity, but their effects are impaired in obese patients. Moreover, immune cells also show defects in their functions. They produce a pro-inflammatory state and contribute to obesity-related diseases. Innate immune system and adaptive immunity are both impaired in obese patients which causes a poor response to infections. In addition, in surgical site infections (SSI), there are local factors that must be considered. The large adipose panicle and visceral adipose tissue increase the surgical technique difficulty and extend the operative time. Besides, the adipose tissue has poor oxygenation and reduces operative field. It has been proven that obesity is associated to surgical site infection irrespective of type of surgery. However, minimal invasive surgery has demonstrated that reducing surgical trauma can diminish the risk for surgical site infection.

Keywords: obesity, surgery, surgical site infection, immune deficiency, surgical complication

1. Introduction

Nowadays, obesity is a serious health problem which affects all countries irrespective of economic status. It is produced by an energy imbalance, and then there is an increase in body-fat mass. A body mass index (BMI) more than 30 kg/m^2 is defined as obesity [1].

There are plenty of diseases that are linked to obesity; the most common are metabolic syndrome, type 2 diabetes mellitus, coronary disease, and hyperlipidemia. Despite not being as well-known as the previous examples, obesity is strongly associated with infection [2].

Obese patients have a higher risk of nosocomial infections because medical care of these patients requires special procedures, equipment, and staff. Moreover, obese patients are usually immobilized which is a risk factor for decubitus ulcers and contributes to increase length of stay [3].

Although there are some controversial studies, an association between caries rates and elevated BMI has been proven. Dietary habits characterized by high consumption of soft drinks, fast food, and refined sugar contribute to dental caries as well as obesity [4]. In addition, it is well-known that severe infections in the face and neck usually have an odontogenic origin and obesity is a risk factor for the infection progression. Besides, an association has been described between the levels of tumor necrosis factor alpha in gingival crevicular fluid and BMI [5]; therefore, there is a systemic effect of obesity in oral health.

Obesity is related to respiratory diseases including nosocomial pneumonia and community-acquired respiratory tract infections [3]. In these patients, a decreased lung volume and a restrictive ventilatory pattern have been noticed. Excess weight on the anterior chest wall, abdominal obesity, and the presence of the adipose tissue in the intra-abdominal visceral tissue increase muscle work in breathing, diminish lung expansion, and increase airway resistance. These mechanical changes and augmented adipose tissue produce an inflammatory state that contributes to metabolic disease [6]. Other respiratory diseases associated to obesity are obstructive sleep apnea, chronic obstructive pulmonary disease, and asthma [6, 7].

On the other hand, obesity is a risk factor for the development of steatosis in patients with chronic hepatitis C infection and biliary disease with infectious complications [3]. Skin and soft tissue infections are also more prevalent in obese patients [2, 3]. The adipose tissue affects the pharmacokinetics and pharmacodynamics of antibiotics. Therefore, some special considerations must be taken when treating an obese patient [8, 9].

Even though there are some important studies that demonstrate obesity is not a risk factor for surgical complications [10], there are still some evidence that contrast with these researches [11]. On the other side, it is well-known that obese patients have a higher risk for surgical site infections (SSI) particularly when open surgery is performed. This phenomenon has been associated to low oxygen tension in the adipose tissue as well as a poor immune response observed in obese patients [3, 10, 11].

In this chapter we will review the available evidence about obesity as a risk factor for surgical infections in most common surgical procedures, considering pathophysiology as well as relevant clinical information.

2. Pathophysiology of infection in obese patients

There are several mechanisms that cause immune dysfunction in obese patients. The adipose tissue produces some cytokines which have effects on immune cells. There are other mechanisms that explain the altered immune response in obese patients.

2.1 Leptin and adiponectin

Nowadays, it is well-known that the adipose tissue has an active role in immunity by producing factors like leptin and adiponectin [3].

Leptin influences hematopoiesis, angiogenesis, and immune homeostasis. It stimulates proliferation and activation of monocytes in vitro and also increases the expression of surface markers. Leptin affects maturation of dendritic cells; deficiency of this cytokine is related to lower levels of tumor necrosis factor alpha and interleukins 12 and 6. It prevents neutrophil apoptosis and stimulates their chemotaxes. Leptin affects immune function of natural killer (NK) cells and T cells. It promotes T-cell proliferation, cytokine secretion, and migration of these cells. Th1-cell immune response is also stimulated by leptin. In addition, B lymphocytes are affected by leptin. It controls their development and can augment their population by suppressing apoptosis and stimulating proliferation of these cells [12–14]. Leptin also plays a role in wound healing. An experimental study has proved that leptin accelerates skin wound healing by increasing proliferation and differentiation of epidermal keratinocytes as well as promoting angiogenesis [15].

Congenital leptin deficiency is rare in humans. Diet-induced obesity is related to high levels of circulating leptin; however, it has been hypothesized that obesity causes some resistance in leptin receptors similar to what happens with insulin resistance [16]. Therefore, in obese patients, leptin cannot produce its effect on the immune system despite high levels of this cytokine.

Adiponectin is another important circulating adipocytokine that plays a role in immunity. It has anti-angiogenic, anti-inflammatory, and anti-apoptotic effects. Adiponectin can inhibit the phagocytic activity of macrophages, reduce the production of tumor necrosis factor alpha and gamma interferon, as well as induce the production of interleukin 10 and interleukin 1 receptor antagonists which are anti-inflammatory molecules. However, serum/plasma levels of adiponectin are higher in immune-mediated diseases [17, 18]. In contrast, in obese patients, adiponectin levels are lower than controls, and it has been observed that production of this adipocytokine increases after weight loss [19].

2.2 Immune cells

Although, in diabetic patients, neutrophils show defects in their functions, in obese patients this phenomenon has not been noticed. Indeed, these cells seem to be chronically primed and contribute to the development of obesity-related diseases [1].

Monocytes and macrophages also take part in immune response. They can change their phenotype getting a pro-inflammatory form (M1 CD11c+) or an anti-inflammatory form (M2 CD11c-) [1]. In obesity, a pro-inflammatory state, adipose tissue macrophages are more prevalent, these cells have M1 phenotype and are considered a factor that increases sepsis mortality. In addition, the percentage of macrophages in the adipose tissue is directly proportional to the adipocyte size [20]. Current evidence suggest that overnutrition causes adipocyte hypertrophy which leads to hypoxia and stimulates macrophage activity [21].

Natural killer cells are lymphocytes of the innate immune system. They are defined as CD3-/CD56+ granular lymphocytes and can be subcategorized based on the level of CD56 expression. $CD56^{dim}$ NK cell (or low density) subset can produce granzymes and perforins and is more cytotoxic than $CD56^{bright}$ (or high density) subset. On the other way, $CD56^{bright}$ NK cells have immunoregulatory effects. In obesity, there is no clear consensus about the effects on peripheral NK cell number. However, there is a study that demonstrates a significant more prevalence of $CD56^{bright}$ NK cells in obese patients as well as these patients also show a decreased percentage of $CD56^{dim}$ NK cells. Therefore, the predominance of $CD56^{bright}$ NK cells could be a cause for the impaired lytic activity NK cells against virus-infected and tumor cells observed in obese patients [22]. Several other studies have shown the impact of obesity on NK cells. An increased expression of activation markers such as CD69 and a decreased expression of other molecules such as NKp30 and NKp44 have been observed. Moreover, NK cells isolated from obese patients fail to engage glycolytic metabolism. They also lose the ability to kill macrophages and augment expression of gamma interferon which stimulates the migration of macrophages [23].

Dendritic cells (DCs) are also affected by obesity. They can activate or suppress immune responses and are characterized as conventional, inflammatory, or plasmacytoid dendritic cells. An increase in inflammatory DCs in the adipose tissue has been described. These cells are created from inflammatory monocytes and contribute to adipose tissue inflammation. However, there is evidence suggesting that conventional dendritic cells also take part in adipose tissue inflammation.

In addition, this study points out that dendritic cells could act independently of monocytes [24]. On the other hand, in obesity DCs failed to upregulate CD83, a marker for maturity. Besides, they produce less IL-12 and more IL-10, suggesting an inability to stimulate T cells [25].

Adaptive immunity is impaired too. Gamma delta T cells, a subset of T cells that takes part in repairing tissue and inducing inflammation, are diminished in obese patients and secrete less gamma interferon, contributing to the persistence of chronic, non-healing wounds [1, 26]. On the other side, memory T cells in the adipose tissue overexpress some cytokines while underexpress other ones. Moreover, obesity increases memory T-cell number which can be related to leptin production. Under healthy circumstances, memory T cells contribute to control infections; however, they can also mediate the pathogenesis in other conditions such as obesity [27]. In contrast, the number of regulatory T cells is reduced in the adipose tissue which promotes inflammation and insulin resistance [1, 26] because these cells participate actively maintaining self-tolerance and suppressing activity of effector T cells. This reduction can be partially explained by the levels of leptin which decreases the proliferation of regulatory T cells [28]. Other affected T cells are Th1 and Th17 cells. The first ones are increased in the visceral adipose tissue of obese patients contributing to inflammation, whereas Th17 cells are increased in the subcutaneous adipose tissue of obese patients and produce IL-17 which promotes inflammation and insulin resistance as well [26].

Relating to humoral immunity, there is no clear consensus. However, there is some evidence that it is impaired in obese patients. Obesity induces pro-inflammatory B cell subsets [29]. In spite of hyperstimulation of B cells and increased number of these, they function suboptimally and antibody production is modified. The most important factors that influence B-cell antibody production are leptin effect and essential fatty acid status [30].

3. Obesity and infection after surgery

Surgical site infection (SSI) is a serious complication that increases morbidity and mortality as well as extends postoperative stay and rises healthcare costs. Indeed, one observational study performed in 7020 patients who underwent colon surgery finds an increased rate of SSI in obese patients (14.5% vs. 9.5%; $p < 0.001$). In this study SSI increases costs in $17,000 because these patients have longer stays and higher rates of hospital readmission [31]. This increased risk for SSI is especially noticeable in clean and clean-contaminated surgeries. In addition, a study described a relation between BMI and the risks for SSI, and then overweight could just be a risk factor for SSI in some kinds of surgery [32].

There are several mechanisms that explain this increased risk. Some of them have already been mentioned. However, there are other ones that are important in surgical site infection. The most important factor is hypoperfusion of adipose tissue which is due to less vascularization of adipose tissue. It causes poor tissue oxygenation and extends wound healing. Moreover, there is more dead space, and antibiotics might not get adequate concentrations in the wound [32, 33].

Other important factors are related to surgery. Obese patients have great adipose panicle which makes open surgery more difficult. In addition, the visceral abdominal tissue is also increased and obligates surgeons to take special considerations on the surgical technique such as longer incisions, prolonged surgery time, and increased mean operative blood loss [32, 33]. Both are known risk factors for surgical site infection.

3.1 Obesity and gastrointestinal surgery

A large study performed in the Netherlands evaluated the relation between obesity and several types of surgery. Laparoscopic appendectomy, laparoscopic cholecystectomy, open colectomy, and laparoscopic colectomy were considered gastrointestinal surgery. The study revealed that the risk of superficial SSI gradually increased with increasing BMI, except in laparoscopic appendectomy. However, deep SSI did not seem related to BMI [32].

A meta-analysis also showed that overweight and obese patients have a 1.2- to 1.5-fold higher odds of developing SSI after colorectal surgery. Moreover, the same study performed a subgroup analysis that included only elective surgery cases, and then the results were similar. The authors highlighted the suboptimal tissue concentrations of antibiotics in obese patients. It is not only related to the increased volume of distribution and altered plasma protein binding; indeed, obese patients have changes in hepatic metabolism and renal excretion, and the prevalence of diabetes is higher in these patients [34].

Another study performed a separate analysis for right colectomy, left colectomy, and rectal resection. Obesity did not affect morbidity and mortality after right colectomy. However, the rate of postoperative intra-abdominal collections was higher in obese patients after left colectomy. Moreover, the study showed that obesity was a risk factor for anastomotic leakage after rectal resection. Therefore, the authors recommended the use of a defunctioning stoma in obese patients when diabetes or ASA > 2 is present [35].

On the other hand, laparoscopic surgery has brought to table other considerations. A meta-analysis showed that the incidence of SSI is significantly less after laparoscopic surgery than after open surgery (70–80% lower risk). These findings could be related to less surgical trauma and smaller incisions that are used in laparoscopic surgery. However, conversion to open surgery has the worst outcomes [36]. Despite the advantages of laparoscopic surgery, it is not always easy to perform it in obese patients. A meta-analysis demonstrated that visceral obesity is associated to longer operative time, less lymph node harvest, and higher conversion rate. Moreover, laparoscopic surgery in obese patients requires technical expertise because of the limited exposure of the surgical field and the thickened mesentery which is difficult to maneuver [37].

In obese children the problem is similar, and there is some evidence that demonstrates that laparoscopy is safe in these patients, although it is related to longer operative time [38].

Laparoscopic surgery is safe in obese patients. However, there are some special considerations: adequate position to expand the surgical field avoiding pressure sores and minimizing nerve compression, adequate entry technique, longer operative time, and thromboprophylaxis [39].

Although there are few studies about obesity and robotic surgery, it has been suggested that it could bring more benefits for obese patients. It has been observed that the length of stay and 30-day readmission rate were lower in patients who underwent robotic surgery than in patients who underwent laparoscopic surgery. It probably happens because of superior stable 3D views and ergonomic wristed instruments that robotic surgery offers [40]. However, it must be considered that robotic surgery is more expensive than laparoscopic surgery and requires appropriate training.

3.2 Obesity and gynecological surgery

In gynecological surgery there is some controversy. Overweight could be a protective factor for SSI in vaginal hysterectomy. However, there is an increased risk for deep SSI in morbidly obese patients [32]. In abdominal hysterectomy, the findings are similar, and the risk for SSI increases linearly with increasing BMI. The same study showed a nonsignificant prevalence of *Enterobacteriaceae* in obese or overweight patients with SSI after abdominal hysterectomy [33].

A large study that included 18,810 patients who underwent hysterectomy for benign indications demonstrated that the risk for superficial and deep wound infection was higher with increasing BMI after total abdominal hysterectomy. However, the risk was not different when minimally invasive surgery (total vaginal hysterectomy, laparoscopic assisted vaginal hysterectomy, total laparoscopic hysterectomy) was performed. In contrast, the operative time was longer with increasing BMI irrespective of the surgical approach [41].

Obesity is a risk factor for leiomyomata, ovulatory dysfunction, and endometrial cancer. All of them are common indications for hysterectomy. Therefore, hysterectomy is a common surgical procedure performed in obese women. In that way, it is recommended to prefer a minimal invasive approach because of its reduced rate of complications. Other aspects to be considered are adequate thromboembolism prophylaxis, antibiotic prophylaxis, and adequate surgical technique [42].

In cesarean section, maternal obesity is also associated with surgical and postoperative risks such as endometritis, intra-abdominal collection, and surgical wound complications. In that way, antibiotic prophylaxis in these patients is different, and the actual recommendation is to administer at least 2 g of cefazolin some 60 minutes before the cesarean section. Another recommendation is to close the subcutaneous tissue layer in obese patients particularly when its depth exceeds 2 cm [43].

Finally, for mastectomy and lumpectomy, it has been observed that the risk of developing SSI augmented with increasing BMI. Moreover, obesity is a risk factor for major and minor complications after mastectomy irrespective of being unilateral or performing reconstruction [44].

3.3 Obesity and orthopedic surgery

Obesity is an important risk factor for SSI after total hip prosthesis. It has been observed that the rate of SSI increased gradually with increasing BMI. Moreover, this association was present in both superficial and deep SSI. However, in partial hip prosthesis, obesity was related to superficial and deep SSI, but overweight only was a risk factor for deep SSI [32]. Another study had similar findings. It showed that members of the *Enterobacteriaceae* were more common among normal-weight patients with hip replacement [33].

On the other hand, among the total knee replacement patients, obesity was a risk factor for deep SSI but not for superficial SSI. Indeed, only a BMI > 40 was a risk factor for superficial SSI [32].

A meta-analysis also demonstrated that the risk of periprosthetic joint infection in obese patients was 1.9-fold higher than non-obese patients. The authors mentioned that this increased risk could be related to prolonged operative time, an increased rate of wound complications, and the presence of medical comorbidities [45].

Finally, a large study that included 161,785 patients showed that obesity was associated to higher rates of complications after total hip arthroplasty than after total knee arthroplasty. The study demonstrated that among the obese and morbidly obese patients who underwent primary total hip replacement, the risk of total complications, wound complications, deep infection, and reoperation was higher than for similar weighted patients who underwent primary total knee arthroplasty. This observed difference would be due to the tendency of the adipose tissue to deposit in the gluteal region [46].

3.4 Obesity and cardiothoracic surgery

Among the patients who undergo cardiothoracic surgery, obesity is a risk factor for SSI. Several studies have shown that the risk for SSI augmented gradually with increasing BMI [32, 33]. In cardiac surgery, however, an obesity paradox has been described. It means that mildly obese or overweight patients may have some benefit instead of an increased risk. Indeed, a large study that included 4740 patients who underwent cardiac surgery demonstrated that extremely obese (BMI > 40 kg/m^2) patients had an increased risk for deep sternal infection, prolonged ventilation after cardiac surgery, and postoperative renal dialysis requirement. In contrast, mildly obese or overweight patients had minor in-hospital mortality, minor operative mortality, and less ICU hours [47]. Another study showed that obesity and underweight were both associated to postoperative adverse events. However, this study did not show differences between extremely and mildly obese patients probably because both studies used different ways to categorize BMI [48].

3.5 Obesity and neurosurgery

A large study performed in the Netherlands failed to demonstrate an association between obesity and surgical site infection after laminectomy [32]. However, another study which included 31,763 patients demonstrated that complications after lumbar spine surgery were associated to obesity. The stratification by BMI established five categories: underweight (BMI < 18.5), normal-overweight (BMI 20.0–29.9), obesity class I (BMI 30.0–34.9), obesity class II (35.0–39.9). and obesity class III (BMI > 40). The study evaluated airway, cardiopulmonary, and infectious complications. They found that obese class I was associated to 4 of the 11 complications analyzed; obesity class II was associated to 6 of the 11 complications analyzed; and obesity class III was associated to 9 of the 11 complications analyzed. In addition, the rate of surgical site infection increased with increasing obesity class [49].

The effect of obesity on cranial surgery is similar to spinal surgery, but the impact on surgical outcomes is lower on cranial surgery. It increases the risk of major medical complications and may increase the risk for SSI after craniotomy. On the other side, in spinal surgery, obesity increases the risk of SSI, venous thromboembolism, and major medical complications [50].

4. Conclusion

Although obesity leads to a pro-inflammatory state, it impairs the immune system and is a risk factor for several infections. Moreover, in surgical site infection, there are local factors related to obesity that must be taken into account: a large adipose panicle with poor oxygenation, a reduced operative field, difficulties in technique, and increased operative time. Therefore, obesity is a proven risk factor for surgical site infection in plenty of surgeries. However, there are some actions that we could take to reduce this risk: performing minimal invasive surgery, ensuring adequate surgical technique, prescribing adequate antibiotic doses, and recommending weight loss.

Acknowledgements

We would like to express our gratitude to Professor Luis Acosta Vega for his guidance and encouragement when we started to research in this field. Finally, we thank our families for their support and encouragement.

Conflict of interest

The authors declare no conflict of interest.

Author details

José Alonso Suclla-Velásquez* and Connie Smedts
Social Health Insurance ESSALUD, Arequipa, Perú

*Address all correspondence to: sucllajose2010inv@gmail.com

IntechOpen

© 2020 The Author(s). Licensee IntechOpen. This chapter is distributed under the terms of the Creative Commons Attribution License (http://creativecommons.org/licenses/by/3.0), which permits unrestricted use, distribution, and reproduction in any medium, provided the original work is properly cited.

References

[1] Frydrych LM, Bian G, O'Lone DE, Ward PA, Delano MJ. Obesity and type 2 diabetes mellitus drive immune dysfunction, infection development, and sepsis mortality. Journal of Leukocyte Biology. 2018;**104**(3):525-534

[2] Ghilotti F, Bellocco R, Ye W, Adami H-O, Trolle Lagerros Y. Obesity and risk of infections: Results from men and women in the Swedish National March Cohort. International Journal of Epidemiology. 10 July 2019;**48**(6):1783-1794

[3] Falagas ME, Kompoti M. Obesity and infection. The Lancet Infectious Diseases. 2006;**6**(7):438-446

[4] Alswat K, Mohamed WS, Wahab MA, Aboelil AA. The association between body mass index and dental caries: Cross-sectional study. Journal of Clinical Medical Research. 2016;**8**(2):147-152

[5] Lundin M, Yucel-Lindberg T, Dahllöf G, Marcus C, Modéer T. Correlation between TNF alpha in gingival crevicular fluid and body mass index in obese subjects. Acta Odontologica Scandinavica. 2004;**62**(5):273-277

[6] Zammit C, Liddicoat H, Moonsie I, Makker H. Obesity and respiratory diseases. International Journal of General Medicine. 2010;**3**:335-343

[7] Mafort TT, Rufino R, Costa CH, Lopes AJ. Obesity: Systemic and pulmonary complications, biochemical abnormalities, and impairment of lung function. Multidisciplinary Respiratory Medicine. 2016;**11**(1):28

[8] Grupper M, Nicolau DP. Obesity and skin and soft tissue infections: How to optimize antimicrobial usage for prevention and treatment? Current Opinion in Infectious Diseases. 2017;**30**(2):180-191

[9] Ihm C, Sutton JD, Timbrook TT, Spivak ES. Treatment duration and associated outcomes for skin and soft tissue infections in patients with obesity or heart failure. Open Forum Infectious Diseases. 7 May 2019;**6**(6):ofz217

[10] Dindo D, Muller MK, Weber M, Clavien P-A. Obesity in general elective surgery. Lancet (London, England). 2003;**361**(9374):2032-2035

[11] STARSurg Collaborative. Multicentre prospective cohort study of body mass index and postoperative complications following gastrointestinal surgery. The British Journal of Surgery. 2016;**103**(9):1157-1172

[12] Procaccini C, La Rocca C, Carbone F, De Rosa V, Galgani M, Matarese G. Leptin as immune mediator: Interaction between neuroendocrine and immune system. Developmental and Comparative Immunology. 2017;**66**:120-129

[13] Abella V, Scotece M, Conde J, Pino J, Gonzalez-Gay MA, Gómez-Reino JJ, et al. Leptin in the interplay of inflammation, metabolism and immune system disorders. Nature Reviews Rheumatology. 2017;**13**(2):100-109

[14] Alti D, Sambamurthy C, Kalangi SK. Emergence of Leptin in infection and immunity: Scope and challenges in vaccines formulation. Front Cell Infect Microbiol. 9 May 2018;**8**:147

[15] Tadokoro S, Ide S, Tokuyama R, Umeki H, Tatehara S, Kataoka S, et al. Leptin promotes wound healing in the skin. PloS One. 23 Mar 2015;**10**(3):e0121242

[16] Myers MG, Leibel RL, Seeley RJ, Schwartz MW. Obesity and leptin resistance: Distinguishing cause from

effect. Trends in Endocrinology and Metabolism: TEM. 2010;**21**(11):643-651

[17] Surendar J, Frohberger SJ, Karunakaran I, Schmitt V, Stamminger W, Neumann A-L, et al. Adiponectin limits IFN-γ and IL-17 producing CD4 T cells in obesity by restraining cell intrinsic glycolysis. Frontiers in Immunology. 2019;**10**:2555

[18] Zhang M-Y, Dini AA, Yang X-K, Li L-J, Wu G-C, Leng R-X, et al. Association between serum/plasma adiponectin levels and immune-mediated diseases: A meta-analysis. Archives of Dermatological Research. 2017;**309**(8):625-635

[19] Nigro E, Scudiero O, Monaco ML, Palmieri A, Mazzarella G, Costagliola C, et al. New insight into adiponectin role in obesity and obesity-related diseases. BioMed Research International. 2014;**2014**:658913

[20] Weisberg SP, McCann D, Desai M, Rosenbaum M, Leibel RL, Ferrante AW. Obesity is associated with macrophage accumulation in adipose tissue. The Journal of Clinical Investigation. 2003;**112**(12):1796-1808

[21] Thomas D, Apovian C. Macrophage functions in lean and obese adipose tissue. Metabolism. 2017;**72**:120-143

[22] Bähr I, Jahn J, Zipprich A, Pahlow I, Spielmann J, Kielstein H. Impaired natural killer cell subset phenotypes in human obesity. Immunologic Research. 2018;**66**(2):234-244

[23] O'Shea D, Hogan AE. Dysregulation of natural killer cells in obesity. Cancers. 23 Apr 2019;**11**(4):573

[24] Cho KW, Zamarron BF, Muir LA, Singer K, Porsche CE, DelProposto JB, et al. Adipose tissue dendritic cells are independent contributors to obesity-induced inflammation and insulin resistance. Journal of Immunology. 2016;**197**(9):3650-3661

[25] Orlandella R, Norian L. Obesity-induced defects in dendritic cell and T cell functions. In: Immunology. Amsterdam: Elsevier; 2018. pp. 171-181. Available from: https://linkinghub.elsevier.com/retrieve/pii/B9780128098196000125

[26] Wang Q, Wu H. T cells in adipose tissue: Critical players in Immunometabolism. Frontiers in Immunology. 2018;**9**:2509

[27] Misumi I, Starmer J, Uchimura T, Beck MA, Magnuson T, Whitmire JK. Obesity expands a distinct population of T cells in adipose tissue and increases vulnerability to infection. Cell Reports. 2019;**27**(2):514-524.e5

[28] Kucharska AM, Pyrżak B, Demkow U, Regulatory T. Cells in obesity. In: Pokorski M, editor. Noncommunicable Diseases. Cham: Springer International Publishing; 2015. pp. 35-40. Available from: http://link.springer.com/10.1007/5584_2015_147

[29] Frasca D, Diaz A, Romero M, Vazquez T, Blomberg BB. Obesity induces pro-inflammatory B cells and impairs B cell function in old mice. Mechanisms of Ageing and Development. 2017;**162**:91-99

[30] Kosaraju R, Guesdon W, Crouch MJ, Teague HL, Sullivan EM, Karlsson EA, et al. B cell activity is impaired in human and mouse obesity and is responsive to an essential fatty acid upon murine influenza infection. Journal of Immunology. 2017;**198**(12):4738-4752

[31] Wick EC, Hirose K, Shore AD, Clark JM, Gearhart SL, Efron J, et al. Surgical site infections and cost in obese patients undergoing colorectal surgery. Archives of Surgery. 2011;**146**(9):1068-1072

[32] Meijs AP, Koek MBG, Vos MC, Geerlings SE, Vogely HC, de Greeff SC. The effect of body mass index on the risk of surgical site infection. Infection Control and Hospital Epidemiology 2019;**40**(9):991-996

[33] Thelwall S, Harrington P, Sheridan E, Lamagni T. Impact of obesity on the risk of wound infection following surgery: Results from a nationwide prospective multicentre cohort study in England. Clinical Microbiology and Infection. 2015;**21**(11):1008.e1-1008.e8

[34] Gurunathan U, Ramsay S, Mitrić G, Way M, Wockner L, Myles P. Association between obesity and wound infection following colorectal surgery: Systematic review and meta-analysis. Journal of Gastrointestinal Surgery. 2017;**21**(10):1700-1712

[35] Benoist S, Panis Y, Alves A, Valleur P. Impact of obesity on surgical outcomes after colorectal resection. American Journal of Surgery. 2000;**179**(4):275-281

[36] Shabanzadeh D, Sørensen L. Laparoscopic surgery compared with open surgery decreases surgical site infection in obese patients: A systematic review and meta-analysis. Annals of Surgery. 2012;**256**(6):934-945

[37] Yang T, Wei M, He Y, Deng X, Wang Z. Impact of visceral obesity on outcomes of laparoscopic colorectal surgery: A meta-analysis. ANZ Journal of Surgery. 2015;**85**(7-8):507-513

[38] Pandian T, Ubl DS, Habermann EB, Moir CR, Ishitani MB. Obesity increases operative time in children undergoing laparoscopic cholecystectomy. Journal of Laparoendoscopic & Advanced Surgical Techniques. 2016;**27**(3):322-327

[39] Afors K, Centini G, Murtada R, Castellano J, Meza C, Wattiez A. Obesity in laparoscopic surgery. Best Practice & Research. Clinical Obstetrics & Gynaecology. 2015;**29**(4):554-564

[40] Panteleimonitis S, Pickering O, Abbas H, Harper M, Kandala N, Figueiredo N, et al. Robotic rectal cancer surgery in obese patients may lead to better short-term outcomes when compared to laparoscopy: A comparative propensity scored match study. International Journal of Colorectal Disease. 2018;**33**(8):1079-1086

[41] Mikhail E, Miladinovic B, Velanovich V, Finan M, Hart S, Imudia A. Association between obesity and the trends of routes of hysterectomy performed for benign indications. Obstetrics and Gynecology. 2015;**125**(4):912-918

[42] Matthews K, Brock E, Cohen S, Chelmow D. Hysterectomy in obese patients: Special considerations. Clinical Obstetrics and Gynecology. 2014;**57**(1):106-114

[43] Ayres-de-Campos D. Obesity and the challenges of caesarean delivery: Prevention and management of wound complications. Best Practice & Research. Clinical Obstetrics & Gynaecology. 2015;**29**(3):406-414

[44] Garland M, Hsu F-C, Clark C, Chiba A, Howard-McNatt M. The impact of obesity on outcomes for patients undergoing mastectomy using the ACS-NSQIP data set. Breast Cancer Research and Treatment. 2018;**168**(3):723-726

[45] Kong L, Cao J, Zhang Y, Ding W, Shen Y. Risk factors for periprosthetic joint infection following primary total hip or knee arthroplasty: A meta-analysis. International Wound Journal. 2017;**14**(3):529-536

[46] DeMik DE, Bedard NA, Dowdle SB, Elkins JM, Brown TS,

Gao Y, et al. Complications and obesity in arthroplasty—A hip is not a knee. The Journal of Arthroplasty. 2018;**33**(10):3281-3287

[47] Gao M, Sun J, Young N, Boyd D, Atkins Z, Li Z, et al. Impact of body mass index on the outcomes in cardiac surgery. Journal of Cardiothoracic and Vascular Anesthesia. 2016;**30**(5):1308-1316

[48] O'Byrne ML, Kim S, Hornik CP, Yerokun BA, Matsouaka RA, Jacobs JP, et al. Effect of obesity and underweight status on perioperative outcomes of congenital heart operations in children, adolescents, and young adults. Circulation. 2017;**136**(8):704-718

[49] Bono OJ, Poorman GW, Foster N, Jalai CM, Horn SR, Oren J, et al. Body mass index predicts risk of complications in lumbar spine surgery based on surgical invasiveness. The Spine Journal. 2018;**18**(7):1204-1210

[50] Castle-Kirszbaum MD, Tee JW, Chan P, Hunn MK. Obesity in neurosurgery: A narrative review of the literature. World Neurosurgery. 2017;**106**:790-805

Chapter 7

Calcium Dyshomeostasis in Neuropathy Diabetes

Shahdevi Kurniawan

Abstract

Diabetes is a ceaseless ailment that is basic in practically all nations. Neuropathy is the most well-known constant difficulty of diabetes and is the underlying reason for ulceration in the legs of lower appendage removals. The predominance of diabetic polyneuropathy shifts from 23 to 29%. Incessant metabolic pressure incited by hyperglycemia, either low insulin creation in type 1 diabetes or diminished fringe affectability to insulin in type 2 diabetes influences cell homeostasis in practically all phone types. Changes in the sign Ca^{2+} have been recognized in different seclusion tissues from creatures initiated to diabetes just as patients with diabetes. Ca^{2+} homeostasis variations from the norm have likewise been found in an assortment of tissues, including bone, heart and smooth muscle, secretory cells, platelets, kidneys and osteoblasts. This variation from the norm by and large shows as an expanded resting centralization of intracellular Ca^{2+} ($[Ca^{2+}]I$), diminished Ca^{2+} transporter movement and diminished boost that produces Ca^{2+} signals. Ca^{2+} flagging issue are likewise found in neuron-sensory from trial creatures with diabetes.

Keywords: neuropathy, diabetes, calcium, intracellular, dyshomeostasis

1. Introduction

Diabetes is a chronic disease that is common in almost all countries. It is estimated that there were around 285 million adults with diabetes in 2010, this number will continue to increase globally due to population aging, population size growth, urbanization and high prevalence of obesity and lifestyle changes [1]. Estimated death rates from diabetes are 3.9 million sufferers worldwide in 2010 and remain a major problem in each country [2–6]. Whereas in Indonesia alone, it was estimated that 7 million people with diabetes mellitus in 2010 became number 9 in the world [7].

Neuropathy is the most common chronic complication of diabetes and is the initial cause of foot ulceration, Charcot type neuroarthropathy and lower limb amputation. Epidemiologically, a study based in Europe, the prevalence of diabetic polyneuropathy varies from 23 to 29%. One third of all diabetic patients have symptoms of neuropathy regardless of deficits or symptoms of neuropathic pain. Neuropathic pain due to diabetes is more common in patients with type 2 diabetes, women, and people from South Asia [7, 8].

Diabetes mellitus in people causes inconveniences in different tissues and organ frameworks, including the heart muscle, retina, secretory organs, kidneys, and fringe nerves. Ceaseless metabolic pressure instigated by hyperglycemia, either low insulin creation in type 1 diabetes or diminished fringe affectability to

IntechOpen

insulin in type 2 diabetes influences cell homeostasis in practically all phone types. Hyperglycemia is generally viewed as the fundamental driver that triggers cell pathology variations from the norm and different downstream instruments, including metabolic worry, with the development of receptive oxygen species (ROS) that harm layers and other cell frameworks. Ongoing exploration uncovers an early decrease of the two intracellular frameworks associated, the Ca^{2+} signal homeostasis and the mitochondrial physiology. The event of these intracellular changes is comparative in each extraordinary cell type and can be viewed as a typical neurotic pathway [9, 10].

Diabetes mellitus in people causes entanglements that influence different tissues and organ frameworks, including the heart muscle, retina, glandular emissions, kidneys, and fringe nerves. Interminable metabolic pressure brought about by hyperglycemia coming about because of either low insulin creation in type 1 diabetes or diminished insulin affectability in type 2 diabetes influences cell homeostasis in practically all phone types. Hyperglycemia is generally viewed as the principle procedure that triggers cell pathology, and different downstream instruments, including metabolic pressure and the arrangement of receptive oxygen species (ROS) that harm cell layers and different frameworks [11].

Changes in the Ca^{2+} signal have been identified in different detachment tissues from creatures prompted into diabetes just as patients with diabetes. Ca^{2+} homeostasis variations from the norm have additionally been found in an assortment of tissues, including bone, heart and smooth muscle, secretory cells, platelets, kidneys and osteoblasts. This issue, for the most part, shows as an expanded resting convergence of intracellular $[Ca^{2+}]I$, diminished movement of the Ca^{2+} transporter (in spite of the fact that not generally) and diminished improvement that creates Ca^{2+} signals. Ca^{2+} flagging issue is likewise found in neuron-sensory from trial creatures with diabetes [11, 12].

Calcium (Ca^{2+}) homeostasis in nerve cells that is upset or irregular happens in different maladies of the sensory system. The most well-known issue of the fringe sensory system, neuropathic torment and diabetes polyneuropathy, were seen as related with weakened articulation and capacity of Ca^{2+}. Likewise found a connection between Ca^{2+} dyshomeostasis and mitochondrial brokenness in neuropathy because of diabetes. The primary impacts of changes in Ca^{2+} flagging happen in the plasma film and in intracellular Ca^{2+} in tactile neurons and are identified with irregularities in the endoplasmic reticulum. Impeded Ca^{2+} axonal motioning in diabetic neuropathy will incite axonal degeneration in fringe neuropathy. The nearness of Ca^{2+} dysregulation is influenced by varieties in waterway structure and Ca^{2+} siphon, this is seen in neuropathic and neuropathic structures, making the Ca^{2+} approach in neurons can be utilized for remedial mediations for neuropathic agony and fringe neuropathy. Neuropathic torment largely affects personal satisfaction and disarranges of physiology and Ca^{2+} waterway articulation have been embroiled in various torments. This investigation will likewise feature the most widely recognized type of fringe neuropathy, which is diabetes polyneuropathy. This issue can incorporate agony as a manifestation and in the long run form into degeneration of fringe nerve strands described by tangible misfortune [11, 13, 14].

Neural harm both horrible and models of harm with specific illnesses, will harm fringe tactile nerves and meddle with essential afferent action. As a rule interruption of essential afferent movement can likewise add to diligent neuropathic pain. The role of Ca^{2+} flux in the formation of axonal potential and release of neurotransmitters by primary sensory neurons will produce Ca^{2+} regulatory abnormalities which in turn contribute to neuropathic pain [15].

Late research has uncovered early aggravations from two intracellular integrative flagging frameworks, specifically Ca^{2+} signal homeostasis and mitochondrial physiology. These progressions happen also in an assortment of totally different cell types, and can be considered as normal neurotic pathways [11, 16, 17].

2. Homeostasis of Ca^{2+} signals in cells

A portion of the systems for keeping up the centralization of Ca^{2+} in intracellularity are through the Ca^{2+} channel, Ca^{2+} transport and including the support. Various Ca^{2+}-sensors (spoke to by Ca^{2+}-controlled proteins) go about as effectors, which make an interpretation of Ca^{2+} signals into physiological reactions. What is significant is that the free Ca^{2+} resting focus in cells can change, going from 50 to 100 nM in the cytosol and near 0.5–1.0 mM in the lumen of the endoplasmic reticulum (ER). Any move from this fixation go, both the overabundance Ca^{2+} in the cytosol and Ca^{2+} exhaustion in the ER will make obsessive results, including activating different kinds of cell demise [11, 13].

2.1 Calcium channel

Transient changes in intracellular calcium levels can be caused by signals from intracellular calcium storage or from extracellular compartments through specific regulations. Electrophysiology of calcium channel sub type with kinetic opening and its conduct can be divided into [18–20]:

a. Type L, the conductance is strong, long lasting inward current, the antagonist is dihydropyridine.

b. Type T, transient inward current.

c. Type N, neither type L or T, many in neurons, are blocked by w-conotoxins GVIA

d. Type P, found mostly in cerebellar Purkinje cells, is blocked by IVA agatoxin.

e. Another type found is type Q and R in Purkinje cells.

Different classifications based on open or closed formations can be differentiated into:

a. VOC (voltage gate channel), the opening depends on the voltage that occurs.

b. ROC (receptor-operated channels), depending on the specific ligand bond.

c. SOC (store operated channels), the activation depends on the depletion of calcium in the ER with the CCE (capacitative calcium entry) mechanism.

The VOC contains four homologous units, each containing six transmembrane regions with conduction holes, voltage sensors, and places to open and regulatory channels, which can be passed by for example protein kinases, toxins and drugs. Dihydropyridine, phenylalanine, and benzodiasepin are attached to sub-unit a1. Three types of ROC canals are known, activated by glutamate and some agonists that can be attached such as KA, AMPA and NMDA, so they are also named as attached agonists. The location is in the synapses post. The canals formed by KA and AMPA receptors are permeable to Na^+ and K^+, some AMPA are also to Ca^{2+}, whereas NMDA is permeable to Na^+ and Ca^{2+}. In neuroendocrine cells, activation by calcium passes through the SOC canal, this channel cannot be known in detail with protein levels but is homologous with transient potential receptors (trp or trp-like) from drosophila. The process of SOC through CCE, where the release of a small number of chemical factors will induce canal opening, and the second possibility is that the physical interaction between ER and plasma membrane stimulates CCE opening [18, 21, 22].

2.2 Calcium pumps

Plasma membranes control the exchange of calcium between intracellular and extracellular. Calcium in small and controlled amounts of calcium can enter cells through specific channels to stimulate intracellular events, including freeing calcium from its storage. An equal amount of calcium must also be excreted extracellularly. There are two known systems, i.e. mostly through the electrical exchange of NA^+ and Ca^{2+}. Another system is through ATPase (PMCA pump) with high affinity but low capacity to remove calcium, so it is also called fine-tuner cellular Ca^{2+}. Calcium also exchanges between the cytoplasm and internal organelles, dominated by mitochondria and ER which have SERCA pumps that have a mechanism similar to PMCA [23, 24].

The total calcium transported in the reticulum depends on the amount of pump available, which is high in the heart and skeletal muscles, but low in non-skeletal muscles. Calcium pumps are also found in low eukaryotes. In mushrooms there are two pumps namely PMR1 and PMC1 which are in the Golgi and Vacuole complex. 40–50% homologous with SERCA and PMCA, PMC1 does not have the calmodulin which is a characteristic of PMCA pumps [23, 24].

2.3 PMCA pumps

The PMCA pump was discovered since 1966 and functions to remove calcium from erythrocytes. It was purified in 1979 with a protein weight of 135 kDa. The architecture of this protein resembles that of the SERCA pump, having 10 transmembrane domains and three large hydrophilic units that protrude into the cytoplasm, what is different is the existence of a long C-terminal tail that contains a place to attach to calmodulin. Calmodulin is the main regulator for PMCA, although polyunsaturated fatty acids, phospholipids, protein kinases A or C also activate these pumps, with the result of reducing the concentration of calcium. After activation, it is dimerized by binding with calmodulin and proteolytic enzymes by removing C terminals. The calmodulin bond at rest will bind to both sides of the cytosol part of the pump, so that the pump will remain obstructed [23, 25].

A Ca^{2+} signalosome signal consists of many Ca^{2+} signal components. Duplication of components is the fact that there are many isoforms that increase the diversity of the Ca^{2+} signal system. Yellow arrows describe the ON reaction that enters Ca^{2+} into the cell, and the blue arrow represents the OFF reaction where Ca^{2+} will exit the cell or return to the endoplasmic reticulum (ER). During a trip through the cytoplasm, Ca^{2+} will temporarily stay in a buffer or inside the mitochondria. For the signal to occur, Ca^{2+} binds to sensors which then use various effectors to stimulate cellular processes. Different and suitable components will produce cell-specific signalosomes [26].

2.4 SERCA pumps

An enzyme that hydrolyzes ATP to transport Ca^{2+} across the SR membrane was discovered 40 years ago, then identified as a pump in the ER in non-muscle cells. The ATPase was then called the SERCA pump as a protein weighing around 100 kDa. SERCA 1a is a major isoform in adult human muscle cells with rapid contraction, while SERCA1b in neonates. SERCA2a is found in heart muscle and muscle with slow contractions, while SERCA2b is found in smooth muscle and almost in non-muscle cells. SERCA3 is expressed only in non-lumen cells [27, 28].

The principle of action of enzymes in calcium pumps is actually almost the same. Calcium is bound to one side of the membrane and this reaction does not require ATP, then ATP attaches and splits into acyl phosphate as an aspartic residue, intermediate formation of phosphorylation is also called a P type pump. After phosphorylation, the pump transitions from E1 to E2 form, on E1 forms calcium-bound pumps with high affinity exposed to the cytosol side; in the E2 form calcium bound with low affinity is exposed to the ER/SR lumen or extracellular part, so that calcium can be released. After ATP and calcium released, enzymes slowly dephosphorylate and return to form E1. The SERCA and PMCA pumps are different in calcium-ATP transport [27, 28].

2.5 Calcium-sodium exchange

Sodium/calcium exchange (NCX, Na^+/Ca^{2+} exchangers) in the plasma membrane (PM, plasma membrane) is an important factor in homeostasis and calcium regulation in almost all cells. The NCX PM was discovered nearly 35 years ago in cardiac cells and neurons by using sodium electrochemical energy gradients, not directly from ATP for calcium transport. So the importance of calcium import or export depends on the NCX coupling ratio, membrane potential and sodium concentration gradient. Potential membranes and sodium gradients are maintained by sodium pumps (Na^+, K^+-ATPase) that are dependent on ATP. Sodium-calcium exchange in the mitochondria has also been identified and works similar to NCX [29–31]. Exchange in heart cells and neurons shows the coupling ratio is 3 Na^+:1 Ca^{2+}.

Sodium-calcium exchange is also present in photoreceptor cells, this cell is also dependent on K^+ and has a coupling ratio of $4Na^+$:($1Ca^{2+}$+K^+) so this exchange is also referred to as Na/(Ca,K) or NCKX exchange. The family of NCX is NCX2, NCX2 and NCX3, most of which are NCX1 with distribution on all networks. In the NCKX family, there are three sub-types namely NCKX1 in photoreceptors, NCKX2 in rods and neurons and NCKX3 expressed in the brain and smooth muscle. Topologically NCKX is almost similar to NKCX which both function on ion attachment and translocation [29–31].

NCX can facilitate the electronic exchange of sodium-sodium or calcium–calcium, also can be for sodium in-calcium exit or sodium in-calcium entry. For calcium- calcium exchange it is activated by nontransported alkaline metal ions. The sodium- calcium exchange reaction is consistent and sequential, where one calcium or three sodium binds to one side of the membrane, then translocates to the other side of the membrane, and dissociates before the other ions are bound to that side. In the exchange of sodium in and out of calcium and sodium in and out of calcium are both rheogenic (related to electric current/current flow) [29–31].

2.6 Calcium buffer

The principle of calcium buffer is that all groups that have negative potential can be a chelator for calcium. In this system many are dominated by small molecular carbosilic groups such as citrate or carbonyl protein groups. Included here are EF-hand protein, annexin and C2 protein. Most calcium buffers are included in the EF-hand protein group. To find out the buffer mechanism in calcium homeostasis, there are several parameters that influence it, namely: cytosolic concentration, affinity for calcium ions or other metal ions, calcium kinetic for attachment and release as well as the mobility of calcium itself. In a simple way buffer works is that once calcium enters the buffer cells will bind calcium and reduce calcium levels. However, a fixed level of calcium concentration is obtained from the calcium balance across the cell membrane, not absolutely from the presence of the buffer itself [32, 33].

2.7 Mitochondria and calcium signaling

Mitochondria are no longer static organs as ATP producers, but also as a store of various lethal proteins which will be released in programmed cell death and this is an important intracellular calcium signal. Since the expression of the calcium transport membrane in the mitochondria has been found, the process of signaling calcium in the mitochondria has become clear [34–36]. Pension movements in the mitochondria are driven by several things such as:

a. Uniporter

b. VDAC (voltage dependent anion channel)

c. Exchange xNa^+/Ca^{2+}

Calcium is inserted into the membrane in the mitochondria by the uniporter. Uniporter activity is influenced by temperature and cation selectivity so that it can almost be called a channel rather than a career. Intake of calcium through uniporters is inhibited by red ruterium (RuR) which also blocks many cation channels including calcium plasmalemma canals, the ER channel which is sensitive to ryanodine to release calcium and vanilloid receptor channels, making it more convincing that the uniporter is a canal. Uniporters are regulated by cytosolic calcium levels and thus require higher levels to increase mitochondrial calcium levels [34–36].

The outer membrane of the mitochondria is permeable to small ions so it is not considered in calcium exchange. However, the outer membrane of the mitochondria has an important role in the modulation of calcium by the uniporter to pass the VDAC filter. VDAC is permeable to calcium and regulated both calcium levels and RuR levels. The most important way for calcium to exit the mitochondria is through the exchange of xNa^+/Ca^{2+}; initially thought to be the electronic exchange of $2Na^+/Ca^{2+}$. It will be doubted because this exchange requires twice as much energy as against the sodium gradient. The entry of calcium into the mitochondria is inhibited by mitochondrial depolarization [34–36].

A progression of proteins in MAMs (for example, PML, AKT, GRP-75, SIG-1R, Mfn-1/-2, BIP, AKT) controls the arrival of Ca^{2+} from ER and Ca^{2+} take-up by mitochondria, bringing about various useful outcomes. Cells produce Ca^{2+} flags through two instruments that utilization inside and outer Ca^{2+} sources. Calcium enters the cell through channels and siphons situated on the plasma layer, this is controlled by voltage (VOC) or outer ambassadors (ROCs). A progression of upgrades that follow up on receptors on the cell surface triggers enactment of the PLC which catalyzes the hydrolysis of 4.5-bisphosphate phosphatidylinositol to IP3 and DAG. IP3 official with IP3R receptors invigorates the arrival of Ca^{2+} ER and subsequently moves Ca^{2+} (red specks) from the ER to the mitochondria. The mitochondrial surface collaborates straightforwardly with the ER through the Ca^{2+} hotspot signal unit. Imports of mitochondrial Ca^{2+} happen through mitochondrial Ca^{2+} uniporters (MCU) and H^+/Ca^{2+} exchangers LETM1; on the other hand, NCLX, mitochondrial Na^+/Ca^{2+}

exchangers, together with PTP, send out Ca^{2+} from the lattice. Ca^{2+} levels come back to resting conditions through a progression of channels and siphons: PMCA and NCX bring about particle expulsion to the extracellular condition, SERCA (situated in the ER) and SPCA (in the Golgi mechanical assembly) make Ca^{2+} levels come back to basal levels in the capacity zone [17].

2.8 Endoplasmic reticulum (ER) and calcium signaling

ER as a widespread flagging organelle, ER works a ton, as a matter of first importance is a spot for protein amalgamation and development. Protein union is completed in harsh ER, though handling of protein after interpretation is orchestrated in escorts some portion of ER, which structures buildings with recently integrated proteins, collapsing them into the last tertiary structure and keep them from accumulating. In the event that the collapsing procedure falls flat, the escorts are still amassed with proteins that neglect to crease, therefore keeping them from continuing through the ER and out into the Golgi complex. Each time the collapsed protein fixation increments extremely high, ER builds up an exceptional response known as ER worry, subsequently, the signs that influence translation are sent to the core, which will control quality articulation as indicated by the earth. Other than blend protein, ER is a position of arrangement of phospholipids, glycosyl-phosphatidylinositols, and leukotrienes. ER can likewise work as a transfer site for different undesirable particles and toxic substances. Since ER has a constant lumen, as an expressway that permits transport of RNA, secretory items, different proteins and particles between enraptured cell parts. This ER is likewise firmly engaged with quick cell signals since it is a powerful stockpiling territory of Ca^{2+} which controls Ca^{2+} cytosol focus and creates Ca^{2+} transition between the cytosol and ER lumen because of extracellular incitement. At last, ER arranges all the different physiological procedures of cells. In this manner, ER is characterized as a multifunctional organelle fit for recognizing and incorporating approaching signs and creating yield flags because of natural changes [37, 38].

The definite system of ER combination is generally unfamiliar, including the focal job of Ca^{2+}. Ca^{2+} is the way in to the info and yield signals from the ER. An expansion in Ca^{2+} cytosol focus influences its fixation in ER, and thusly the exit and passage of Ca^{2+} in the ER influences the cytosolic Ca^{2+} focus. Various intra-ER escorts, for example, calreticulin, calnexin, grp78/BiP, endoplasmin (or glucose managed protein, grp94), are Ca^{2+} restricting proteins, and changes in free Ca^{2+} focuses in ER lumens extraordinarily influence their practical movement. In this manner, changes in Ca^{2+} content in the ER can give a connection between quick signals and moderate cell versatile reactions [38, 39]. The essential physiology of ER as calcium stockpiling is known in different volatile and non-sensitive cells. ER goes about as a powerful stockpiling of Ca^{2+} alongside the action of Ca^{2+} directs and transporters in the endomembranes, and intraluminal Ca^{2+} restricting protein, which works as a high limit Ca^{2+} cradle framework. Ca^{2+} that leaves the ER is controlled by two Ca^{2+} channels, Ca^{2+}-gated Ca^{2+} channels which are normally known as ryanodine receptors (RyRs) and InsP3-gated channels which are regularly known as InsP3 receptors (InsP3Rs). The aggregation of Ca^{2+} into the ER lumen is the consequence of Ca^{2+} siphon action from the sarco (endo) plasmic reticulum Ca^{2+}-ATPase (SERCA) [37, 38].

The Ca^{2+} flagging framework in certain cell types is regularly not single, yet comprises of various pathways, which are identified with produce cell-explicit frameworks in various cell types. A portion of the primary modules utilized by cells are [26]:

1. Agonists, for example, glutamate synapses and ATP act straightforwardly on channel-worked receptors (ROCs) in the plasma layer to permit outside Ca^{2+} to enter the cell.

2. Second couriers, for example, diacylglycerol (DAG), cyclic AMP, cyclic GMP and arachidonic corrosive work on the cytoplasmic side when opening SMOCs in the plasma layer.

3. Film depolarization (V) enacts VOC in the plasma layer for permits the passage of outside Ca^{2+} rapidly.

4. Film depolarization (V) enacts certain VOC isoforms, in particular, the L-type CaV1.1 channel, which actuates the receptor ryanodine 1 (RYR1) in the skeletal muscle through an immediate coupling compliance system.

5. The depolarizing film (V) enacts VOC in the plasma layer for permits the passage of outside Ca^{2+} to trigger Ca^{2+} enacting ryanodine 2 receptor (RyR2) to trigger the arrival of Ca^{2+} stores in the sarcoplasmic reticulum (SR) through the Ca^{2+} incited Ca^{2+} (CICR) discharge process. This component is found in the heart muscle and neurons.

6. Agonists following up on the outside of receptor cells produce 1,4,5-trisphosphate inositol, which at that point diffuses into the cell to enact the InsP3 (InsP3R) receptor to discharge Ca^{2+} from the ER.

CICR (calcium-induced calcium release) causes the release of Ca^{2+} from its storage site, the endoplasmic reticulum (ER). Canals that are sensitive to Ca^{2+} namely the ryanodine (R) receptor and the InsP3 (I) receptor are in the ER. CICR has two stages, namely the first is the transfer of signals from the plasma membrane to the channel receptors in the ER, starting from the opening of the VOC canal due to depolarization in the plasma membrane then Ca^{2+} will enter, diffuse then activate the R and I receptors, the second is with the Ca^{2+} process will be released from one canal to the next canal to release Ca^{2+} again so that the Ca^{2+} wave will arise which will increase the concentration of Ca^{2+} in the cytosol. Increasing the concentration of Ca^{2+} cytosol will activate the ON system thus activating intracellular signals [26, 39].

3. Dyshomeostasis Ca^{2+} in neurons

Signal unsettling influences and Ca^{2+} fixations have been recognized in different diabetic creature cell disengagement explores just as from diabetic patients. Ca^{2+} homeostasis variations from the norm have been found in most trial tissues, including bone, heart and smooth muscle, discharge cells, platelets, kidneys and osteoblasts. Diminished (in spite of the fact that not generally) and diminished upgrade evoked Ca^{2+} signals. Ca^{2+}-dealing with disarranges have additionally been found in tangible neurons from creatures with diabetes [11, 40, 41].

3.1 Increase in $[Ca^{2+}]$I break

A huge increment in resting $[Ca^{2+}]$ in diabetic tangible neurons is a typical finding, despite the fact that there are a few contrasts between kinds of neurons. Research shows an expansion in resting $[Ca^{2+}]$ in dorsal root ganglion neurons

(DRG) of rodents with type 1 and type 2 diabetes. Centralization of $[Ca^{2+}]$I breaks 30% higher in disconnection of DRG neurons in streptozotocin (STZ)-C57Bl/6, (type 1 diabetes model) contrasted with controls (205 ± 16 nM versus 156 ± 16 nM). The expansion in $[Ca^{2+}]$I in little neurons is more noteworthy in db/db mice (type 2 diabetes model). There was no distinction in $[Ca^{2+}]$I in huge neurons in the two mouse models. In another examination in Wistar-diabetic mice with STZ 8–14 weeks there was an expansion of 2- to 2.5-overlay resting $[Ca^{2+}]$I in seclusion of enormous and little DRG neurons from L4-L6 lumbar, however expanded $[Ca^{2+}]$ I rest was not influenced in neurons from the ganglion in the more elevated levels of the spinal line (C3-L3). This distinction connects with the lumbar DRG tactile neuron vulnerability and the long axon of diabetic neuropathy. A portion of these distinctions are identified with contrasts in estimation of $[Ca^{2+}]$I between considers with different models and term of diabetes, maybe likewise because of contrasts in different sub-populaces of neurons from the degree of DRG in the spine [11, 40].

3.2 Disruption of Ca^{2+} entry plasmalemma

The section of Ca^{2+} into the cytoplasm through the voltage-gated Ca^{2+} channel of plasmalemma is a significant part of the Ca^{2+} signal in sensitive cells. Tangible neurons have a few kinds of voltage-gated Ca^{2+} channels including low-edge (type T) and high-edge (type N and L), which vary in conductance, voltage-reliance and pharmacology. The measure of Ca^{2+} flows at both high and low edges is accounted for to increment in diabetic creatures by 40–100%. In any case, the adequacy of transient depolarization which is Ca^{2+} prompted in the separation of DRG neurons from diabetic and sound creatures is commonly not influenced, just discouraging in disengagement of little DRG neurons from L4-L6. This distinction can be clarified by an expansion in resting $[Ca^{2+}]$, though an increment in waterway Ca^{2+} flow might be redressed [42, 43].

3.3 Ca^{2+} homeostasis in ER

ER works as a dynamic Ca^{2+} stockpiling, fit for amassing, appropriating and discharging Ca^{2+} particles. Ca^{2+} ER homeostasis is accomplished within the sight of Ca^{2+} siphons spoke to by sarco (endo) plasmic reticulum Ca^{2+} ATP-ases (SERCAs) and Ca^{2+} trenches for discharge, including rianudin receptors (RyR), inositol triphosphate receptor (InsP3R) and Ca^{2+} adenine receptors for discharge, including rianudin receptors (RyR), inositol triphosphate receptors (InsP3R) and nicotinic adenic corrosive receptors. Dinucleotide phosphate (NAADP) in the endomembrane. The grouping of free Ca^{2+} in the ER lumen ($[Ca^{2+}]$L) is high, around 0.5–1.0 mM. The degree of $[Ca^{2+}]$L is practically significant in light of the fact that it will control the speed of SERCA-subordinate Ca^{2+} take-up, actuation of the Ca^{2+} discharge channel, the Ca^{2+} sponsor and give tight power over different ER capersons for collapsing post-translational proteins. In this way, any long haul changes in $[Ca^{2+}]$L will have significant sign, practical and adjustment results [44, 45].

ER additionally assumes a job in the quick reaction of neuronal Ca^{2+} through commencement (by means of metabotropically controlled InsP3-actuated Ca^{2+} discharge), enhancement (through Ca^{2+}-actuated Ca^{2+} discharge), engendering (by both regenerative initiation of Ca^{2+} and Ca^{2+} ER channels) and end (with SERCA-intervened Ca^{2+} uptake in the ER lumen. These procedures are directed by $[Ca^{2+}]$ I and $[Ca^{2+}]$L fixations and second emissary digestion including InsP3, cyclic-ADP-ribose and NAADP. Diabetes will disturb Ca^{2+} ER homeostasis in tangible neurons by diminishing the measure of Ca^{2+} in the ER, in this way decreasing the plentifulness of the arrival of Ca^{2+}.The measure of Ca^{2+} discharged from ER is altogether decreased in DRG neurons with diabetes. The evacuation of Ca^{2+} is prompted by low-portion ionomycin, caffeine (RyRs actuation) or by ATP (metabotropic initiation from diabetes). InsP3Rs), Ca^{2+} use diminishes essentially in the disconnection of tactile neurons from diabetic creatures after STZ administration. The decrease in the measure of Ca^{2+} ER is more prominent in DRG neurons and L1-L6 lumbar ri contrasted and cervical and cylinder DRG. Direct estimations of $[Ca^{2+}]L$ and $[Ca^{2+}]I$ indicated a huge reduction in cytosolic-instigated cytosolic Ca^{2+}. Decrease of $[Ca^{2+}]L$ and the pace of take-up of Ca^{2+} in diabetic neurons is related with diminished SERCA articulation in the homogenate of DRG L4-L5 from diabetic creatures [45, 46].

The focus of Ca^{2+} homeostasis regulation has shifted from pericarion/soma to axons. In sensory neuron culture from diabetic rats, axons appear to be far more susceptible to neurodegeneration because of high glucose levels. Adult sensory neurons isolated from diabetic rats after STZ administration for 3–5 months can grow in vitro 1–4 days. High-level glucose delivery triggers oxidative stress leading to an increase in 4-hydroxy-2-nonenal staining (ongoing lipid peroxidation measurement), axonal development to be suboptimal and the appearance of axonal structural abnormalities similar to axonal dystrophy/axonal degeneration in animal and human models with human diabetes. But pericarions/soma from neuron culture do not show clear signs of oxidative stress or degeneration. Axon toxicity due to glucose induced is only seen in neurons from diabetic animals and neurons that grow from control mice that match their age do not have sensitivity to high glucose levels [11, 45].

Research on Ca^{2+} homeostasis in axons utilizing continuous confocal imaging with Fluo4-AM under high amplification (X100) to investigate Ca^{2+} drifters in the seclusion of grown-up tactile neurons with diabetic rodents after STZ 4–5 months organization.

3.4 Ca^{2+} termination signal

End of the Ca^{2+} signal is activated during the time of cell action, this is finished by expelling Ca^{2+} in the plasmalemma (siphon Ca^{2+} ATP-ase plasmalemma, PMCA, Na^{+}/Ca^{2+} exchanger) or retention of Ca^{2+} to the ER and/or mitochondria. In the segregation of neurons from diabetic creatures, the practical limit of the expulsion framework has all the earmarks of being hindered as showed by the easing back down of the arrival of $[Ca^{2+}]I$ after incitement. This might be because of a lessening in PMCA siphon articulation. Simultaneously, prolongation/high Ca^{2+} levels are likewise connected with diminished Ca^{2+} take-up by intracellular organelles, for example, ER and mitochondria. Diminished SERCA articulation is likewise found in the core of diabetic creatures with STZ. In neurons, diminished SERCA action is showed by an abatement in the ingestion pace of Ca^{2+} after direct estimation of $[Ca^{2+}]L$. Moreover, mitochondrial buffering Ca^{2+} additionally debilitates in neurons with diabetes [47, 48].

3.5 Mitochondrial depolarization in diabetes

Endothelial cell culture shows that high intracellular glucose levels energize extreme electron gifts in the electron transport chain in the mitochondria which will result in mitochondrial hyperpolarization and expanded ROS creation. The procedure in the mitochondria is a focal arbiter of oxidative worry as a confusion of diabetes. This hypothesis recommends that high glucose focuses in the objective tissue as a type of diabetes confusions lead to an expansion in the inventory of NADH in the mitochondria which will additionally build the quantity of electrons and/or immersion, this can prompt a fractional decrease of oxygen and superoxide radicals in the proximal piece of the electron transport chain. An expansion in ROS will at that point empower tissue degeneration. The capability of the inward mitochondrial layer depolarizes as opposed to hyperpolarization. Mitochondrial depolarization in STZ-diabetes can be forestalled by controlling low-portion insulin or NT-3 [49, 50].

Concentrates in the way of life of tactile neuron incipient organisms show that high glucose levels cause ceaseless mitochondrial depolarization followed by apoptosis. High glucose focuses do not execute neuronal incipient organisms from the passable portion for grown-ups in vitro or grown-up tangible neurons (for about a month at 50 mM glucose in vitro). Moreover there are no basic variations from the norm in mitochondrial neurons/axons or nerve cell passing in tangible ganglia in people with diabetes or autonomic neuropathy. In creature models of type 1 diabetes found unmyelinated little neuron cell misfortune however there is no data of apoptosis or variations from the norm in mitochondrial structure in DRG. Be that as it may, morphology and axonal development are upset by high glucose because of high oxidative pressure which brings about axonal degeneration [49, 50].

Adult sensory neurons from diabetic rodents with STZ 3–5 months were refined for 1 day, at that point given tetramethylrhodamine methyl ester (TMRM) and a color used to identify mitochondrial film depolarization. The outcomes demonstrated that axons from ordinary neurons encountered a pace of mitochondrial depolarization much sooner after expansion of uncoupler carbonylcyanide p-trifluoromethoxyphenylhydrazone (FCCP). Before the expansion of FCCP, mitochondrial axons were more energized than the diabetic neuron bunch [11].

3.6 Mitochondrial dysfunction and Ca^{2+} dyshomeostasis

Disarranges of Ca^{2+} homeostasis and mitochondrial film depolarization in grown-up tactile neurons happen prior (3–14 weeks) in test diabetes type 1 (STZ) and type 2 (db/db), this can be key in tangible neuropathy. The determinant factor for mitochondrial brokenness is not the nearness of hyperglycemia yet the nonattendance of insulin-subordinate neurotropic help, this is seen in vivo and in vitro. Insulin organization of 1 nM for 6–24 h of solid DRG societies essentially builds the capability of the mitochondrial layer and expands the degree of ATP generation contrasted with societies without insulin. Giving 50 mM glucose within the sight of insulin in culture has no impact on the layer potential in the mitochondria. Comparative outcomes were gotten in vivo, STZ-diabetic rodents given insulin focuses low which did not influence hyperglycemia. Insulin organization completely standardizes mitochondrial layer polarization, resting [Ca^{2+}] level and speed of tangible and engine nerve conductance [49, 51, 52].

Mitochondrial polarization and Ca^{2+} homeostasis in tangible neurons from diabetic creatures additionally become ordinary after organization of the neurotropic factor, NT-3. Giving neighborhood insulin to the spinal line at the degree of the lumbar (intrathecal) or fringe nerve (little osmotic siphon) or intranasally expands nerve conduction and epidermal nerve fiber thickness in STZ-diabetic rodents. Different investigations have indicated the job of phosphoinositide 3-kinase (PI3-kinase) and protein kinase B (Akt) in guideline of film potential in the mitochondria. This pathway is managed by insulin plasmalemma receptors (α and β subunit receptor insulin communicated in DRG neurons) and neurotrophin receptors. PI3/Akt association is checked whether DRG neurons are directed with a particular PI3-kinase inhibitor (LY294002), which will hinder insulin-subordinate and neurotrophin-subordinate, therefore repressing the guideline of mitochondrial and insulin-subordinate layer potential to build ATP levels [14, 16].

Several cell types are with specific Ca^{2+} signals. The four cells in **Table 1** are very different in spatial and temporal terms of the Ca^{2+} pathway, for example striped

	Skeletal muscle cell	Cardiac atrial cell	Ca1 Neuron	T cell
Receptors	—	ET-1R/α1R AngIIR	mGluR1 M1	TCR
PLC	—	PLCβ	PLCβ	PLCγ1
Entry channels	$Ca_v1.1$	$Ca_v1.2$	$Ca_v1.2/Ca_v2.1$ $Ca_v2.2$/NMDAR	ORAi1
Release channels	RYR1	RYR2 $InsP_3$ R2	RYR2 $InsP_3$ R2	$InsP_3$ R2
PMCAs	PMCA1a, 1c, 1d	PMCA1c, 1d, 2a	PMCA1a, 2a, 3a	PMCA4b
SERCAs	SERCA1a, 1b	SERCA2a	SERCA2b,3	SERC2b,3
Na^+/Ca^{2+} exchanger	NCX	NCX1	NCX1,3	—
Buffers	Parvalbumin	—	Parvalbumin Calbindin 28 K	—
Sensors	Troponin C Calmodulin	Troponin C Calmodulin	Calmodulin	Calmodulin

Table 1.
Ca^{2+} signals in various cells [1].

muscle cells use a specific pathway to deliver Ca^{2+} quickly for activation of muscle contraction, whereas T cell signals have a slower pathway component that is useful.

3.7 Dysregulation of Ca^{2+} and release of neurotransmitters

Signal contribution from the essential afferent into the spinal line includes the arrival of excitation synapses from the nerve terminal to the dorsal horn. Many mechanisms of neuropathic pain along with spinal cord sensitization in response to primary afferent activity in a state of persistent pain. The arrival of synapses from essential afferents is activated by potential activity, nearby film depolarization and enactment of high-voltage Ca^{2+} channels. The passage of Ca^{2+} will begin docking of vesicles containing excitation synapses and modulators, for example, glutamate, substance P and CGRP in the presynaptic layer and arrival of this particle into neural connections. Obstructing the passage of Ca^{2+} into the prespinal terminal forestalls the section of fringe contribution to the spinal rope, this piece of the sedative component hinders the impression of torment by restraining the passage of Ca^{2+} moderator into little tactile neurons through the actuation of narcotic receptors (sub-type) in the essential afferent terminal turns into an option in contrast to the objective of hindering the arrival of synapses from neurons. Peptides that are specific inhibitors of type N channels have been recognized in snails, conotoxins, which can square agony receptors in mice [8, 11].

4. Conclusion

In the fringe nerve, diabetes quite often influences the tactile nerve which brings about even tangible neuropathy. At first, diabetes will decrease the speed of nerve conduction and patients can likewise encounter an assortment of tactile manifestations going from torment to reflex issue. The cell and atomic pathophysiology of diabetes polyneuropathy stays dubious and a few pathways are related with hyperglycemia, including the polyol pathway, oxidative pressure, protein glycosylation and impeded help from neurotropics. Elective components for starting the beginning of diabetic neuropathy are those identified with changes in mitochondrial work and cell Ca^{2+} homeostasis that are not legitimately brought about by hyperglycemia, however are activated by disabled sign falls identified with insulin receptors and neurotropic elements. The underlying pathogenesis of diabetes neuropathy is diminished insulin receptor incitement. This triggers mitochondrial brokenness and diminished ATP generation. The diminished ATP bolster will influence the component of Ca^{2+} homeostasis, the most evident aggravations are in the plasmalemma and the Ca^{2+} siphon in the ER. Diminishing Ca^{2+} take-up in the ER will decrease the Ca^{2+} focus in intra-ER, causing an ER stress condition. ER worry thus impacts union, post-translational alteration and protein transport, which thusly diminishes the stock of protein to the voltage-gated channel to the axon, bringing about an abatement in nerve conduction speed. These procedures can happen all the more effectively found in axons. This is exacerbated by constant hyperglycemia so degenerative neuropathy and extreme tactile nerve brokenness will happen.

Author details

Shahdevi Kurniawan
Medical Faculty, Neurology Department, Brawijaya University, Malang, Indonesia

*Address all correspondence to: shahdevinandar@ub.ac.id

IntechOpen

© 2020 The Author(s). Licensee IntechOpen. This chapter is distributed under the terms of the Creative Commons Attribution License (http://creativecommons.org/licenses/by/3.0), which permits unrestricted use, distribution, and reproduction in any medium, provided the original work is properly cited.

References

[1] Zhang P, Zhang X, Brown J, Vistisen D, Sicree R, Shaw J, et al. Diabetes Research and Clinical Practice. 2010;**87**(3):293-301. DOI: 10.1016/j.diabres.2010.01.026

[2] Alqurashi KA, Aljabri KS, Bokhari SA. Prevalence of diabetes mellitus in a Saudi community. Annals of Saudi Medicine. 2011;**31**(1):19-23. DOI: 10.4103/0256-4947.75773

[3] Metelko Ž, Pavlić-Renar I, Poljičanin T, Szirovitza L, Turek S. Prevalence of diabetes mellitus in Croatia. Diabetes Research and Clinical Practice. 2008;**81**(2):263-267. DOI: 10.1016/j.diabres.2008.04.016

[4] Gupta S, Singh Z, Purty A, Kar M, Vedapriya DR, Mahajan P, et al. Diabetes prevalence and its risk factors in rural area of Tamil Nadu. Indian Journal of Community Medicine. 2010;**35**(3):396. DOI: 10.4103/0970-0218.69262

[5] Chang CH, Shau WY, Jiang YD, Li HY, Chang TJ, Sheu WH-H, et al. Type 2 diabetes prevalence and incidence among adults in Taiwan during 1999-2004: A national health insurance data set study. Diabetic Medicine. 2010;**27**(6):636-643. DOI: 10.1111/j.1464-5491.2010.03007.x

[6] Aekplakorn W, Chariyalertsak S, Kessomboon P, Sangthong R, Inthawong R, Putwatana P, et al. Prevalence and management of diabetes and metabolic risk factors in Thai adults. Diabetes Care. 2011;**34**(9):1980-1985. DOI: 10.2337/dc11-0099

[7] Zhou B, Lu Y, Hajifathalian K, Bentham J, et al. Worldwide trends in diabetes since 1980: A pooled analysis of 751 population-based studies with 4·4 million participants. The Lancet. 2016;**387**(10027):1513-1530. DOI: 10.1016/S0140-6736(16)00618-8

[8] Abbott CA, Malik RA, van Ross ERE, Kulkarni J, Boulton AJM. Prevalence and characteristics of painful diabetic neuropathy in a large community-based diabetic population in the U.K. Diabetes Care. 2011;**34**(10):2220-2224. DOI: 10.2337/dc11-1108

[9] Giacco F, Brownlee M. Oxidative stress and diabetic complications. Circulation Research. 2010;**107**(9):1058-1070. DOI: 10.1161/CIRCRESAHA.110.223545

[10] Volpe CMO, Villar-Delfino PH, Dos Anjos PMF, Nogueira-Machado JA. Cellular death, reactive oxygen species (ROS) and diabetic complications. Cell Death & Disease. 2018;**9**(2):119. DOI: 10.1038/s41419-017-0135-z

[11] Fernyhough P, Calcutt NA. Abnormal calcium homeostasis in peripheral neuropathies. Cell Calcium. 2010;**47**(2):130-139. DOI: 10.1016/j.ceca.2009.11.008

[12] Lambert R, Srodulski S, Peng X, Margulies KB, Despa F, Despa S. Intracellular Na^+ concentration ($[Na^+]i$) is elevated in diabetic hearts due to enhanced Na^+-glucose cotransport. Journal of the American Heart Association. 2015;**4**(9):e002183. DOI: 10.1161/JAHA.115.002183

[13] Pinton P. Mitochondria-associated membranes (MAMs) and pathologies. Cell Death & Disease. 2018;**9**(4):413. DOI: 10.1038/s41419-018-0424-1

[14] Verkhratsky A, Fernyhough P. Mitochondrial malfunction and Ca^{2+} dyshomeostasis drive neuronal pathology in diabetes. Cell Calcium. 2008;**44**(1):112-122. DOI: 10.1016/j.ceca.2007.11.010

[15] Voitenko NV. Role of calcium signalling in the development of pain syndromes. Neurophysiology.

2005;**37**(2):166-171. DOI: 10.1007/s11062-005-0061-z

[16] Calì T, Ottolini D, Brini M. Mitochondrial Ca^{2+} and neurodegeneration. Cell Calcium. 2012;**52**(1):73. DOI: 10.1016/J.CECA.2012.04.015

[17] Patergnani S, Suski JM, Agnoletto C, Bononi A, Bonora M, De Marchi E, et al. Calcium signaling around mitochondria associated membranes (MAMs). Cell Communication and Signaling: CCS. 2011;**9**:19. DOI: 10.1186/1478-811X-9-19

[18] Kawamoto EM, Vivar C, Camandola S. Physiology and pathology of calcium signaling in the brain. Frontiers in Pharmacology. 2012;**3**:61. DOI: 10.3389/fphar.2012.00061

[19] Gardete-Correia L, Boavida JM, Raposo JF, Mesquita AC, Fona C, Carvalho R, et al. First diabetes prevalence study in Portugal: {PREVADIAB} study. Diabetic Medicine. 2010;**27**(8):879-881. DOI: 10.1111/j.1464-5491.2010.03017.x

[20] Prakriya M, Lewis RS. Store-operated calcium channels. Physiological Reviews. 2015;**95**(4):1383-1436. DOI: 10.1152/physrev.00020.2014

[21] Lüscher C, Malenka RC. NMDA receptor-dependent long-term potentiation and long-term depression (LTP/LTD). Cold Spring Harbor Perspectives in Biology. 2012;**4**:6. DOI: 10.1101/cshperspect.a005710

[22] Huettner JE. Glutamate receptor pores. The Journal of Physiology. 2015;**593**(1):49-59. DOI: 10.1113/jphysiol.2014.272724

[23] Brini M, Carafoli E. The plasma membrane Ca^{2+} ATPase and the plasma membrane sodium calcium exchanger cooperate in the regulation of cell calcium. Cold Spring Harbor Perspectives in Biology. 2011;**3**:2. DOI: 10.1101/cshperspect.a004168

[24] Carafoli E, Lim D. Plasma membrane calcium ATPase. In: Handbook of Neurochemistry and Molecular Neurobiology. Boston, MA: Springer US; 2009. pp. 581-596

[25] Niggli V, Carafoli E. The plasma membrane Ca^{2+} ATPase: Purification by calmodulin affinity chromatography, and reconstitution of the purified protein. Methods in Molecular Biology (Clifton, N.J.). 2016;**1377**:57-70

[26] Berridge MJ. Module 2: Cell signalling pathways. Cell Signalling Biology. 2014;**6**:csb0001002. DOI: 10.1042/csb0001002

[27] Sacchetto R, Bertipaglia I, Giannetti S, Cendron L, Mascarello F, Damiani E, et al. Crystal structure of sarcoplasmic reticulum Ca^{2+}-ATPase (SERCA) from bovine muscle. Journal of Structural Biology. 2012;**178**(1):38-44. DOI: 10.1016/j.jsb.2012.02.008

[28] Vandecaetsbeek I, Vangheluwe P, Raeymaekers L, Wuytack F, Vanoevelen J. The Ca^{2+} pumps of the endoplasmic reticulum and Golgi apparatus. Cold Spring Harbor Perspectives in Biology. 2011;**3**:5. DOI: 10.1101/cshperspect.a004184

[29] Noble D, Herchuelz A. Role of Na/Ca exchange and the plasma membrane Ca^{2+}-ATPase in cell function. Conference on Na/Ca exchange. EMBO Reports. 2007;**8**(3):228-232. DOI: 10.1038/sj.embor.7400914

[30] Ottolia M, Torres N, Bridge JHB, Philipson KD, Goldhaber JI. Na/Ca exchange and contraction of the heart. Journal of Molecular and Cellular Cardiology. 2013;**61**:28-33. DOI: 10.1016/j.yjmcc.2013.06.001

[31] Wang Y-C, Chen Y-S, Cheng R-C, Huang R-C. Role of Na+/

Ca^{2+} exchanger in Ca^{2+} homeostasis in rat suprachiasmatic nucleus neurons. Journal of Neurophysiology. 2015;**113**(7):2114-2126. DOI: 10.1152/jn.00404.2014

[32] Schwaller B. Cytosolic Ca^{2+} buffers. Cold Spring Harbor Perspectives in Biology. 2010;**2**(11):a004051. DOI: 10.1101/cshperspect.a004051

[33] Kreutz MR, Naranjo JR, Koch K-W, Schwaller B. The neuronal functions of EF-hand Ca^{2+}-binding proteins. Frontiers in Molecular Neuroscience. 2012;**5**:92. DOI: 10.3389/fnmol.2012.00092

[34] Britti E, Delaspre F, Tamarit J, Ros J. Mitochondrial calcium signalling and neurodegenerative diseases. Neuronal Signaling. 2018;**2**:4. DOI: 10.1042/NS20180061

[35] Bradshaw RA, Dennis EA. Handbook of Cell Signaling. 2nd ed. Vol. 1. USA: Academic Press; 2010

[36] Supnet C, Bezprozvanny I. Neuronal calcium signaling, mitochondrial dysfunction, and Alzheimer's disease. Journal of Alzheimer's Disease. 2010;**20**(s2):S487-S498. DOI: 10.3233/JAD-2010-100306

[37] Verkhratsky A. Endoplasmic reticulum calcium signaling in nerve cells. Biological Research. 2004;**37**(4):693-699. DOI: 10.4067/s0716-97602004000400027

[38] Popugaeva E, Bezprozvanny I. Role of endoplasmic reticulum Ca^{2+} signaling in the pathogenesis of Alzheimer disease. Frontiers in Molecular Neuroscience. 2013;**6**:29. DOI: 10.3389/fnmol.2013.00029

[39] Kawano H, Mitchell SB, Koh J-Y, Goodman KM, Harata NC. Calcium-induced calcium release in noradrenergic neurons of the locus coeruleus. bioRxiv. 2019;**1729**:853283. DOI: 10.1101/853283

[40] Ghorbani ML, Nyborg NCB, Fjalland B, Sheykhzade M. Calcium activity of upper thoracic dorsal root ganglion neurons in Zucker diabetic fatty rats. International Journal of Endocrinology. 2013;**2013**:532850. DOI: 10.1155/2013/532850

[41] Shpakov AO, Derkach KV, Berstein LM. Brain signaling systems in the Type 2 diabetes and metabolic syndrome: Promising target to treat and prevent these diseases. Future Science OA. 2015;**1**(3):FSO25. DOI: 10.4155/fso.15.23

[42] Deleuze C, David F, Behuret S, Sadoc G, Shin H-S, Uebele VN, et al. T-type calcium channels consolidate tonic action potential output of thalamic neurons to neocortex. Journal of Neuroscience. 2012;**32**(35):12228-12236. DOI: 10.1523/jneurosci.1362-12.2012

[43] Gemes G, Bangaru MLY, Wu H-E, Tang Q, Weihrauch D, Koopmeiners AS, et al. Store-operated Ca^{2+} entry in sensory neurons: functional role and the effect of painful nerve injury. The Journal of Neuroscience. 2011;**31**(10):3536-3549. DOI: 10.1523/JNEUROSCI.5053-10.2011

[44] Burdakov D, Petersen OH, Verkhratsky A. Intraluminal calcium as a primary regulator of endoplasmic reticulum function. Cell Calcium. 2005;**38**(3-4):303-310. DOI: 10.1016/j.ceca.2005.06.010

[45] Zherebitskaya E, Schapansky J, Akude E, Smith DR, Van der Ploeg R, Solovyova N, et al. Sensory neurons derived from diabetic rats have diminished internal Ca^{2+} stores linked to impaired re-uptake by the endoplasmic reticulum. ASN Neuro. 2012;**4**:1. DOI: 10.1042/AN20110038

[46] Nedergaard M, Verkhratsky A. Calcium dyshomeostasis and pathological calcium signalling in neurological diseases. Cell Calcium. 2010;**47**(2):101-102. DOI: 10.1016/j.ceca.2009.12.011

[47] Gerbino A, Ruder WC, Curci S, Pozzan T, Zaccolo M, Hofer AM. Termination of cAMP signals by Ca^{2+} and Gαi via extracellular Ca^{2+} sensors: A link to intracellular Ca^{2+} oscillations. Journal of Cell Biology. 2005;**171**(2):303-312. DOI: 10.1083/jcb.200507054

[48] Boulware MJ, Marchant JS. Timing in cellular Ca^{2+} signaling. Current Biology. 2008;**18**:17. DOI: 10.1016/j.cub.2008.07.018

[49] Wang CH, Wei YH. Role of mitochondrial dysfunction and dysregulation of Ca^{2+} homeostasis in the pathophysiology of insulin resistance and type 2 diabetes. Journal of Biomedical Science. 2017;**24**(1):70. DOI: 10.1186/s12929-017-0375-3

[50] Haider SZ, Sadanandan NP, Joshi PG, Mehta B. Early diabetes induces changes in mitochondrial physiology of inner retinal neurons. Neuroscience. 2019;**406**:140-149. DOI: 10.1016/j.neuroscience.2019.02.026

[51] Farmer KL, Li C, Dobrowsky RT. Diabetic peripheral neuropathy: Should a chaperone accompany our therapeutic approach? Pharmacological Reviews. 2012;**64**(4):880-900. DOI: 10.1124/pr.111.005314

[52] Kann O, Kovács R. Mitochondria and neuronal activity. American Journal of Physiology. Cell Physiology. 2007;**292**(2):C641-C657. DOI: 10.1152/ajpcell.00222.2006

Chapter 8

Hyponatremia and Psychiatric Diseases

Ermal Bojdani, Flavia De Souza, Aishwarya Rajagopalan, Anderson Chen, Alesia A. Cloutier, Troy R. Nold and Dil Tahera

Abstract

Eating disorders, psychotic illnesses, and substance use disorders are some of the more common psychiatric conditions encountered in clinical practice that are associated with hyponatremia. The mechanisms that lead to hyponatremia vary, and at times hyponatremia may be a result of a drug side effect or drug-drug interaction. Additionally, hyponatremia from a non-psychiatric condition may lead to psychiatric symptomatology. Given the potential for hyponatremia to cause significant morbidity and potential mortality, clinicians are urged to consider screening for plasma sodium in patients at risk of hyponatremia, such as patients in the three categories of psychiatric conditions described above. Treatment of hyponatremia consists of various acute interventions, with consideration that treatment of the underlying psychiatric condition may help to diminish or eliminate the frequency of hyponatremic episodes in the long run.

Keywords: hyponatremia, anorexia nervosa, bulimia nervosa, psychosis, alcohol use disorder

1. Introduction

Sodium abnormalities can be seen in various psychiatric diseases. Common conditions include eating disorders, psychotic illnesses, and certain substance use disorders. Additionally, hyponatremia of any cause, including from drug side effects in patients being treated for psychiatric illnesses, can cause or worsen psychiatric conditions and may lead to medical comorbidities. References used in this chapter include articles from an online PubMed search of hyponatremia and psychosis spanning the past 50 years, and various Up-to-date review articles. In this chapter we dissect these conditions and open with a typical patient case.

1.1 Case

Lucia is a 19 year old junior majoring in Mathematics and Literature. She runs cross-country and has fainted multiple times while training with her teammates. On the recommendation of her coach she went to the student medical center for a wellness check. She looks thin and athletic. Vital sign checks show postural hypotension and orthostatic increase in pulse rate. Her BMI is calculated at 18 kg/m^2. She reports otherwise good health and no psychiatric concerns. She is doing well in school and excelling on the cross-country team.

1. What additional questions might you ask to elucidate the cause of her syncopal episodes? 2. What additional investigation would you find helpful?

2. Eating disorders and hyponatremia

2.1 Three main types of eating disorders

Eating disorders are characterized by a disturbance in eating or eating related behavior and body image associated with substantial distress and psychosocial impairment and/or jeopardizing physical health [1]. Anorexia Nervosa, Bulimia Nervosa, and Binge Eating Disorder are the most well-known and best understood eating disorders. Other recognized eating disorders include avoidant/restrictive food intake disorder, pica, and rumination disorder. This classification scheme is mutually exclusive, such that during one-episode patients can carry only one diagnosis at a time. In this chapter we discuss the diagnostic categories that lead to hyponatremia and then focus on detecting and treating hyponatremia in the eating disordered patient [2].

Anorexia Nervosa is distinguished by severe restriction in nutritional intake leading to a BMI that is less than 18.5 kg/m^2 in adults, an intense fear of becoming fat, gaining weight, and distortion in body shape and image. This is accompanied by behaviors that continue to interfere with weight gain and that stimulate weight loss. These behaviors include exercising, restricting food, eating low calorie foods, or purging by using laxatives or diuretics to lose weight.

As defined by DSM-5 [1], anorexia nervosa—restricting subtype describes an individual whose weight loss has been accomplished primarily by dieting and fasting and has not engaged in recurrent episodes of binge eating or purging in the last 3 months. In Anorexia nervosa—binge-eating/purging subtype, the individual meets criteria for anorexia nervosa and has engaged in episodes of binge-eating and purging over the last 3 months.

Bulimia Nervosa is characterized by recurrent episodes of binge eating and compensatory behavior aimed at preventing weight gain, occurring at least once a week for at least 3 months. Like in the binge-purge subtype of Anorexia Nervosa, these purging behaviors may include self-induced vomiting, misuse of diuretics, or laxatives, or excessive exercise. Patients may also restrict by fasting.

2.2 Electrolyte disturbances

If untreated and persistent, these two types of eating disorders result in electrolyte and acid-base disturbances, affecting serum and urine sodium, potassium, and chloride, and serum bicarbonate and pH [3]. Common electrolyte disturbances include hypokalemia and hyponatremia [4]. Hyponatremia is defined by a serum sodium concentration of <135 mEQ/L. Patients who purge consistently lose sodium through fluid output; self-induce vomiting, laxatives abuse leading to diarrhea; and diuretic abuse, leading to excessive urination. This decrease in effective circulating vascular volume stimulates the release of antidiuretic hormone (ADH) from the pituitary gland leading to water reabsorption through the kidneys. The body's attempt to preserve volume leads to dilution of the sodium already present in circulation. Hyponatremia in our eating disordered patients can be associated with low, normal or high serum tonicity. Hyponatremia associated with hypovolemia is as a result of low serum tonicity. Hyponatremia may also result from excessive water intake or impaired renal sodium reabsorption due to chronic starvation.

2.3 Identifying hyponatremia

A quick screen can be utilized to investigate eating disordered patterns. Clinicians should use a validated eating disorder questionnaire, like the Eating Disorder Questionnaire Online (EDQ-O) or the SCOFF (Sick Control, One, Fat, Food) questionnaire to assess for the presence of an eating disorder [5]. On physical examination, patients who purge consistently or who restrict may appear volume depleted with orthostatic decreases in blood pressure, increases in pulse rate and decreased skin turgor. In addition to a basic metabolic panel, urine electrolyte screens should be completed to help elucidate the etiology of the hyponatremia. Patients who misuse prescribed diuretics or who use copious amounts of over the counter diuretics will not have low urine sodium. On the other hand, patients who self-induce vomiting or diarrhea will have low urinary sodium because of increased sodium retention through the kidneys.

2.4 Treatment

Treatment depends on the severity of hyponatremia. In the case of patients with eating disorders, psychiatrists and nutritionists should be consulted and involved in treatment and care to facilitate discontinuation of purging, and excessive water drinking [6]. Some hospitals have developed protocols for treating such patients, including observed meals and caloric counting to ensure a smooth recovery when food is re-introduced and for prevention of refeeding syndrome [7].

3. Psychotic illnesses, bipolar illnesses, and obsessive-compulsive disorder (OCD) affecting serum sodium

3.1 Psychotic illnesses

One of the most common psychotic illnesses that affect serum sodium is schizophrenia. As defined by DSM-5 [1], schizophrenia is characterized by two of more of the following symptoms including delusions, hallucinations, disorganized speech, grossly disorganized or catatonic behavior, and negative symptoms (i.e. diminished emotional expression) that are present for a significant portion of a 1-month period and continuous signs of disturbance in functioning level present for at least 6 months. Patients with schizophrenia can experience primary psychogenic polydipsia (PPD), characterized by an increase of fluid intake along with excretion of excessive amounts of dilute urine exceeding 40–50 mL/kg of body weight [8]. It is hypothesized that this occurs in patients with schizophrenia due to elevated levels of dopamine that stimulate the thirst center [8]. In patients with schizophrenia, polydipsia prevalence is estimated at 6–20%, and complications can include not just hyponatremia but rhabdomyolysis as well [9]. Severe water intoxication has also been reported in a patient with delusional skin infestation leading to hyponatremia [10].

3.2 Bipolar illness

PPD has also been implicated in psychiatric patients with bipolar I disorder in a manic state whose increase in fluid intake can lead to hyponatremia [8]. As defined by DSM 5, a manic episode is a distinct period of abnormally and persistently elevated, expansive or irritable mood with increased activity or energy lasting at least 1 week that is not attributable to physiological effects of substances with three or more of the following symptoms present including inflated self-esteem, decreased need for sleep, pressured speech, flight of ideas, distractibility, increased goal directed activity, and excessive involvement in activities that have a high potential for painful consequences such as gambling, sexual indiscretions, and unrestrained buying sprees. The presence of mania distinguishes bipolar I from bipolar II; in bipolar I a patient must meet criteria for a manic episode, which may have been preceded or followed by a hypomanic or major depressive episode. Additionally, as defined by DMS 5 [1], bipolar disorder type II is diagnosed when the individual meets criteria for a current or past hypomanic episode and a current or past major depressive episode. A hypomanic episode is defined by DSM 5 [1] as a distinct period of abnormally and persistently elevated, expansive or irritable mood with increased activity or energy lasting at least 4 days with three or more of the following symptoms present including inflated self-esteem, decreased need for sleep, pressured speech, flight of ideas, distractibility, increased goal directed activity, and excessive involvement in activities that have a high potential for painful consequences such as gambling, sexual indiscretions, and unrestrained buying sprees. Major depressive episode includes 5 or more of the following symptoms over a 2-week period that represent a change from previous functioning such as depressed mood, diminished interest in activities, significant change in weight, insomnia or hypersomnia, psychomotor agitation or retardation, loss of energy, feelings of worthlessness, decreased ability to concentrate, and recurrent thoughts of death.

3.3 Obessive compulsive disorder (OCD)

Obsessive-compulsive disorder as defined by DSM 5 [1] is characterized by the presence of obsessions, compulsions or both. Obsessions are recurrent or persistent intrusive thoughts that cause marked anxiety or distress that individuals try to ignore or suppress by performing compulsions such as repetitive behaviors or mental acts including hand washing, praying, or checking behaviors. The obsessions and compulsions are time consuming, and distressing, and are not attributed to another medical condition. An interesting case of an Indian woman has been reported in the literature, where her behaviors of excessive water intake, intrusiveness, excessive washing, cleaning, checking and perfectionism led to a diagnosis of OCD. She had experienced recurrent seizures with no benefit from antiepileptic medication, and only after further assessment it was discovered that her urge to drink excessive water led to consumption of 7 L of water producing hyponatremia and seizure [11]. This case is important because it highlights how a psychiatric condition (OCD) can present as a neurological emergency [11].

4. Low serum sodium from other medical conditions contributing to mental health conditions

Exclusive relationships between hyponatremia, depression symptoms, and cognitive impairments have been reported in patients with chronic kidney disease who are also undergoing hemodialysis [12]. In DSM-5 [1], major depressive disorder is defined as a change from previous functioning that includes 5 or more of the following symptoms over a 2-week period of time such as depressed mood, diminished interest in activities, significant change in weight, insomnia or hypersomnia, psychomotor agitation or retardation, loss of energy, feelings of worthlessness, decreased ability to concentrate, and recurrent thoughts of death. Major neurocognitive disorder is characterized by significant cognitive decline from a previous level of functioning in one or more cognitive domains including complex attention, executive function, learning and memory, language, perceptual motor, or social cognition that interfere with independence in everyday activities.

Hyponatremia has also been reported in association with catatonia and delirium, highlighting the profound effect that hyponatremia can have on one's mental status [13]. As defined by DSM 5 [1], catatonia includes a clinical picture dominated by three or more of the following symptoms including stupor, catalepsy (passive induction of posture held against gravity), waxy flexibility (slight, even positioning by examiner), mutism, negativism (opposition or no response), posturing, mannerism (odd, circumstantial caricature of normal actions), steryotypy (repetitive, abnormally frequent, non-global directed movements), grimacing, agitation, echolalia (mimicking another's speech), and echopraxia (mimicking another's movements). Mechanisms of hyponatremia leading to catatonia are not well elucidated. Based on case reports, it has been demonstrated multiple times that catatonia and delirium do occur in the context of hyponatremia. Some hypothesize that vasopressin regulation mediates the development of hyponatremia when one has catatonia with psychosis. While others argue that because only some Addison's disease patients develop hyponatremia (potential implication of aldosterone as regulator of sodium and water balance in the distal tubules and collecting ducts of the kidneys) and only some of those develop catatonia that therefore there is a presence of susceptibility of unknown reasons with hyponatremia causing catatonia [13]. DSM 5 [1] defines delirium as a disturbance in attention, awareness, and cognition that develops over a short period of time and tends to fluctuate in severity over the course of the day.

5. Drug side effects and drug-drug interactions affecting serum sodium in patients being treated for psychiatric conditions

5.1 Antidepressants and non-steroidal anti-inflammatory drugs (NSAIDs) implicated in hyponatremia

Among the classes of medications used to treat psychiatric conditions there are many side effects and interactions that may alter serum sodium. This is a critical consideration as many of the symptoms of hyponatremia, particularly generalized malaise and alterations in appetite can mimic symptoms of depression. A recent case report documented duloxetine induced hyponatremia, including symptoms such as "unsteady gait, dizziness, nausea, general malaise and poor appetite," resolved by discontinuing duloxetine [14]. Serotonin Norepinephrine Reuptake Inhibitors (SNRIs), such as duloxetine, have been associated with syndrome of inappropriate antidiuretic hormone (SIADH) with resulting hyponatremia. Hyponatremia results from an inappropriately high release of antidiuretic hormone (ADH) from the posterior pituitary, which results in an excess retention of water and a low serum osmolality. In particular SNRIs act primarily to inhibit the reuptake of both serotonin and noradrenaline, and in experimental models it has been shown that both serotonin and noradrenaline can result in the increased release of ADH (in rat models serotonin (5-HT) activated 5-HT1A receptors cause sympathoexcitation of 5HT1C and 5HT2 receptors and the release of ADH; also stimulation of the paraventricular and supraoptic nuclei with norepinephrine can increase release of ADH within the serum) [14]. Therefore, through these mechanisms it is hypothesized that SNRIs cause SIADH in patients, a life-threatening side effect that must be monitored for by clinicians.

A case report of a patient diagnosed with schizophrenia, taking desmopressin and meloxicam identified that NSAIDs can significantly augment hyponatremia by "increas[ing] water retention" [15]. Notably, the worsened water retention is particularly problematic for patients on desmopressin, and complete resolution of symptoms occurred after desmopressin was tapered and meloxicam stopped, with normalization in plasma sodium [15] (**Figure 1**, used with permission from authors).

5.2 Other medications and interactions implicated in hyponatremia

Fabrazzo et al. [16] discuss three cases involving delorazepam, olanzapine and fluvoxamine, respectively, in which patients with various presentations of bipolar disorder were hospitalized, and hyponatremia was discovered on admission. Workup revealed SIADH. Multiple interventions were trialed, including administration of hypertonic saline, and decreasing doses of various medications. It was not until the offending medications were removed that patients demonstrated resolution of their hyponatremia. Notably, olanzapine, fluvoxamine and delorazepam were being administered in conjunction with other medications that may have contributed to the hyponatremia. In the case of the patient taking delorazepam, they also were prescribed oxcarbazepine, which ultimately was replaced with gabapentin. In the case of the patient taking olanzapine, he also was taking delorazepam and oxcarbazepine. Likewise, the patient on fluvoxamine was also taking oxcarbazepine. These medications in conjunction with one another appear to have an additive property on hyponatremia.

5.3 Additional considerations for antipsychotics and hyponatremia

Antipsychotic medications alone have been reported in the literature to be associated with hyponatremia; however, recently, the long-acting risperidone injectable treatment has been implicated in hyponatremia as well. In this case, the patient did not improve simply with the removal of risperidone, due to the extended half-life, and ultimately required Tolvaptan administration [17]. The half-life of these medications may be an important factor in determining the management of subsequent hyponatremia. Along a similar vein, Fabrazzo et al. [16] detail that hyponatremia and other electrolyte derangements are often only detected in patients with psychiatric diagnoses when they are hospitalized. This is a critical consideration for clinicians in terms of practice, particularly whether there is an impetus for psychiatrists

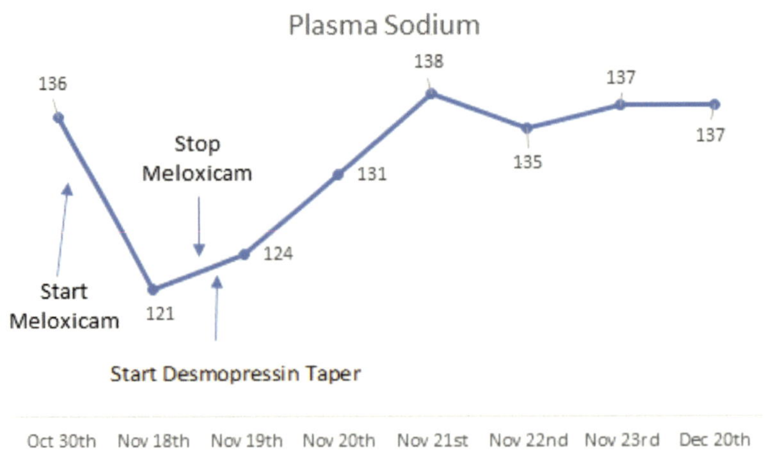

Figure 1.
Plasma sodium levels over time.

to consider routinely monitoring electrolytes of patients on longstanding medications with the potential for these derangements, especially in patients with bipolar disorder.

5.4 Practice considerations

There currently are no routine guidelines for screening of electrolyte abnormalities among patients with psychiatric diagnoses and this should be further evaluated given the range of dangerous consequences of hyponatremia, including seizure, as demonstrated in at least one of the cases delineated above [15].

6. Alcohol and other substance use disorders affecting serum sodium

6.1 Alcohol and hyponatremia

Substance use is also implicated in derangements of serum sodium, particularly among patients who abuse alcohol and MDMA. As defined by DSM 5 [1], alcohol use disorder is a pattern of alcohol use within the past 12 months that has led to significant impairment in one's life characterized by at least two of the following including alcohol taken in larger amounts, persistent desire to cut down, increased time obtaining alcohol, cravings, continued use despite recurrent impairment in social functioning, developed tolerance, and withdrawal symptoms present when alcohol use is ceased. As delineated in previous sections, there are profound potential consequences of hyponatremia, particularly because of sodium's role in maintaining nerve impulse conduction and neuromuscular excitability. Michal et al. [18] observed that in patients with likely alcohol use disorder, the level of derangement in serum sodium was associated with the worsening of physical and psychological quality of life; that is to say, patients with severe hyponatremia (<120 mmol/L) were likely to have worse quality of life than patients with low hyponatremia (<135 mmol/L) [18]. The specific causal pathways are not delineated; however, beer potomania is an observed phenomenon in which dietary insufficiency of protein, coupled with dietary sodium results in a sort of dilutional hyponatremia. It is possible that patients with more severe hyponatremia may be further in their disease course, ultimately consuming more alcohol.

6.2 MDMA (3,4-methylenedioxymethamphetamine) and hyponatremia

Stimulant use disorder in DSM-5 [1] is defined as a pattern of stimulant use within the past 12 months that has led to significant impairment in one's life characterized by at least two of the following including the stimulant is taken in larger amounts, persistent desire to cut down, increased time obtaining the stimulant, cravings, continued use despite recurrent impairment in social functioning, developed tolerance, and withdrawal symptoms present when stimulant use is ceased. MDMA (3,4-methylenedioxymethamphetamine), a stimulant, is thought to be associated with hyponatremia because of increased diaphoresis, yielding sodium loss, and compensatory water intoxication. It is not a common side effect of MDMA use; however, Armitage et al. [19] presented a case report of an 18-year-old woman who had a generalized tonic-clonic seizure in the setting of hyponatremia from MDMA intoxication. This woman's serum sodium was 121, notably close to what many would argue is severe hyponatremia. Notably, MDMA related hyponatremia with seizure is more common among young women under 30 years of age, particularly because of estrogen inhibiting the Na+-K+-ATPase. This ultimately inhibits a known compensatory mechanism for cerebral edema, which may place young women at increased risk of neurological impacts of hyponatremia with MDMA use. Further, a metabolite of MDMA, 4-hydroxy-3-methoxymethamphetamine (HMMA), is documented to stimulate ADH release, which can worsen hyponatremia. These are vital considerations given the potential sequela of seizure, and the urgency of its management.

7. General treatment considerations for hyponatremia in psychiatric illnesses

Here, we aim to describe general considerations of hyponatremia by going over symptoms, treatment, and cautions.

7.1 Summary of general symptoms of hyponatremia

Symptoms of hyponatremia can be thought of as severe, moderate, and mild. Severe symptoms are red flag signs that include seizure and changes in cognition that can rapidly progress to coma and death. These symptoms are classically correlated with serum levels of less than 120. As such, these are the constellation of symptoms that would require hospitalization. Moderate and mild symptoms differ in severity but include flu like symptoms of headache, myopathy, and general malaise; these symptoms are observed mostly with sodium serum level ranges from 120 to 135. Lastly, there are patients who have low serum levels but are generally asymptomatic, with minimal changes in gait or sensorium [20].

7.2 Treatment of hyponatremia and cautions

When treating hyponatremia, it is important to recognize that there is a high risk of morbidity and mortality in conditions where hyponatremia develops within 48 h, post-op hyponatremia in female and pediatric populations, patients with history of cerebral pathology, as well as those presenting with psychosis (because they could have ingested large amounts of water). Regardless of symptom severity, it is important to note that increasing serum sodium level by 4–6 mEq/L in 24 h can reverse symptoms, and the rate should never exceed 8 mEq/L in a day, as rates faster than this can increase risk of demyelination [20]. Asymptomatic hyponatremia, if mild, may be left untreated.

Interventions commonly used in the context of treating hyponatremia include fluid restriction, increasing dietary salt, potassium replacements, hypertonic saline, and vasopressin antagonists, with selection based on the etiology and severity of the hyponatremia. Fluid restriction is most helpful in the context of volume overload (such as heart failure or cirrhosis), SIADH, renal failure, or if the patient has polydipsia. The amount of fluid restriction is determined often with nutritional consultation; this is the gold standard approach in treatment of SIADH. Patients may initially start with fluid restriction to 500 mL/d. Pharmacotherapy is typically considered if serum sodium has not improved with fluid restriction over 48 h [21].

Pharmacotherapy includes a broad range of options, including dietary salts and oral salt tablets, potassium replacements and vasopressin antagonists. Dietary salts and oral salt tablets are generally utilized for patients with mild to asymptomatic symptoms with SIADH. Potassium replacements are helpful when patients are developing conditions that are causing hypokalemic states as well, such as inappropriate diuretic uses and excessive vomiting. These may be associated with feeding and eating disorders, and additional considerations for the treatment of those disorders may include 1:1 supervision for prevention of continued vomiting, and consultation with nutrition to minimize risk of refeeding during early hospitalization. Vasopressin antagonists will cause water loss, making it non-ideal for patients with volume deficits.

The clinician must always be wary of any contributing factors causing the hyponatremia; for example, if the patient has adrenal insufficiency, glucocorticoid replacement will be crucial. In this case, endocrinology consultation may be appropriate. Likewise, if the patient has drug induced SIADH, it is important to re-visit the necessity of the drugs and to find replacements if able; common culprits include SSRIs like fluoxetine and sertraline [20]. The clinician and the patient should have a conversation about the risks, benefits, and alternatives to continuing treatment with an offending agent and informed consent should be documented whether the medication is maintained or switched. In patients with psychogenic polydipsia associated with antipsychotic medication use, treatment of the underlying psychotic disorder coupled with behavioral intervention to limit water intake may decrease the frequency of hyponatremic episodes and lessen morbidity. In patients with substance use disorders, particularly alcohol use disorder, psychoeducation and motivational interviewing surrounding their substance use disorder and risks of hyponatremia, including increased risk of seizure, may be a helpful part of decreasing use of substance. These patients should also be offered medication assisted treatment for their substance use disorder when appropriate and desired by the patient.

In sum, hyponatremia in psychiatric conditions is best treated in a comprehensive, multi modal approach. With many etiologies, including SIADH, endocrine pathologies, feeding and eating disorders, and delirium, consultation with different medical specialties and nutritional teams may augment and improve the treatment of hyponatremia. Regardless of etiology, psychoeducation and involvement of the patient in shared decision making is essential in understanding the future course of treatment.

8. Conclusion

Hyponatremia is a complex electrolyte disturbance which can both manifest with psychiatric symptoms, and can be associated with psychiatric disease itself. Eating disorders, psychotic illnesses, and substance use disorders are some of the more common psychiatric conditions encountered in practice that are associated with hyponatremia. The mechanisms that lead to hyponatremia vary, and at times hyponatremia may be a result of a drug side effect or drug-drug interaction. Given the potential for hyponatremia to cause significant morbidity and potential mortality, clinicians are urged to consider screening for plasma sodium in patients at risk of hyponatremia, such as patients in the three categories of psychiatric conditions described above. Treatment considerations include: (1) understanding the underlying etiology of the hyponatremia, (2) asymptomatic mild hyponatremia may not need treatment, (3) fluid restriction is the initial treatment of choice for SIADH, (4) hypertonic saline is used to correct moderate-severe hyponatremia, but should be done only under the guidance of medical teams to avoid demyelination syndromes, (5) there may be other considerations, such as 1:1 supervision for feeding-eating disorders, (6) specialty consultation may be appropriate in determining course of treatment, such as nutrition for advancement of diet, or endocrinology for concomitant adrenal pathology. Treatment of hyponatremia consists of various acute interventions, with consideration that treatment of the underlying psychiatric condition may help to diminish or eliminate the frequency of hyponatremic episodes in the long run.

9. Case consideration

1. The patient should have a comprehensive assessment, which includes a medical interview, physical exam, and tests as needed. This assessment should include questions about diet, alcohol and drug use, exercise regimen, and past and current medical and psychiatric histories.

2. Additional investigations can include checking blood electrolytes and an EKG. In patients with eating disorders, one can see derangements in sodium and potassium (usually hyponatremia or hypokalemia or both). EKG may show QT prolongation.

Author details

Ermal Bojdani[1,2,3*], Flavia De Souza[4,5,6], Aishwarya Rajagopalan[1,2,3], Anderson Chen[1,2,3], Alesia A. Cloutier[1,2,3], Troy R. Nold[1,2,3] and Dil Tahera[2,3]

1 Harvard South Shore Psychiatry Residency Training Program, Brockton, MA, United States

2 VA Boston Healthcare System, Brockton, MA, United States

3 Department of Psychiatry, Harvard Medical School, Boston, MA, United States

4 Yale Psychiatry Residency Training Program, New Haven, CT, United States

5 Yale Public Psychiatry Fellowship, New Haven, CT, United States

6 Department of Psychiatry, Yale School of Medicine, New Haven, CT, United States

*Address all correspondence to: ermal.bojdani2@va.gov

IntechOpen

© 2019 The Author(s). Licensee IntechOpen. This chapter is distributed under the terms of the Creative Commons Attribution License (http://creativecommons.org/licenses/by/3.0), which permits unrestricted use, distribution, and reproduction in any medium, provided the original work is properly cited.

References

[1] Diagnostic and Statistical Manual of Mental Disorders. Diagnostic and Statistical Manual of Mental Disorders, Fifth Edition (DSM-5). Arlington, VA: American Psychiatric Association; 2013

[2] Taylor D, Paton C, Kapur S. Prescribing Guidelines in Psychiatry. 12th ed. UK: Wiley Blackwell; 2015

[3] Mehler PS. Electrolyte and acid-base abnormalities associated with purging behaviors. The International Journal of Eating Disorders. 2016;**49**(3):311-318. DOI: 10.1002/eat.22503

[4] Miller KK, Grinspoon SK, Ciampa J, Hier J, Herzog D, Klibanski A. Medical findings in outpatients with anorexia nervosa. Archives of Internal Medicine. 2005;**165**(5):561-566. DOI: 10.1001/archinte.165.5.561

[5] Cotton MA, Ball C, Robinson P. Four simple questions can help screen for eating disorders. Journal of General Internal Medicine. 2003;**18**(1):53-56. DOI: 10.1046/j.1525-1497.2003.20374.x

[6] https://www.uptodate.com/contents/anorexia-nervosa-endocrine-complications-and-their-management?search=hyponatremia%20and%20anorexia&source=search_result&selectedTitle=1~150&usage_type=default&display_rank=1

[7] Skipper A. Refeeding syndrome or refeeding hypophosphatemia. Nutrition in Clinical Practice. 2012;**27**:34-40. DOI: 10.1177/0884533611427916

[8] Parag S, Espiridion ED. Hyponatremia presenting with recurrent mania. Cureus. 2018;**10**(11):e3645. DOI: 10.7759/cureus.3645

[9] Chen LC, Bai YM, Chang MH. Polydipsia, hyponatremia and rhabdomyolysis in schizophrenia: A case report. World Journal of Psychiatry. 2014;**4**(4):150-152. DOI: 10.5498/wjp.v4.i4.150

[10] Lai J, Lu Q, Xu Y, Hu S. Severe water intoxication and secondary depressive syndrome in relation to delusional infestation. Neuropsychiatric Disease and Treatment. 2016;**12**: 517-521. DOI: 10.2147/NDT.S102993. eCollection 2016

[11] Dar MA, Wani RA, Rather YH, Kawoos Y, Hussain A, Margoob MA, et al. Obsessive compulsive disorder presenting as neurological emergency. Indian Journal of Psychological Medicine. 2015;**37**(4):467-469. DOI: 10.4103/0253-7176.168611

[12] Fan SS, Lin LF, Chen VC, Hsieh CW, Hsiao HP, McIntyre RS, et al. Effects of lower past-year serum sodium and hyponatremia on depression symptoms and cognitive impairments in patients with hemodialysis. Therapeutic apheresis and dialysis. 2019. DOI: 10.1111/1744-9987.13395. [Epub ahead of print]

[13] McGuire E, Yohanathan M, Lally L, McCarthy G. Hyponatraemia-associated catatonia. BMJ Case Reports. 2017;**2017**. pii: bcr-2017-219487. DOI: 10.1136/bcr-2017-219487

[14] Sun CF, Chen YL, Li YH, Kumaraswamy M, Lo YC, Chen YT. Duloxetine-induced hyponatremia in an elderly male patient with treatment-refractory major depressive disorder. Case Reports in Psychiatry. 2019;**2019**:4109150. DOI: 10.1155/2019/4109150. eCollection 2019

[15] Bojdani E, Chen A, Buonocore S, Li K, Gurrera R. Meloxicam-desmopressin drug-drug interaction producing hyponatremia. Psychiatry Research. 2019;**279**:284-286. DOI: 10.1016/j.

psychres.2019.05.009. pii: S0165-1781(19)30250-1. [Epub ahead of print]

[16] Fabrazzo M, Fuschillo A, Perris F, Catapano F. The unmasking of hidden severe hyponatremia after long-term combination therapy in exacerbated bipolar patients: A case series. International Clinical Psychopharmacology. 2019;**34**(4):206-210. DOI: 10.1097/YIC.0000000000000265

[17] Chowdhury W, Lodhi MU, Kuzel AR, Johnson P, Rahim U, Rahim M. Management of persistent hyponatremia induced by long-acting injectable risperidone therapy. Cureus. 2018;**10**(5):e2657. DOI: 10.7759/cureus.2657

[18] Michal O, Magdalena MZ, Halina M, Magdalena BZ, Tadeusz N, Elzbieta M, et al. Hyponatremia effect in patients with alcohol dependence on their physical and mental health status. Alcohol. 2016;**57**:49-53. DOI: 10.1016/j.alcohol.2016.10.002. Epub 2016 Oct 5

[19] Armitage MC, Bryant RJ, Page CB. Severe hyponatremia complicated by seizure following 3,4-methylenedioxy-methamphetamine ingestion. Emergency Medicine Australasia. 2018;**30**(5):730-731. DOI: 10.1111/1742-6723.13159. Epub 2018 Aug 14

[20] Sterns RH, Emmett M, Forman JP. Overview of the treatment of hyponatremia in adults. UpToDate 2019. Available from: https://www.uptodate.com/contents/overview-of-the-treatment-of-hyponatremia-in-adults?search=hyponatremia&source=search_result&selectedTitle=1~150&usage_type=default&display_rank=1

[21] Verbalis JG, Goldsmith SR, Greenberg A, Korzelius C, Schrier RW, Sterns RH, et al. Diagnosis, evaluation, and treatment of hyponatremia: Expert panel recommendations. American Journal of Medicine. 2013;**126**(10 Suppl 1):S1-S42. [Medline]

Chapter 9

Effect of Foot Morphology and Anthropometry on Bipedal Postural Balance

Charmode Sundip Hemant

Abstract

Maintenance of accurate postural balance is imperative to avoid falls and incapacities especially in overweight and older population. Normal postural balance is affected by various factors like age, gender, body characteristics like lean muscle mass, soft tissue mass, stature, foot anthropometry, etc. A cross-sectional study was conducted among 1000 young population of north Karnataka in which human stature, weight, body mass index, foot anthropometric parameters, etc. along with postural sway were measured. The correlation of these parameters with human stature, weight and postural sway was studied. Data obtained were tabulated, graphically represented and statistically analyzed. Correlation coefficient was formulated for each variable. Foot length and width showed positive significant correlation with height, weight and other variables. Study observations were compared with those obtained from previous studies. The study observations will enable us to understand the influence of foot anthropometry on postural balance and help researchers to formulate weight transfer strategies, thereby facilitating management and rehabilitation of patients with postural instability.

Keywords: anthropometry, bipedal posture, postural stability, gait, body mass

1. Introduction

Postural balance is dynamic and demands constant amendments to adapt to external disturbances, by using vision, muscle activity, articular positioning and proprioception, and the vestibular system to prevent falls [1, 2]. Awareness of the body's position in space is determined by the integration of the visual, vestibular and somatosensory systems [3, 4]. The study of postural control is imperative for diagnosing balance disorders, as well as for assessing the effects of both therapeutic interventions and fall prevention programs. Postural stability is determined by mechanical factors that include both individual and environmental characteristics. This chapter focuses on various factors influencing the bipedal postural stability and provides an insight into the measures to facilitate improvement in the accuracy of diagnosis and quality of treatment and rehabilitation, thereby preventing falls and incapacities.

2. Evolution of bipedal posture

Our ancestors would have probably become extinct if they had not developed their bipedal posture including the corresponding transitional behavioral constraints. "Bipedalism evolved more as a terrestrial feeding posture than as a walking adaptation" [5]. The adapted bipedal posture brought various disadvantages like decreased velocity, increased time for social interaction, more chances of injuries from fall, more energy consumption, etc.

Advantages of bipedal posture could be many, namely freeing of hands, the visual advantage of being able to survey the surrounding, ability to acquire the skill of throwing, ability to carry infants while running, ability to reach out for food, ability for carrying food or provisioning, etc. But the most important hypothesis is that the ability to venture into shallow water made the ancestors to adapt bipedal posture.

3. Biomechanics of bipedal posture

Upright postural balance describes the dynamics of body posture to prevent falling over a relatively small base of support under gravitational field. As for postural balance without stepping, the stable balancing condition can be analyzed using the following equation under assumption that a one link inverted pendulum describes human sway motions.

$$\text{Fy.xcop–Mg.xcom} = \text{I}\ \theta\text{a}. \qquad (1)$$

where Fy is vertical reaction force, Mg is human total weight, xcop is the center of pressure (COP), xcom is the horizontal component of the center of mass (COM) (e.g., the center of gravity (COG)), I is the moment of inertia of the total body about the ankle joint, and θa is the ankle joint angle [6].

Two basic models for biped locomotion are walking and running. A gait of walking consists of stance and swing phases and a gait of running consists of stance and flight phases. Stance phase describes the period when a foot remains on the ground, and either swing or flight describes the period when a foot does not touch the ground. At midstance, the COM is at its highest point and gravitational potential energy is at maximal and kinetic energy at minimal. The exchange between kinetic and gravitational potential energies is cyclical over gaits. On the other hand, a running leg acts as a spring; therefore, a simple running model is a mass-spring system. At the braking phase during stance, the spring gets compressed and energies are stored as elastic energy. At midstance, the COM reaches its lowest point. The stored elastic energy recoils the spring at propulsive phase during stance to produce kinetic and gravitational potential energies. Both models principally exchange and store energies repeatedly to produce forward thrust and stability [6].

4. Factors affecting postural balance

Numerous determinants like age, gender and body characteristics like body mass, height and body mass index affect postural stability. Anthropometric parameters of ankle joint and foot also affect bipedal and unipedal postural stability.

4.1 Effect of age and gender on postural balance

Vijada Raiva et al. [6] stated that females have more postural stability than males. Hageman et al. [7] stated that compared to younger population, older generation showed more tendency to sway. Older adults performed the timed movement task much slower than the younger adults. Longer response times by the elderly have been attributed to slower event detection and impaired sensorimotor integration. Greve et al. [8] stated that women showed less movement on Biodex Balance System than men did, and these findings were similar to those of Rozzi et al. [9] who evaluated basketball and American football players using the same equipment. Lee and Lin [10] studied children and observed that girls presented better postural balance than boys. This could be due to anthropometric factors (greater in men), but other factors such as neuromuscular (flexibility) and neurophysiologic (processing of inferences), as well as the habit of using higher heels, may also account for the differences.

4.2 Effect of body mass on postural balance

Ledin and Odkvist [11] demonstrated that a 20% increase in body mass reduced the ability to make adjustments in response to external perturbations in the orthostatic position, with a consequent increase in postural instability. Chiari et al. [12] and Molikova et al. [13] in their respective studies conducted on individuals with normal or slightly higher than normal BMI have shown low correlations between body mass and balance. Majority of studies indicate that there was a direct relationship between obesity and increased postural instability, as evaluated by means of various tools and methods. Greve et al. [14] showed that in young adult males, the higher the BMI, the worst the postural balance, needing more postural adjustments to maintain balance in single leg stance. Greve et al. [8] proposed that the male group demonstrated stronger correlations for overall, anteroposterior and mediolateral stability index with body mass index (BMI) compared to women. They stated that there was a need for greater movements to maintain postural balance. Hue et al. [15] found that body mass was responsible for more than 50% of balance at speed and Chiari et al. [12] demonstrated a strong correlation between body mass, anteroposterior movements and the area of detachment. McGraw et al. [16] reported that greater postural adjustments are necessary to maintain an erect posture when there is a build-up of adipose tissue, thus causing a reduction in balance and an increase in injuries and falls. Due to the high degree of correlation between balance and body mass, we can safely infer that the mechanical factor of body mass inertia requires greater musculoskeletal force to balance it against the force of gravity, and therefore, to maintain balance, obese individuals require greater movement from the center of gravity to remain in the orthostatic position.

4.3 Impact of stature on postural balance

There is a consensus that the greater the height, the worse the balance. Berger et al. [17] and Alonso et al. [3] stated that ankle displacements and the response of the gastrocnemius increased with increasing height. Allard et al. [18] and Lee and Lin [10] reported that tall individuals present greater postural sway than do short individuals, and they attributed this to the higher position of the center of mass. Kejonen et al. [19] and Hue et al. [15] have found that body stability is inversely related to the height of the center of gravity and that, for this reason, posturography measurements are affected by individuals' anthropometric characteristics.

4.4 Role of foot anthropometry in maintaining postural balance

The architecture of the vertebral column, upper and lower appendages, and organs and tissues that attach to or are suspended from the spinal column affects postural stability. Very few studies are available on correlation of foot parameters with unipedal and bipedal postural balance [18].

4.5 Effect of muscle strength and fatigue on postural balance

As the age advances particularly after forties, the muscle mass goes on decreasing so does the muscle strength. Muscle fatigue, which is a common condition affecting the elderly population, can result in mobility, postural and gait deficiencies. The state of mind can influence the activity of the muscular system, that is, the muscular tonus. The muscular activation or, in the contrary case, the muscular relaxation influences postures adopted by people. The body height and the lower limb length constitute partly to weight transfer strategy. The trunk-cephalic length does not correlate to the postural sway. Body mass is located above the hips, so it is not the main factor for the mediolateral sway. The weight transfer strategy for men depends on the size of the basis of support and their lean mass, while, for women, only the lengths (whole body and lower limbs) are important. Lower basis of supports leads to higher postural sway in the ML direction (Chiari et al. [11]; Chou et al., [20]), and to control the increase in body sway, it is necessary to increase the lean mass, probably and mainly the muscle mass to be able to generate more muscle force. The increase in body height affects the body mass and soft tissue mass (lean and fat masses) increases the postural sway. The increase in body mass indeed enlarges the postural sway.

5. Research study

A study was conducted in central population of northern Karnataka on 1000 young adult population in which foot anthropometry was measured and correlated with stature, weight, body mass index and bipedal posture stability [21].

6. Methodology

Study design: Descriptive cross-sectional study.

Setting: Anthropometric section of department of Anatomy, ESIC Medical College and Hospital, Gulbarga, Karnataka.

Duration of study: 14 months; from 31 October 2017 to 31 December 2018.

Sample size: 1000 participants included medical, dental and nursing students aged between 18 and 21 years of age.

Inclusion criteria: Medical, dental and nursing students aged between 18 and 21 years of age in ESIC Medical College, Gulbarga.

Exclusion criteria: Students of NRI quota and students with poorly defined wrist creases, deformities of vertebral column and limbs, contractures, missing limbs, history of trauma to hand and foot, with features suggestive of dysmorphic syndromes, chronic illness and hormonal therapy were excluded from the study.

Sample selection: Simple random sampling method [13] as we selected 1000 participants out of total 3000 medical, dental and nursing students in our institute satisfying the inclusion criteria. As subjects belonging to the first to third year, they were easily accessible and also represented the young adult age group.

6.1 Data collection procedure

Foot length: Each subject will stand on a calibrated foot board with his/her back against the wall in such a manner that the posterior most point of the heel will

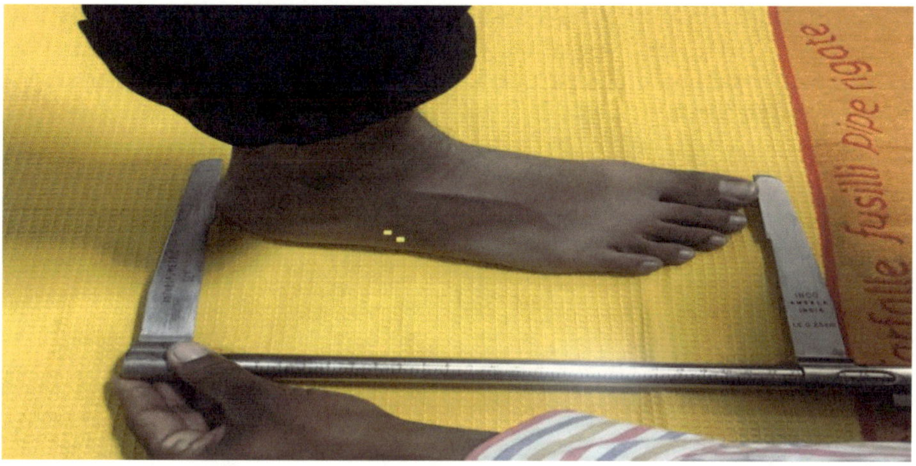

Figure 1.
Measurement of foot length.

gently touch the wall. A vertical stop was placed against the anterior most point of the foot. The distance between the posterior most point of the heel and the anterior most point of the foot was measured as the foot length [22] (**Figure 1**).

Foot breadth: It will be measured as distance between metatarsal tibiale (point projecting most medially on the head of the 1st metatarsal bone) and metatarsal fibulare (point projecting most laterally on the head of the 5th metatarsal bone) [23].

Height: Standing height will be measured to the nearest centimeters (cm) using a stadiometer with the subject standing erect on a horizontal resting plane bare footed having the palms of the hands turned inward and the fingers pointing downwards. The height will be measured from the sole of the feet to the vertex of the head as recommended by International Biological Program [23].

Body weight: It will be taken using the Mechanical Weighing Balance to the nearest kg according to the standard procedures A. Ibegbu, David et al. [24].

Body mass index: It will be calculated by dividing weight by height squared [weight/height squared (kg/m^2)] David et al. [24].

6.2 Data collection tools

Vernier slide calipers, calibrated foot board, stadiometer, regular weight machine, questionnaire for collection of personal details, academic scores, lead pencils, stationary, etc. Data collected were tabulated, graphically represented and statistically analyzed.

7. Observations

In our study, mean foot length was observed as 24.34 cm on the right side and 24.32 cm on the left side. Mean body mass index was calculated as 20.97. Correlation between foot length and body mass index was done. No statistically significant correlation between BMI and foot length of the right and left sides ($P > 0.05$) was observed. For further details, refer to **Table 1**.

In the present study, mean foot breadth was observed as 8.95 cm on the right side and 8.96 cm on the left side. Mean body mass index was calculated as 20.97. Correlation between foot length and body mass index was done. There was a statistically significant correlation between BMI and foot breadth of the right and left sides ($P < 0.01$). The observations in the study stated that foot breadth of both sides was considerably more in participants who had higher body mass index. Linear regression coefficient was derived. For further details, refer to **Table 2, Figure 2.**

Variables	Minimum	Maximum	Range	Mean	SD	N	Correlation r	P value
Body mass index (kg/m^2)	12.22	40.61	28.39	20.97	4.66	1000	—	—
Foot length right (cm)	21.0	28.9	7.9	24.34	1.54	1000	r = 0.073	P > 0.05 NS
Foot length left (cm)	21.5	29.0	7.5	24.32	1.50	1000	r = 0.024	P > 0.05 NS

Table 1.
Correlation of foot length and body mass index.

Variables	Minimum	Maximum	Range	Mean	SD	N	Correlation r	P value
Body mass index (kg/m^2)	12.22	40.61	28.39	20.97	4.66	1000	—	—
Foot breadth right (cm)	7.5	10.9	3.4	8.95	0.78	1000	r = 0.124	P < 0.05 S
Foot breadth left (cm)	7.7	11.5	3.8	8.96	0.68	1000	r = 0.115	P < 0.05 S
Linear regression equation	BMI = 19.306 + 0.168 (foot breadth right)							
Linear regression equation	BMI = 17.214 + 0382 (foot breadth left)							

Table 2.
Correlation of foot breadth and body mass index.

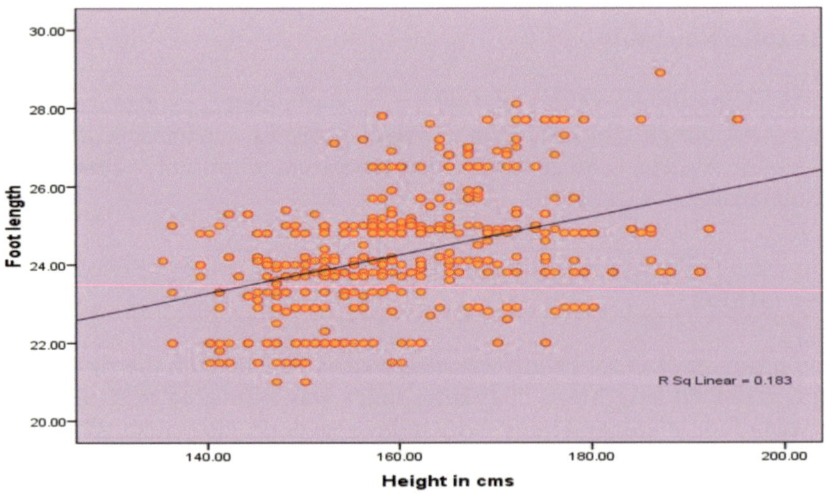

Figure 2.
Correlation between foot length and body mass index.

Variables	Minimum	Maximum	Range	Mean	SD	N	Correlation r	P value
Height (cm)	135.2	195.2	60.0	161.88	13.45	1000	—	—
Foot length right (cm)	21.0	28.9	7.9	24.34	1.54	1000	r = 0.428	P < 0.01 HS
Foot length left (cm)	21.5	29.0	7.5	24.32	1.50	1000	r = 0.516	P < 0.01 HS
Linear regression equation	Height = 71.391 + 4.782 (foot length right)							
Linear regression equation	Height = 49.706 + 4.786 (foot length left)							

Table 3.
Correlation of foot length and human stature.

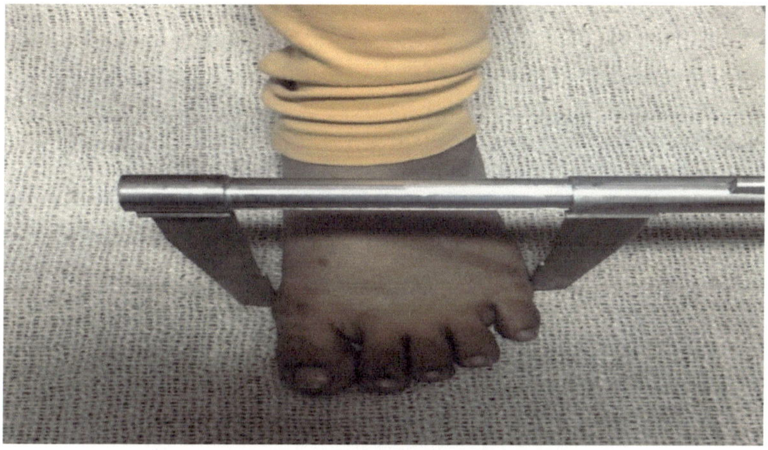

Figure 3.
Measurement of foot breadth.

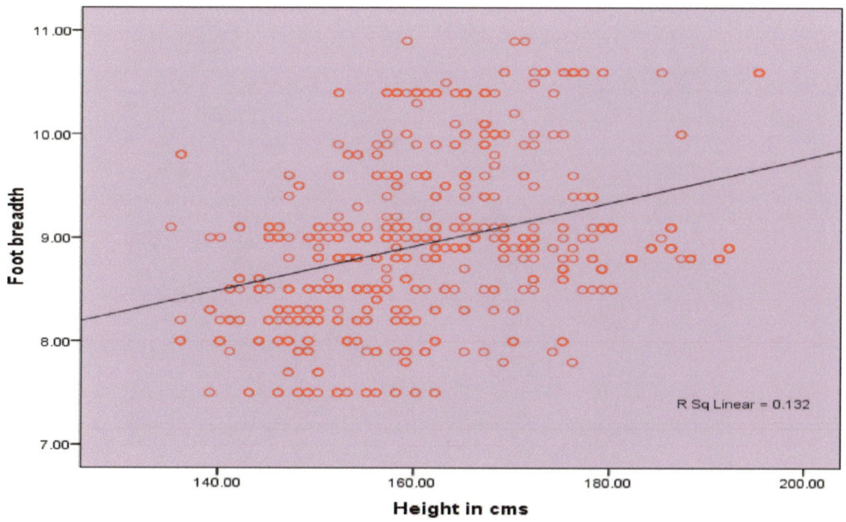

Figure 4.
Correlation between foot breadth and body mass index.

Variables	Minimum	Maximum	Range	Mean	SD	N	Correlation r	P value
Height (cm)	135.2	195.2	60.0	161.88	13.45	1000	—	—
Foot breadth right (cm)	7.5	10.9	3.4	8.95	0.78	1000	r = 0.364	P < 0.01 HS
Foot breadth left (cm)	7.7	11.5	3.8	8.96	0.68	1000	r = 0.367	P < 0.01 HS
Linear regression equation	Height = 106.01 + 6.240 (foot breadth right)							
Linear regression equation	Height = 96.843 + 7.253 (foot breadth left)							

Table 4.
Correlation of foot breadth and human stature.

We also observed foot length on both sides. Mean foot length on the right side was observed as 24.34 cm, and on the left side, it was 24.32 cm. Correlation of foot length was conducted with human stature. Linear regression equation was derived for both sides. Statistically highly significant positive correlation was observed between height and foot length of both sides (P < 0.01). **Table 3** reveals that foot length of both sides was also significantly more among those having more height (**Figures 3** and **4**).

Foot breadth was observed on both sides. Mean foot breadth on the right side was observed as 8.95 cm, and on the left side, it was 8.96 cm. Correlation of foot breadth was conducted with human stature. Linear regression equation was derived

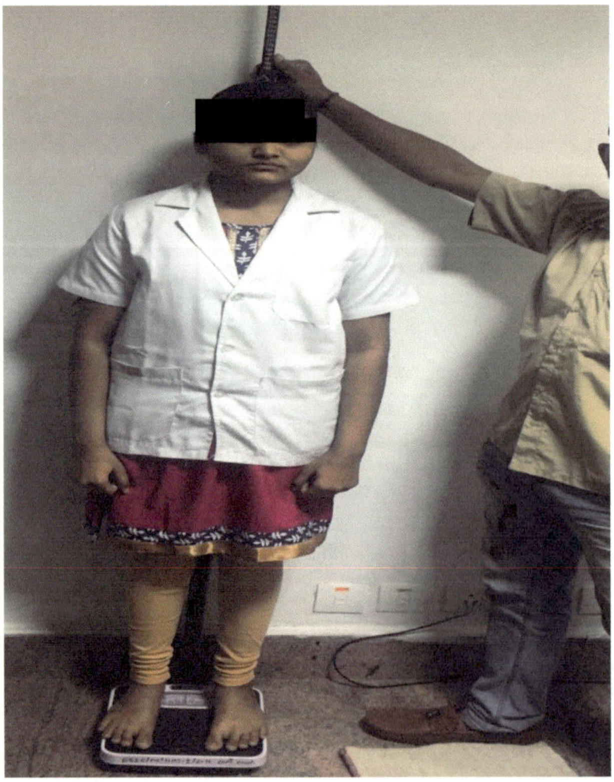

Figure 5.
Measurement of human stature.

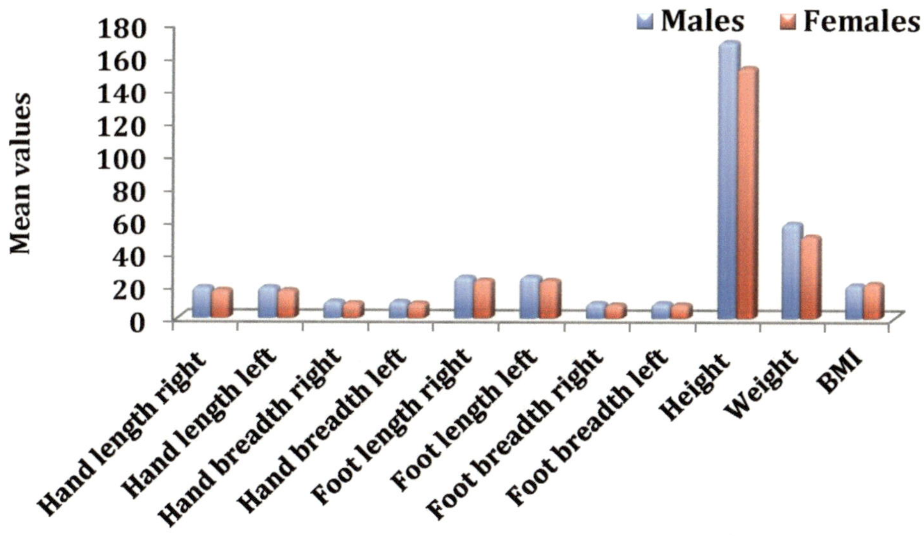

Figure 6.
Correlation between foot length and stature.

Variables	Male (N = 500) Mean ± SD	Female (N = 500) Mean ± SD	Z-test value	P value and significance
Foot length right (cm)	25.18 ± 1.32	23.39 ± 1.19	Z = 30.07	P < 0.001, VHS
Foot length left (cm)	25.31 ± 1.16	23.19 ± 0.96	Z = 31.19	P < 0.001, VHS
Foot breadth right (cm)	9.39 ± 0.71	8.45 ± 0.52	Z = 22.97	P < 0.001, VHS
Foot breadth left (cm)	9.35 ± 0.59	8.52 ± 0.47	Z = 23.21	P < 0.001, VHS
Height (cm)	169.28 ± 11.75	153.42 ± 9.75	Z = 22.26	P < 0.001, VHS
Weight (kg)	58.21 ± 11.91	50.14 ± 9.85	Z = 11.21	P < 0.001, VHS
BMI (kg/m^2)	20.58 ± 4.94	21.41 ± 4.27	Z = 2.53	P < 0.05, S

NS, not significant; S, significant; HS, highly significant; VHS, very highly significant.

Table 5.
Gender-wise comparison of parameters.

for both sides. Statistically highly significant positive correlation was observed between height and foot breadth of both sides ($P < 0.01$). **Table 4** reveals that foot breadth of the right or left side was significantly more in those participants whose height was more (**Figures 5** and **6**).

Gender-wise comparison of observations was done. We observed very highly significant difference in foot length, foot breadth, height and weight among males and females. The foot length, foot breadth, height and weight were significantly more in males compared to females, whereas body mass index was significantly more in females as compared to males. The observations have been tabulated in **Table 5, Figures 7** and **8**.

Postural sway was measured in the participants both male and female in anteroposterior and mediolateral direction (**Figure 9**). Correlation of postural sway with foot length and foot breadth was conducted. Mediolateral postural sway amplitude was the same, that is, −0.3 cm in both males and females.

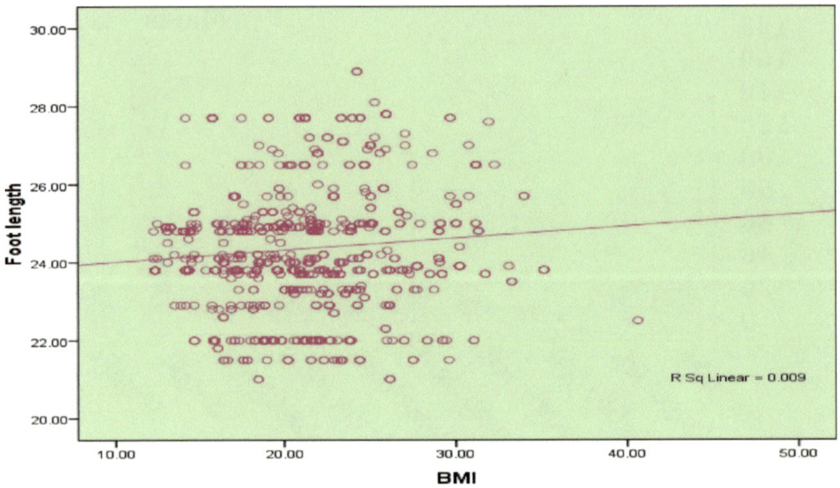

Figure 7.
Correlation between foot breadth and stature.

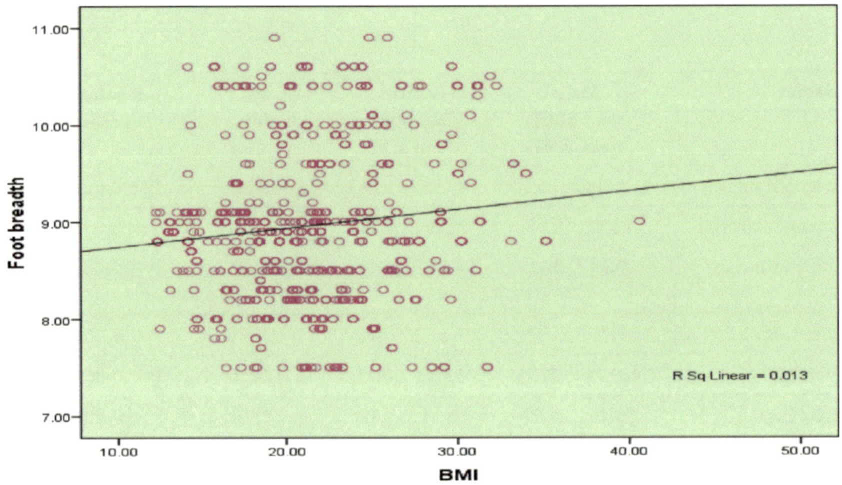

Figure 8.
Multiple bar diagram represents gender-wise comparison of variables.

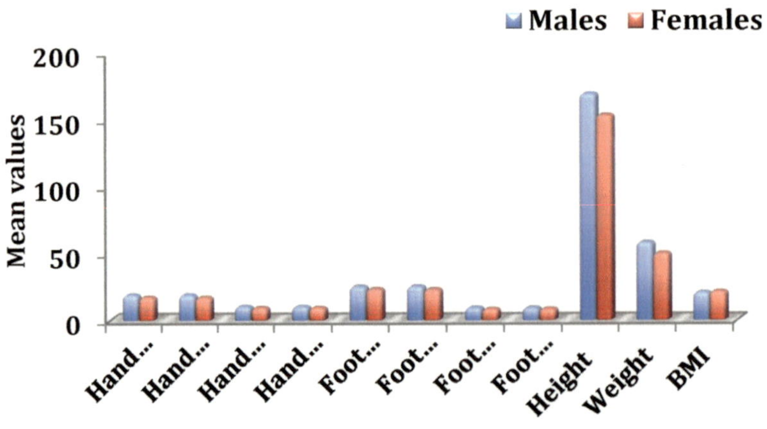

Figure 9.
Gender-wise comparison of parameters.

Variables	Foot length (cm) r(p)	Foot breadth (cm)	Angle (°)
Female			
Mediolateral sway (cm)	0.01 (0.88)	0.01 (0.80)	−0.01 (0.89)
Mediolateral ampl sway (cm)	0.05 (0.54)	0.01 (0.82)	−0.03 (0.70)
Anteroposterior sway (cm)	0.07 (0.43)	0.05 (0.53)	−0.12 (0.21)
Anteroposterior ampl sway (cm)	0.09 (0.35)	−0.11 (0.25)	−0.95 (0.35)
Sway velocity (cm/s)	0.05 (0.56)	−0.12 (0.22)	0.11 (0.25)
Sway area (cm^2)	0.67 (0.50)	−0.24 (0.80)	−0.12 (0.22)
Male			
Mediolateral sway (cm)	0.32 (0.00)	0.02 (0.84)	−0.04 (0.68)
Mediolateral ampl sway (cm)	0.27 (0.00)	0.02 (0.83)	−0.03 (0.69)
Anteroposterior sway (cm)	0.29 (0.00)	0.00 (0.94)	−0.11 (0.24)
Anteroposterior ampl sway (cm)	0.27 (0.00)	−0.06 (0.52)	−0.10 (0.31)
Sway velocity (cm/s)	0.15 (0.13)	−0.08 (0.42)	−0.09 (0.37)
Sway area (cm^2)	0.36 (0.00)	0.02 (0.78)	−0.10 (0.32)

Spearman's correlation, $^*p \leq 0.05$. ampl, amplitude.

Table 6.
Correlation between foot anthropometric measurements and postural balance.

Anteroposterior sway amplitude was −.95 cm in females and − .10 cm in males. **It was observed that men exhibited more postural sway compared to females in anteroposterior direction**. The findings were statistically significant. Refer to **Table 6** for details.

8. Discussion

Few studies have worked on the relationship of foot anthropometry with balance. Clarke [25] analyzed the angle of foot. Swanenburg et al., [26] examined static posturography using the center of pressure (COP) oscillation on a force platform. Our study suggested association between greater foot length and higher stabilometric parameters only in the male group. Our study observations matched with those of Alonso et al. [27], Kejonen et al., [19] and Molikova et al., [13]. Previous studies by Alonso et al., [3] and Chou et al., [20] also demonstrated that an increase in the size of the support base can improve the balance.

Our study states that neither the foot length nor the foot width influences postural balance. These observations matched with Alonso et al., [28], but they had conducted the study using unipedal standing balance task. Our findings contradicted with those of Chiari et al.[12] in which foot width showed positive correlation with postural balance. They conducted the study by bipedal standing balance task. They stated that the increase in lean mass correlates to the decrease of the amplitude of the postural sway. They added that the percentage of fat mass explains part of the anteroposterior postural sway in men, but not in women.

Mainenti et al. [29] showed that elderly women with more fat mass had larger balance sway and Winters and Snow [30] reported that 31% of postural sway variability in premenopausal women was caused by the fat mass. Hence, it can be concluded that the effect of fat mass on the postural control is age dependent.

The increase in body height indeed increases the postural sway. Hence, in our study, the greater height in the male group may have been the reason for the greater influence of this parameter on COP in comparison to the female participants.

In our study, conducted among young adults, without major health diseases or other abnormalities, the anthropometric measurements showed gender-related differences.

9. Conclusions

1. Bipedal postural sway shows sexual dimorphism.

2. Significance of body composition in maintenance of postural sway also shows sexual dimorphism.

3. Lean muscle mass is inversely proportional to the degree of postural sway.

4. Soft tissue mass is directly proportional to the degree of postural sway.

5. Human height is directly proportional to the degree of postural sway.

6. Foot length and foot width do not influence postural balance.

7. Overweight individuals require greater movement from the center of gravity to remain in the orthostatic position.

10. Suggestions

1. Gender-related variations in factors maintaining postural balance should be considered during ankle and weight transfer strategies.

2. Foot anthropometric parameters should be taken into consideration while facilitating diagnosis, treatment and rehabilitation of patients with postural instability.

Author details

Charmode Sundip Hemant
Department of Anatomy, All India Institute of Medical Sciences, Ministry of Health and Family Welfare of India, Gorakhpur, India

*Address all correspondence to: sundip.charmode@yahoo.com

IntechOpen

© 2020 The Author(s). Licensee IntechOpen. This chapter is distributed under the terms of the Creative Commons Attribution License (http://creativecommons.org/licenses/by/3.0), which permits unrestricted use, distribution, and reproduction in any medium, provided the original work is properly cited.

References

[1] Prado JM, Stoffregen TA, Duarte M. Postural sway during dual tasks in young and elderly adults. Gerontology. 2007;**53**(5):274-281

[2] Alonso AC, Greve JMDA, Camanho GL. Evaluating the Centre of gravity of dislocations in soccer players with and without reconstruction of the anterior cruciate ligament using a balance platform. Clinics. 2009;**64**(3):163-170

[3] Alonso AC, Luna NM, Mochizuki L, Barbieri F, Santos S, Greve JMDA. The influence of anthropometric factors on postural balance: The relationship between body composition and posturographic measurements in young adults. Clinics. 2012;**67**(12):1433-1441

[4] Riemann BL, Myers JB, Lephart SM. Comparison of the ankle, knee, hip, and trunk corrective action shown during single-leg stance on firm, foam, and multiaxial surfaces. Archives of Physical Medicine and Rehabilitation. 2003;**84**: 90-95

[5] Jo S. Hierarchical Neural Control of Human Postural Balance and Bipedal Walking in Sagittal Plane. Department of Electrical Engineering and Computer Science. Massachusetts institute of technology; May 2006

[6] Raiva V, Wannasetta W, Gulsatitporn S, Aksaranugraha S. Age and gender effects on postural stability and static balance in Thai community dwelling adults. Journal of the Medical Association of Thailand. 2004;**87** (Suppl. 2):S112-S116

[7] Hageman PA, Leibowitz JM, Blanke D. Age and gender effects on postural control measures. Archives of Physical Medicine and Rehabilitation. 1995;**76**:961-965

[8] Julia Maria D, Greve A, Cug M, Dulgeroglu D, Brech GC, Alonso AC. Relationship between anthropometric factors, gender, and balance under unstable conditions in young adults. BioMed Research International. 2013; **2013**:1-5. Article ID: 850424

[9] Rozzi SL, Lephart SM, Gear WS, Fu FH. Knee joint laxity and neuromuscular characteristics of male and female soccer and basketball players. American Journal of Sports Medicine. 1999;**27**(3):312-319

[10] Lee AJY, Lin WH. The influence of gender and somatotype on single-leg upright standing postural stability in children. Journal of Applied Biomechanics. 2007;**23**(3):173-179

[11] Ledin T, Odkvist LM. Effects of increased inertial load in dynamic and randomized perturbed posturography. Acta Oto-Laryngologica. 1993;**113**(3): 249-252

[12] Chiari L, Rocchi L, Cappello A. Stabilometric parameters are affected by anthropometry and foot placement. Clinical biomechanics. 2002;**17**(9–10): 666-677

[13] Molikova R, Bezdickova M, Langovaetal K. The relationship between morphological indicators of human body and posture. Biomedical Papers of the Medical Faculty of the University Palacky, Olomouc, Czechoslovakia. 2006;**150**(2):261-265

[14] Greve JMDA, Alonso AC, Bordini ACPG, Camanho GL. Correlation between body mass index and postural balance. Clinics. 2007;**62**(6):717-720

[15] Hue O, Simoneau M, Marcotte J, et al. Body weight is a strong predictor of postural stability. Gait and Posture. 2007;**26**(1):32-38

[16] McGraw B, McClenaghan BA, Williams HG, Dickerson J, Ward DS.

Gait and postural stability in obese and non-obese prepubertal boys. Archives of Physical Medicine and Rehabilitation. 2000;**81**(4):484-489

[17] Berger W, Trippel M, Discher M, Dietz V. Influence of subjects' height on the stabilization of posture. Acta Oto-Laryngologica. 1992;**112**(1):22-30

[18] Allard M, Nault L, Hinse S, LeBlanc R, Labelle H. Relationship between morphologic somatotypes and standing posture equilibrium. Annals of Human Biology. 2001;**28**(6):624-633

[19] Kejonen P, Kauranen K, Vanharanta H. The relationship between anthropometric factors and body-balancing movements in postural balance. Archives of Physical Medicine and Rehabilitation. 2003;**84**(1):17-22

[20] Chou SW, Cheng HK, Chen JH, Ju YY, Lin YC, Wong MKA. The role of the great toe in balance performance. Journal of Orthopaedic Research: Official Publication of the Orthopaedic Research Society. 2009;**27**(4):549-554

[21] Charmode SH, Pujari DK, Shivappa KH, et al. Correlation of foot dimensions with body mass index: A study in young population of Central India. Indian Journal of Anatomy. 2020; **9**(1):61-68

[22] Oommen A, Mainker A, Oommen T. A study of the correlation between hand length and foot length in humans. Journal of the Anatomical Society of India. 2005;**54**(2):55-57

[23] Tandon R, Yunus SM, Faruqi NA, Asghar A. Measurements of hand and foot – A predictor of stature in adult human population of Uttar Pradesh. International Journal of Anatomy, Radiology and Surgery. 2016;**5**(1):12-15

[24] Ibegbu AO, David ET, Hamman WO, Umana UE, Musa SA. Association of hand length with height in Nigerian school children. Journal of Biology and Life Science. 2013;**4**(2): 83-94

[25] Clarke HH. An objective method of measuring the height of the longitudinal arch in foot examinations. Research Quarterly. 1993;**4**(3):99-107

[26] Swanenburg J, Bruin ED, Favero K, Uebelhart D, Mulder T. The reliability of postural balance measures in single and dual tasking in elderly fallers and non-fallers. BMC Musculoskeletal Disorders. 2008;**9**:162

[27] Alonso AC, Mochizuki L, Luna NMS, Canonica AC, Souza RR, Maifrino LBM, et al. Men and women do not have the same relation between body composition and postural sway. Journal of Morphological Sciences. 2015; **32**(2):93-97

[28] Alonso AC, Peterson M, Duganieri MR, Garcez-Leme LE, Mochizuki L, Bocalini DS, et al. The effects of foot morphology and anthropometry on unipodal postural control. Motriz: Revista de Educação Física Rio Claro. 2016;**22**(1):94-98

[29] Mainenti MR, Rodrigues EC, Oliveira JF, Ferreira AS, Dias CM, Silva AL. Adiposity and postural balance control: Correlations between bioelectrical impedance and stabilometric signals in elderly Brazilian women. Clinics. 2011;**9**:1513-1518

[30] Winters KM, Snow CM. Body composition predicts bone mineral density and balance in premenopausal women. Journal of Women's Health & Gender-Based Medicine. 2000;**9**(8): 865-872

Section 3

Eating Disorders - A Therapeutic Challenge

Chapter 10

Discretion or Disorder? The Impact of Weight Management Issues on the Diagnosis and Treatment of Disordered Eating and Clinical Eating Disorders

Abigail H. Natenshon

Abstract

Eating disorders, the most lethal of all the psychiatric disorders, are frequently misdiagnosed as benign weight management problems, which contribute to their being underdiagnosed and under-reported. Though eating disorders are typically first identified through easily discernible weight change, their unseen origins lie in genetic propensities, neurobiology, environmental and family influences, inborn temperament, and trauma. Non-integrative, behaviorally based weight management solutions that call for dieting and meal plans alone, by ignoring the psychological underpinnings and neurobiological origins of dysfunctions driving these disorders, can potentially lead to loss of life and/or life quality. Conversely, generic psychotherapy protocols typically fail to address and enforce the behavioral prerequisite to re-feed the malnourished eating disordered brain and body, which is required to optimize therapy outcomes. It is for the intuitive and skillful diagnostician to determine whether the patient's desire for weight change is based on healthful autonomous discretion or on the dictates of compulsions based in life-threatening pathology, thus informing treatment. Eating disorders are disorders of the core Self of self-regulation, self-perception, self-esteem and self-care, affecting life spheres far exceeding eating-lifestyle and weight management. Healing weight management problems requires integrative diagnosis and care, re-establishing one's healthy relationship with food, weight, and eating, as well as with one's re-integrated core self.

Keywords: weight management, diets, dieting, obesity, disordered eating, eating disorders, anorexia nervosa, bulimia nervosa, obsessive compulsive disorder, binge eating disorder, purging, food restriction, healthy eating, exercise bulimia, refeeding edema, diabulimia

1. Introduction

Most individuals seeking advice about weight management issues approach healthcare professionals with the intention of improving their health, well-being, and appearance by losing weight and altering their metabolic function. Typically, first responders, be they parents, nutritionists, physicians, nurses, coaches, or personal trainers, offer non-integrative behavioral approaches to weight management in the form of prescriptive diet plans. In the absence of underlying pathology or compulsions that may drive dysfunctional eating behaviors, such simple solutions may be adequate. But when the origin of an individual's desire and efforts to lose weight resides in underlying eating pathology, purely behavioral solutions can mask potentially life-threatening dysfunctions. Sometimes hiding in plain sight, otherwise benign disordered eating (DE) habits may ultimately take on an element of compulsivity, leading to chronic illnesses such as heart disease, diabetes, and/or as heart disease or diabetes and/or the eventual onset of a life-threatening clinical eating disorder (ED) in genetically susceptible individuals. It is for the astute and intentional diagnostician to sniff out, intuit, or otherwise identify the potential for pathological origins within a constellation of seemingly benign weight management dysfunctions by determining whether a patient's desire for weight change is based on healthful, autonomous discretion or on the dictates of a tyrannical and potentially lethal eating disorder. Overlooking the nature and severity of DE behaviors or warning signs of a clinical ED can carry dire consequences. By partnering with the patient to affirm or negate a diagnostic hunch, the clinician informs appropriate treatment, promoting disease prevention or the achievement of a timely and sustainable problem resolution.

2. The continuum of healthy eating

The nature and quality of eating patterns reside along a continuum that includes eating behaviors and self-care. Along the span of this continuum, healthy eating patterns may evolve into disordered eating patterns, potentially leading to deadly ED in genetically susceptible individuals. At one end of the continuum, healthy eating behaviors mark the achievement of a fit and effectively functional body capable of sustaining its own ideal set point weight through healthy eating and self-care (**Figure 1**). At the opposite end of the continuum, life-threatening ED represent the tip of an underlying emotional, physiological, and neurobiological iceberg. A clinical ED marks the fragmentation or loss of the core self and, with it, the patient's lost capacity for self-regulation, self-trust, self-esteem, and self-care. Feelings of guilt and of shame typically foster secrecy, denial, and reluctance to seek or sustain care. Ambiguous and inconstant DE behaviors exist somewhere between the polarities of healthy eating and potentially life-threatening ED. Some DE patterns that may appear to be pathological may actually represent variations of normal and benign behaviors, being shared by otherwise healthy eaters. As an example, healthy eaters who choose to indulge excessively in the lavish offerings of dessert buffets, typically consider such an opportunity benign and not-to-be-missed, guilt-free, gastronomic sensory and aesthetic delight.

The evolution of dysfunction along the eating continuum is influenced by the melding of eating lifestyle with genetic propensities, inborn temperament, value

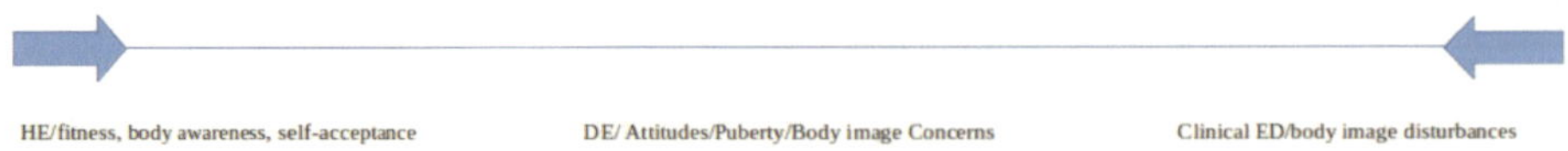

Figure 1.
Along the continuum of healthy eating, the evolution of healthy eating to DE, and from DE to a clinical ED, represents a journey of developing pathology; likewise, recovery from eating pathology represents a journey in the opposite direction, towards developing health.

systems, developmental life stages, and self-concept issues culminating in body image perception and preoccupations. The confluence of normal child development and early bodily maturation, environmental triggers gleaned through social media, attitudes in the home, and peer pressure can lead to high-risk responses in teens and young adults which might include dieting, excessive exercise, abuse of diet pills, purging, food restriction, or eating only when hungry/skipping meals. In response to a societal disconnect between biology and culture, as girls grow older, they are expected to grow smaller. Studies show that 42% of first to third grade girls wish to be thinner [1] and, in the attempt to change one's natural body shape and size, 81% of 10-year-old girls feel better about themselves when they are dieting [2], creating a greater risk of obesity in adulthood. 25% of American men and 45% of American women are dieting on any given day [3], giving rise to cravings, malnutrition, metabolic dysfunction, and increased overweight once the individual "falls off the dieting wagon." It has been reported that 35% of "occasional dieters" progress to pathological dieting and DE, and as many as 25% progress to partial or full syndrome eating disorders [4].

It is for the perceptive and responsive diagnostician to determine at what point, along the healthy eating continuum, eating behaviors cross the thin line between normal eating and various forms and degrees of eating pathology and compulsions. A patient of mine with binge eating disorder (BED) assumed that she was in "remission" until, "It suddenly occurred to me that this was not just about having an extra piece of pie ... this was starting to feel like an all-out binge." Pathology exists when food, exercise, or the abuse of dietary substances is used to resolve emotional problems or in response to posttraumatic stress; when food serves purposes other than satiating hunger, fueling the body, or sociability; when the act of eating evokes guilt and fear; when eating habits become inflexible, immoderate, imbalanced, and excessive; when compulsive thoughts, such as calculating caloric intake, and preoccupations about becoming fat preclude other thinking, interfering with learning and normal daily function; and when attitudes and beliefs about food and eating are misguided.

> *When a child who is a healthy eater runs out the door without breakfast because (s)he is late for the school bus, she will surely want to snack during the morning or eat a bigger lunch to make up for the calories lost. The child with an ED who runs out the door without breakfast does so because (s)he would otherwise be wracked with fear, anxiety, and guilt that the calories she might ingest would make her fat. This child would feel compelled to calculate how many calories (s)he can allow herself to ingest throughout the rest of the day so as not to gain a single ounce.*

3. Weight management diagnosticians face multiple challenges

In the face of weight management issues, information that patients communicate to clinicians is often not accurate or comprehensive; and what patients request of health professionals is frequently not what they need. Falling between the cracks of accurate assessment and appropriate treatment, DE and potentially lethal ED all too frequently remain misunderstood, underdiagnosed, and undertreated [5] by myopic, underinformed physicians, psychotherapists, and nutritionists who lack an integrative "big picture" perspective of the possible existence of underlying, co-occurring diagnoses that need to be revealed, monitored, and treated. The diagnosis of a clinical ED remains elusive, with more than one half of all cases remaining undetected [6].

A patient of mine had been treated by a psychiatrist for 7 years, during which time, she never told him that she vomited 30 times a day, for fear of his finding her "disgusting" and therefore refusing to treat her. This physician failed to "read between the lines" of her symptoms and to intuit and investigate the presence of an ED from the constellation of personality traits, temperament, and behaviors that she did reveal to him. Through our work together, she came to understand her problem and her self. The quality of our relationship led to the improvement of all her significant relationships—with food, with her self, and with others.

The unique requirements of weight management issues demand the uniquely specialized skills of an informed, intentional, and intuitive diagnostician, capable of hearing what has not yet been spoken. Within the context of initial history-taking, the nature of weight-related dysfunctions is likely to remain elusive in the absence of an active probe for problem origins in pathology. The diagnostician's enlightened line of questioning will substantiate, or negate, such a presence, revealing the subtleties of distinctions between the nature of eating behaviors as they reside along the healthy eating continuum. When eating behaviors do appear to cross the line into pathology, the diagnostician takes on the role of crisis interventionist, through immediate responsiveness to the needs of the moment through an investigation into the past. Because the patient's quality of life may depend upon assessment accuracy, the obligation for first responders or clinicians to detect, explore, and interpret issues yet to be unearthed becomes a unique challenge within the confines of the limited timeframe of a single-session weight management consultation. On high alert for potentially unseen issues, the proactive first responder must be prepared to offer psychoeducation, a plan of action, and, where appropriate, referrals to collaborating experts and/or higher-level treatment milieus. If it looks like a duck and acts like a duck, it is for the responsible practitioner to treat it like a duck, unless proven otherwise, even before the assignment of a definitive diagnosis.

Esther was a 29-year-old woman who came to treatment for depression, poor self-esteem, and relationship problems. In response to her description of her college days during which she spoke of herself as perfectionistic, highly compulsive, anxious, and depressed, I chose to wonder aloud if she had ever struggled with an ED or other eating-related issues. "My God!" she responded. "How did you know? I have never told a soul!" By understanding the nature of her personality structure and recognizing characteristics of her emotional functioning, I was able to intuit and surmise the possible existence of a past ED, which upon inquiry, I discovered had yet to be fully resolved. Following the tenet of John Muir, "If we try to pick out anything by itself, we find it hitched to everything else in the universe." By following my hunch and having made this discovery, I was able to launch the ED treatment process immediately.

Where the clinician's depth and breadth of understanding of weight management issues is limited and non-integrative, the patient is liable to leave the treatment office with a diet plan in hand, yet without a practicable and sustainable solution for pressing weight-related concerns. More significantly, the loss of a timely and poignant opportunity for the patient to discover unknown problem origins and aspects of self and personality represents a lost opportunity for self-reflection, self-awareness, and self-integration, all leading to healthier lifestyle choices.

Factors further clouding the differential diagnosis of eating-related pathology include the elusive assessment of evolving and ambiguous DE patterns, and the widespread misunderstanding and erroneous information surrounding the issues of eating, weight control, and ED. In asking my ED patients what triggered the onset of their ED, a frequently heard response is that they "started to diet in an effort to lose weight, and ultimately found themselves feeling compelled to eat 'healthier and healthier.'" The term "healthy eating" not infrequently becomes a euphemism for food restriction, or 'clean eating,' potentially triggering the onset of orthorexia in ED individuals. Further complicating the diagnostic process, ED symptoms vary appreciably from patient to patient, with; every ED a 'thumbprint.' Fully half of the ED population suffers from the difficult-to-identify condition called "other specified feeding or eating disorder" (OSFED), previously known as "eating disorder not otherwise specified" (EDNOS) [7]. OSFED describes atypical AN (without low weight) and atypical BN or BED (with lower frequency of behaviors, purging disorder, and/or night eating syndrome). Patients who do not meet the strict diagnostic cutoffs for full criteria for AN and BN often remain undiagnosed despite the seriousness of their illness, foregoing or delaying necessary treatment [8]. Patients with clinical ED are often reticent, within a diagnostic interview, to divulge a stigmatized disorder. A recent discovery, important for its potential to reduce the degree of stigma that is associated with ED nondisclosure revealed that 20% of the neurobiology of AN could be derived from metabolic genes (possibly activated by a state of starvation) [9].

3.1 Myths and misconceptions regarding clinical ED abound

Consider the following examples of decoys to the recogntion and understanding of ED:

- People mistakenly assume that AN is easy to spot, believing that "all anorexic individuals are exceedingly thin."
- It is a commonly believed misconception that an AN individual's full restoration of weight marks a full recovery from an ED. In fact, ED recovery is marked by neurobiological, emotional, cognitive, and behavioral changes that lead to the reintegration of the individual's core self and the normalization of body fat mass and sexual hormones, which have a widespread impact on the body and multiple pathways in the brain [10].
- Despite the widely accepted misconception that ED represent an incurable "life sentence," about half of those individuals with AN or BN attain a full recovery, 30% achieve a partial recovery, and 20% show no substantial improvement [11].

3.1.1 The physician's role in weight management detection

Though early detection of ED warning signs is pivotal in disease prevention and/or promoting a timely recovery, the medical community has been known to overlook opportunities for early disease recognition.

- Because signs of an ED rarely appear in blood tests until advanced stages of disease, normal test results in early stages of ED are often misconstrued to represent a "clean bill of health."
- Pediatricians frequently overlook the significance of precipitous weight loss in children when their numbers fall within the range of normal on the growth charts, precluding early disease prevention.
- Gynecologists regularly prescribe birth control pills for ED patients with amenorrhea, erroneously assuming that hormone replacement will counteract or reverse bone loss and improve reproductive functionality [12].

- Cardiologists, in the face of a co-occurring activity disorder that takes the form of excessive and compulsive exercise, frequently miss an ED diagnosis by attributing a low heart rate and amenorrhea to "healthy athleticism."

When driven by the fear of weight gain, individuals who suffer from ED, co-occurring anxiety, and obsessive-compulsive disorders (OCD), are particularly susceptible to developing activity disorders. Also known as anorexia athletica, exercise bulimia, or exercise addiction, ED individuals engage in such compensatory compulsions with the intention of burning calories. Between 40% and 80% of AN patients are prone to excessive exercise in their efforts to avoid putting on weight [13].

Binny ran 10 miles a day, followed by 2 hours of working out. She ate no more than 750 calories a day while training regularly for countrywide marathon races. One 26.2-mile event landed her in a hospital, where her legs swelled and she required an emergency blood transfusion. Because her eating and running regime provided her with a sense of being "alive," upon release from the hospital she felt incapable of curtailing the compulsive behaviors that threatened her life. Her emergency room doctors attributed her blood disorder and amenorrhea to her athleticism, failing to recognize both conditions as signs of ED pathology.

4. Gaining clarity through defining terms

"The beginning of wisdom is to call things by their right names."
Chinese Proverb

4.1 Understanding weight management

Barring origins in genetic, metabolic, or hormonal dysfunctions, weight management dysfunctions typically originate in an individual's unhealthy relationship with food, leading to a disordered eating lifestyle. The term "weight management" describes the techniques and physiological processes that contribute to attaining and maintaining an individual's ideal weight. Healthy weight management techniques encompass long-term lifestyle strategies promoting healthy eating and daily physical activity, fostering sustainable change and well-being. In contrast, unhealthy weight management strategies, lacking an integrative treatment perspective, fail to achieve sustainable weight goals. Examples of unhealthy weight management include dieting, skipping meals, food restriction, eating only when hungry, and forms of purging that may include vomiting, spitting, compulsive exercise, and the abuse of laxatives, diet pills, and diuretics. Multiple studies have found that dieting for purposes of weight management is associated with greater weight gain and increased rates of binge eating in both boys and girls [14].

4.2 Understanding healthy eating

Healthy eating is guilt-free, balanced, and fearless eating, with flexibility in accommodating the parameters of the dining moment. Healthy eating includes three meals daily, each including all the nutritionally-dense food groups, as well as snacks. There are no bad foods. What is bad is extremism, compulsivity, and unhealthy attitudes about food and eating, i.e., how we feel about what we eat. What is worse than eating Oreos is never eating Oreos, as forbidding a child to eat Oreos can ultimately lead to sneaking, hiding, or stealing food. Healthy eating results in healthy weight maintenance naturally, through the inherent wisdom of a body which, when fed healthfully, and having reached its ideal set point weight, will predictably sustain that appropriate weight-to-height ratio indefinitely, through its own natural functions. In most cases, the healthfully fed and exercised body with a healthfully functioning metabolism needs no help from arbitrarily devised dietary interventions to sustain a healthy weight throughout one's lifetime.

4.3 Understanding disordered eating

At times we are all a little eating dysfunctional. Bombarded by nutritional research and food fads in an age of pervasive social media, "normal" eating (i.e., eating all food groups, including moderate amounts of processed foods and sugar) is no longer considered to be "healthy" eating. Certain patterns of DE, in light of their prevalence, are becoming increasingly difficult to recognize as pathological. A study found that nearly 91% of female college students use dieting as a weight control mechanism [15], putting many of them at risk to develop a clinical ED. The prevalence of AN and BN is relatively rare among the general population [16], affecting 1% to 4% of adolescents and young adult women [17]; DE, however, which has been defined as a psychological illness, [18], and the misguided attitudes about food and weight management that lead to them, are widespread and prevalent among all age groups. The consequences of DE, which include rampant dieting and body image obsessions, can be devastating; though not the cause of eating disorders, they are often precursors to their onset. Occasional DE, as well as certain behaviors that manifest themselves in clinical ED, are not in themselves abnormal. Differentiating normalcy from pathology is best accomplished by assessing the patient's attitudes towards food and eating. Benign forms of DE are fully discretionary, dependent upon the individual's capacity for self-awareness, self-regulation, and choice-making through their own free will.

Picky eating syndrome is a DE pattern that originates in early childhood. Typically indicative of a sensory processing disorder (SPD), food choices tend to be limited to bland "white" foods (containing sugar and flour) of specific textures. Picky eating often results in overweight. Studies show that 40% of overweight girls and 37% of overweight boys are teased/bullied about their weight by peers or family members and that traumatic experiences such as these during the formative years are predictive of weight gain, binge eating, and extreme weight control measures [14]. DE patients have experienced a higher frequency of traumas (childhood adversities in particular), especially in circumstances related to childhood obesity [18]. Childhood picky eaters who do not grow out of the condition and who become malnourished because of the limited variety of foods that they eat qualify for a diagnosis of avoidant restrictive food intake disorder (ARFID), a condition which typically extends into adulthood.

Rising obesity rates, the result of DE lifestyles, clinical ED, and hereditary factors have become a major concern worldwide, especially in North America, where more than 2 in 3 adults (70.2%) are considered to be overweight or obese [19]. Obesity, DE, and ED are considered major health problems among adolescents because of their increasing prevalence in this age group and their potentially serious physical and psychosocial consequences [20, 21]. Dieting and unhealthful weight control practices lead to eating psychopathology in DE, ED, and obesity, particularly when associated with variables such as personality characteristics like perfectionism or anxious temperament, a microbial imbalance, or a genetic predisposition to be influenced by an obesogenic environment. Other possible causal mechanisms linking dieting to later problems are neurophysiological mechanisms associated with food restriction (e.g., effects on neurotransmitters that could increase risks for either obesity or ED via influences on food regulation processes) [21]. In the face of a genetic, hormonal, or metabolic predisposition to obesity, following a healthy lifestyle in which the individual learns to eat differently, not less, may counteract gene-related risks. Individuals with obesity and co-occurring eating disorders are at higher risk for several medical and psychosocial complications than individuals with either condition alone [22]. Because obesity may become a precursor to an ED, and vice versa, collaborative exchanges of experiences and specialized knowledge between healthcare professionals working in the fields of obesity and eating disorders are essential [22].

4.4 Understanding clinical eating disorders

ED onset is an integrative process, stimulated by contributing factors that include genetics, neurobiological vulnerability, physiology, co-occurring mood and emotional disorders, past trauma, and familial and cultural influence. For the individual with AN, BN, BED, or OSFED, behavioral and emotionally based compulsions become etched in neuronal pathways, impacting the structure and function of the brain. ED patients consider their disorder to be a survival tool, an adaptive coping mechanism that they cannot live without. Underlying the clinical ED is the primordial fear of becoming fat. For the ED individual, food is "fattening," and fat, the enemy of a body that can never be too thin, becomes a "feeling," a sensation, a perception. ED are self-regulatory dysfunctions. All types of ED share a great number of symptoms and issues, as aspects of the same disease syndrome; however, ED victims vary in the basic structure and function of personality and emotional makeup, and treatment needs to vary, reflecting these differences. BN behaviors tend to be marked by impulsivity, followed by "undoing" practices, such as various forms of purging. AN behaviors reflect behaviors and attitudes marked by rigidity, restriction, and containment.

Though ED are essentially not about food, their successful healing depends upon the resumption and maintenance of a healthy weight and relationship with food [22]. ED are disorders of the core self, characterized by diminished self-control, self-regulation, self-attunement, self-trust, self-agency, self-reliance, self-perception, self-sensing, and self-worth. A full ED recovery is defined by several factors, including the return of a healthy and sustainable eating lifestyle and relationship with food; the reintegration of the mind, brain, and body, reconstituting a fully integrated self; the arrival at one's set point weight; and a full restoration of healthful physiological functioning leading to the natural resumption of menstruation. Observable weight change is typically the factor that brings ED patients to treatment. Once in treatment, additional predictive assessment factors include the ED mentality, marked by perfectionistic, obsessive, black-and-white thinking, cognitive rigidity, the compulsive quality of behaviors, the intolerance of uncertainty, and the fear of gaining weight and becoming fat. It is important to note that many individuals with various forms of ED maintain a normal weight, a phenomenon observed particularly in BN and BED because of "weight cycling," where patients alternate between starvation and gorging or compulsive bingeing followed by compensatory forms of purging.

ED do not stand still; any ED that is not in the process of healing is becoming increasingly entrenched in the brain and nervous system, destroying life quality, if not taking lives.

> *Pamela suffers from BED. She is not overweight, as might be expected, the result of yo-yoing between gorging and starvation for days on end. Aware of her illness and her need for professional help, she spoke of her frustration in not having been able to get the attention of her family or the healthcare professional community, who refused to acknowledge that she had an ED because her weight was "normal." Having been denied treatment, compassion, much needed support and attention, upon arrival at my office, she spoke of feeling depressed, isolated, and hopeless.*

5. Weight management assessment as a form of crisis intervention

In looking beyond simple, nonlinear solutions for weight management problems, the single-session diagnostic assessment needs to become a discovery process, uncovering the possibility of underlying sources of symptoms in eating pathology or past trauma. In establishing a direction for future treatment, the assessment of DE or ED requires treatment tools of subtle refinement that investigate the patient's current disease and recovery status, as well as the history of past efforts to heal. Following Abraham Maslow's hierarchy of human needs [23], the weight management diagnostician attends to the needs of the patient in a sequence designed first to save lives through medical stabilization, then to remediate life quality through emotional stabilization. For ED patients, the need to refeed body and brain becomes a first priority in minimizing the patient's physiological risk, augmenting receptivity to the therapeutic process and to an environment conducive to the use of medication. Physiological or emotional instability that could result in self-harm or death demands an immediate referral to higher levels of care.

Psychoeducation lies at the core of the patient's engagement in the healing process as a mainstay of support, rectifying distorted attitudes and cognitive belief systems; introducing a deeper understanding of weight management problems and their implications; opening the patient's eyes and mind to insights and self-reflection; and creating the patient's sense of trust in the clinician and the clinical process as well as hope for a full recovery. Psychoeducation emphasizes the importance of maintaining a healthy eating and activity lifestyle to insure short-term and long-term goals for unified mind, brain, and body health. A psychoeducational explanation of the set point weight theory becomes critical in assuaging the AN patient's fear of excessive weight gain during refeeding by describing the wisdom of the human body, which, once having restored optimized bodily functioning, will sustain a constant weight. The AN patient also learns to anticipate that the natural course of ED recovery will involve countless trials and setbacks in regaining lost weight, with the recognition that every movement representing progress or regression represents "grist for the learning mill." Patients and clinicians need to anticipate the emergence of previously buried feelings during the refeeding process, evoking states of psychophysiological fear and/or emotional distress. Psychoeducation is also of great benefit for the parents of eating dysfunctional children or young adults living at home. Through family therapy, parents become knowledgeable about the complexities and risks involved with their child's eating dysfunctions and the urgent need for total healing. As advocates for their ED child's recovery, skillfully coached parents become, and remain, effective agents for positive change throughout an ever-changing treatment and recovery landscape.

Aside from psychoeducation, the work of the initial diagnostic session or series of early sessions needs to be richly flecked with trust-building and relationship building, along with an action plan, devised even prior to the development of a definitive diagnosis. The assignment of tasks such as journaling, requests for ongoing open and honest personal feedback, and contingency contracts all foster the patient's learning, trust, and treatment engagement. The initial session may include professional referrals to prospective members of a treatment team, as needed, initiating an integrative treatment process. Evoking motivation for change, the quality of the initial patient/clinician connection awakens the patient's recognition and acceptance of oneself, of co-occurring diagnoses that may require attention, and of the need for commitment to a treatment process that can accomplish full and sustainable healing. Aside from identifying current behaviors, levels of function, and past treatment and recovery efforts, history-taking needs to assess the patient's internal strengths, external resources, environmental influences and mood dysfunctions, always with attention to the possibility of past or current trauma. Studies that include partial or subclinical forms of posttraumatic stress disorder (PTSD) show that well over half of individuals with BN have PTSD or significant PTSD symptoms [24]. In light of the prevalence of trauma in the background of ED patients, trauma investigation needs to become a central focus within the initial inquiry. The diagnostician does well to become self-aware of personal propensities towards countertransference responses or cultural biases (reflecting weightism). The latter are forces which might preclude the clinician's recognition that many overweight and genetically large individuals who eat healthfully and exercise regularly are physically fit, healthy, and strong.

6. Medical ramifications of weight management in the treatment of DE and ED

A heavy burden of medical comorbidities across multiple body systems, attributable to both the malnutrition of AN and the purging behaviors of BN, contribute to the high mortality rates of these illnesses [25]. Restoration of weight and nutritional status are key elements in the treatment of AN [26]. Nutritional and medical treatment of extreme undernutrition present two very complex and conflicting tasks: the need to avoid "refeeding syndrome" caused by a too fast correction of malnutrition and "underfeeding" caused by a too cautious refeeding [27]. Metabolic, endocrinological, and gastronomic consequences that may develop during the refeeding process for ED individuals in recovery need to be understood and addressed in treatment. For the most part, but not in all cases, adverse consequences are reversible with recovery:

- Efforts of AN patients to restore weight within the refeeding process risk derailment due to the irrational fear that normal eating behaviors will ultimately lead to overweight or obesity following weight restoration. A psychoeducational discussion of optimal set point weight can potentially diminish fears through the knowledge that the body will maintain this optimized weight by using the same energy intake as had been needed for weight restoration. With metabolic normalization and biological functions coming back on line after their dormancy during weight restriction, the extra energy used previously for weight gain becomes expended on usual day-to-day functions [28].

- During initial phases of weight restoration, particularly for restricting ED patients who begin treatment at lower weights, the metabolic rate may overshoot normal levels in a "hypermetabolic" phase in which patients easily lose weight and need to eat an even larger amount of food to gain and sustain weight. This phenomenon is due to increased diet-induced thermogenesis (with calories dissipated as heat) as well as a variety of neuroendocrine alterations [26]. Despite the urgent need for the body to use restored energy efficaciously to replenish fat reserves and repair tissues in the early weeks and months of refeeding following prolonged semi-starvation, metabolic function may not normalize for 3–6 months following weight restoration [28].

- Target weights offer invalid markers of metabolic normalization, providing false indicators of ED recovery progress. It has been shown that ED patients forced to gain weight in hospital settings typically plan to lose it upon discharge [29]. Attempting to attain a target weight that is not reflective of the body's self-determined set point is predictive of a poor long-term prognosis.

Establishing and maintaining a goal-weight range is but one of many integrative physiological, neurobiological, nutritional, cognitive, emotional, and environmental factors contributing to a complete and sustainable ED recovery.

- Weight gain from edema (swelling or bloating) can be caused by hormonal changes brought on by starvation. AN can lead to kidney-related issues that include severe electrolyte disturbances (hypokalemia, hypophosphatemia, etc.), nephrolithiasis, and alterations in water metabolism (with hyponatremia and edema.) Patients with the binge eating/purging subtype of AN are more likely to have kidney disorders, particularly electrolyte disturbances and volume depletion, than those with the restrictive subtype. 'Refeeding edema' occurs during the process of weight restoration [30].

- Weight gain is a common side effect for people who take insulin to manage type 1 diabetes. The deliberate insulin underuse with type 1 diabetes for the purpose of controlling weight is known as diabulimia, a condition leading to a threefold increase in mortality risk [27].

- Sarcopenia, the loss of muscle mass in moderate to severe AN is frequently overlooked by clinicians. Appropriate exercise is required to restore muscle mass and strength [31].

- The strongest predictors of osteoporosis include low body weight and amenorrhea. Hormonally based bone softening and/or bone loss may never become restored to a state of normalcy, even following weight restoration.

- AN has consistently been associated with reduced gray matter and white matter brain volumes. It remains unclear if gray matter alterations are present following recovery from AN [32].

Issues complicating the achievement of full weight restoration matter a great deal, as halting the process of weight restoration at much lower levels than needed for full and sustainable recovery increases the rate of treatment dropout [33] and relapse [34]. The restoration of nutrient status and weight needs to start slowly and gradually, accelerating as tolerated. The refeeding process needs to focus on modifying the disordered dietary patterns that AN patients commonly practice, which might include slow and irregular eating, vegetarianism, and the consumption of a restricted range of foods. Severely malnourished AN patients often need to be admitted to a hospital in order to receive more aggressive treatment, with extra care and monitoring required to prevent the occurrence of refeeding syndrome [26], a clinical complication involving kidney dysfunction [30]. A person may finally be considered "in remission" after maintaining a stable weight for a number of years and experiencing the natural resumption of mensuration, as well as other normal hormonal, metabolic, and gastroenterological processes. Sustained remission is marked by the return of the reintegrated core self, following its fragmentation by the encroachment of the ED "pseudo-self."

7. Discovering and managing the roots of weight management problems in current or past trauma

Trauma in the form of sexual abuse occurs in 30–65% of women with ED [35]. The vast majority of women and men with AN, BN, and BED report a history of interpersonal trauma, with approximately one-third of women with BN meeting criteria for lifetime PTSD [36]. Unresolved trauma and/or PTSD can be an important perpetuating factor in the maintenance of ED symptoms [24]. DE and ED behaviors typically serve the patient as coping tools and distractions that numb the ongoing effects of traumatic memories. A trauma-focused approach to ED treatment facilitates the resolution of traumatic experience that lies at the root of behavioral, emotional, and neurobiological dysfunctions [37].

Unprocessed traumatic memories stored in the mid-brain region become recycled when triggered, creating undischarged energy in the nervous system. Any traumatic assault on, or insult to, the brain impairs brain integration. High stress levels that lead to an overactive amygdala and hippocampus suppress the activities of the prefrontal cortex, the thinking brain that helps to regulate emotions. Body dysmorphic disorder, a common occurrence in ED individuals traumatized by sexual abuse, represents a mind, brain, and body disconnection within the disparate nervous system. BN and AN pathology reflects the disintegration of the structure of the self within the distributed nervous system, resulting in the patient's inaccurate sensing of self-based experience and perception of self. Psychosomatic expressions of traumatic experience are held as bodily sensations. ED heal in the same way as trauma heals, through the neurophysiological and neurobiological reintegration of the distributed nervous system, marking the return of the patient's reintegrated core self [38]. Because traumatic memories are encoded subcortically, the process of healing ED that originate in trauma requires accessing, and gaining leverage within, the structural coding of the brain and nervous system.

Neurophysiological effects of past trauma that are revealed in the present become accessible and available for remediation [38]. Trauma resolution lies in creating a psychophysiological state associated with decreased adrenergic activity, decreased muscular neuromuscular arousal, and cognitive quieting [39]. The introduction of neurophysiological (sensorimotor) and neurobiological (interpersonal, attachment-based) treatment interventions into mainstream clinical treatment for ED increases exposure to mindful embodied movement experience, fostering mind, brain, and body connectivity. By stimulating integrative neuronal firing and synaptic activity, these "top-down" and "bottom-up" transactions enhance acuity in self-sensing, self-perception, and body image coherence, supporting the unification of the disparate self [38].

Trauma resolution becomes enhanced through a mindful, quality connection between the therapist and patient. Rapid resolution therapy (RRT) is a body-based talk therapy technique shown to alleviate negative effects of trauma and PTSD without requiring the patient to recollect painful memories [40]. Trauma resides in the limbic system and in the perceptual world within a neural network, which has sufficient functional boundary thresholds to largely "disintegrate" it from the rest of the nervous system. When negative feelings become dissociated or "split off" (as they do within the bulimic "pseudo-self"), the potential exists to reintegrate them through the patient's connection with his/her best and resourceful self, through solution discovery, or rediscovery, both past and present [40]. Trauma resolution accesses neuroplasticity, through which neural networks that become lit-up at the same time as the neural network associated with the problem result in the problem's loss of definition. This dynamic allows for a free flow of communication with the rest of the nervous system, as the brain reinterprets new combinations of neural connections to create meaning [40]. By creating connections within the distributed nervous system in the context of a trusted human relationship, the technique connects problems to solutions through consolidating memories of human strengths and resourcefulness.

For decades under the care of dietitians treating Charles' disordered eating, dieting efforts failed, leaving him intractably obese at 100 pounds overweight. Still "feeling fat" following bariatric surgery, he came to therapy struggling to lose weight through old patterns of food restriction, leading to junk food binges. At the start of our treatment, history-taking revealed past trauma at the root of his current eating dysfunction. Since childhood, Charles' family had been forced to flee a war-torn country with only a day's notice, leaving their previously comfortable lives and extended family behind. Moving from country to country, they struggled to survive as refugees, grieving their losses and experiencing years of fear, hunger, and social isolation. In response to the combined work of ED recovery and trauma resolution, within the context of our quality therapy relationship, Charles began to experience a sense of grounded integration and selfhood, evidenced in his growing capacity for self-regulation and self-care. Within several months of treatment, he became a normalized healthy eater and started to exercise regularly. Change in his distorted body image perception as a fat person became apparent when he reported, "During an exercise class, I noticed myself in the mirror and thought, 'Who is that normal weight person? Could that be me?' Despite his weight management problems and eating compulsions, the healthy personality at his core had resurfaced through psychotherapy. In completing his treatment, he described himself as having become "a happy and gratified human being, enjoying a fulfilled existence."

In some instances, a skilled practitioner may be capable of discovering trauma and shepherding the start of the trauma resolution process within the context of the initial time-extended single-session weight management assessment.

It was the sudden recurrence of compulsive bingeing habits that she'd assumed were "in remission" that brought this middle-aged woman with BED to treatment. "This is the one area of my life that has always remained just beyond my grasp .... all I know is that my hunger is insatiable." In probing for the possibility of past trauma, our discussion during that initial session uncovered the source of her erratic eating compulsions in feelings of shame, emptiness, and emotional lability originating in early childhood trauma, a connection that had remained outside of her consciousness for 45 years. Her memories of neglect, alienation, and hunger that she suffered at the hands of her parents throughout her growing-up years, having been buried for decades within her limbic brain, now began to surface. Her brain's rapidly firing neuronal connections brought forth immediate new insights into herself, her current feelings, and past emotions, evoking an enlightened clarity about her previously "incomprehensible, over-reactive responses" (sobbing tears, sleeplessness, irrational fears) in the face of certain types of stressful experiences throughout her life. She wept with relief and gratitude upon leaving, recognizing that significant and sustainable change for her would now be in the offing.

8. Conclusion

Weight management anomalies signify the patient's unhealthy relationship with food, potentially giving rise to chronic disease or the onset of genetically predisposed clinical eating disorders and the metabolic, endocrinological, or gastrointestinal consequences that characterize them. Uncovering the origins of weight management dysfunctions in DE or ED pathology, in providing a direction for treatment, enhances the efficacy and sustainability of healing. From the perspective of a hammer, all things look like a nail; in assessing weight management issues through a purely behavioral lens, first responders who fail to investigate and probe an underlying emotional landscape are likely to recommend a non-integrative solution, such as dieting, missing the opportunity to address the full complement of impinging psychological, neurobiological, and neurophysiological factors that contribute to weight management dysfunctions. Dieting, and particularly the use of unhealthful weight control behaviors, increase risk for weight gain and later eating- and weight-related problems [21].

It is through a unique use of self within the diagnostic moment that the knowledgeable and informed first responder approaches the uniquely challenging arena of weight management. By "listening with a third ear," the clinician with clear intention and exquisite sensitivity to implied and unspoken issues intuits and then skillfully addresses the possibility of a yet unknown and unnamed condition as part of a wider constellation of symptoms. The proactive diagnostician fosters the patient's self-reflection, self-acceptance, and incentive to heal dysfunctions sustainably at their source; increased self-esteem and positive body image have been shown to be best achieved through self-acceptance rather than weight reduction [41].

Research justifies the need for long-term implementation of interventions that aim to simultaneously prevent the onset of obesity and ED through the prevention of dieting behaviors and the promotion of healthful eating and physical activity as ongoing lifestyle behaviors [21]. Research reveals that fitness center employees, ideally placed to observe clients who exhibit an addiction-like relationship with exercise in an effort to lose weight as part of an ED, require detailed guidelines for intervention, including ways to start conversations to this end [42]. Bottom line, first responders need to determine whether the patient's desire for weight change is based on healthful choices and discretion, or on the dictates of pathological compulsions that underlie and drive dysfunctional eating behaviors. In either case, the diagnostician sets the stage for the patient's immediate and compelling engagement in integrative treatment, creating the potential to save lives and promote life quality.

Acknowledgments/Thanks

Heartfelt thanks, love, and gratitude to my husband Lou, who edited this chapter with devotion and enthusiasm.

Conflict of interest

The authors declare no conflict of interest.

Acronyms and abbreviations

DE	disordered eating
ED	eating disorders, eating disordered
BED	binge eating disorder
OSFED	other specified feeding or eating disorder
EDNOS	eating disorder not otherwise specified
OCD	obsessive-compulsive disorder
ARFID	avoidant restrictive food intake disorder
SPD	sensory processing disorder
PTSD	posttraumatic stress disorder
RRT	rapid resolution therapy

Author details

Abigail H. Natenshon
Eating Disorder Specialists of Illinois: A Clinic Without Walls, Highland Park, Illinois, United States

*Address all correspondence to: abigailnatenshon@gmail.com

IntechOpen

© 2020 The Author(s). Licensee IntechOpen. This chapter is distributed under the terms of the Creative Commons Attribution License (http://creativecommons.org/licenses/by/3.0), which permits unrestricted use, distribution, and reproduction in any medium, provided the original work is properly cited.

References

[1] Collins ME. Body figure perceptions and preferences among pre-adolescent children. International Journal of Eating Disorders. 1991;**10**:199-208

[2] Mellin L, McNutt S, Hu Y, Schreiber GB, Crawford P, Obarzanek E. A longitudinal study of the dietary practices of black and white girls 9 and 10 years old at enrollment: The NHLBI growth and health study. Journal of Adolescent Health. January 1997;**20**(1):27-37

[3] Smolak L. National Eating Disorders Association/Next Door Neighbors Puppet Guide Book. New York, NY; 1996

[4] Shisslak CM, Crago M, Estes LS. The spectrum of eating disturbances. International Journal of Eating Disorders. 1995;**18**(3):209-219

[5] Hudson JI, Hiripi E, Pope HG, Kessler RC. The prevalence and correlates of eating disorders in the National Comorbidity Survey Replication. Biological Psychiatry. 2007; **61**(3):348-358. DOI: 10.1016/j.biopsych.2006.03.040

[6] Becker AE, Grinspoon SK, Klibanski A, Herzog DB. Eating disorders. The New England Journal of Medicine. 1999;**340**:1092-1098

[7] Anorexia Nervosa and Associated Disorders. ANAD.org

[8] Stanford University Medical Center. Eating disorder cutoffs miss some of sickest patients, study finds. ScienceDaily. 19 April 2010. Available from: www.sciencedaily.com/releases/2010/04/100412075434.htm

[9] Reddy, S. A new genetic explanation for anorexia. The Wall Street Journal. Life and Arts: Your Health. 30 July 2019: A12

[10] Ayton A. The importance of restoring body fat mass in the treatment of anorexia nervosa: An expert commentary. Journal of Population Therapeutics and Clinical Pharmacology. 2019;**26**(3):e9-e13. DOI: 10.15586/jptcp.v26i3.629

[11] Keel PK, Mitchell JE, Miller KB, Davis TL, Crow SJ. Long-term outcome of bulimia nervosa. Archives of General Psychiatry. 1999;**56**(1):63-69

[12] Robinson E, Bachrach LK, Katzman DK. Use of hormone replacement therapy to reduce the risk of osteopenia in adolescent girls with anorexia nervosa. Journal of Adolescent Health. 2000;**26**(5):343-348

[13] Berczik K, Szabó A, Griffiths MD, Kurimay T, Kun B, Urbán R, et al. Exercise addiction: Symptoms, diagnosis, epidemiology, and etiology. Substance Use & Misuse. 2012;**47**(4): 403-417. DOI: 10.3109/10826084.2011.639120

[14] Golden NH, Schneider M, Wood C. Preventing obesity and eating disorders in adolescents. Pediatrics. 2016;**138**(3): 14-16. DOI: 10.1542/peds.2016-1649

[15] Kurth CL, Krahn DD, Nairn K, Drewnowski A. The severity of dieting and bingeing behaviors in college women: Interview validation of survey data. Journal of Psychiatric Research. 1995;**29**(3):211-225

[16] Smink FRE, van Hoeken D, Hoek HW. Epidemiology of eating disorders: Incidence, prevalence and mortality rates. Current Psychiatry Reports. 2012;**14**(4):406-414. DOI: 10.1007/s11920-012-0282-y

[17] Couturier J, Isserlin L, Norris M, et al. Canadian practice guidelines for the treatment of children and

adolescents with eating disorders. Journal of Eating Disorders. 2020;**8**:4. DOI: 10.1186/s40337-020-0277-8

[18] Malinauskiene V, Malinauskas R. Lifetime traumatic experiences and disordered eating among university students: The role of posttraumatic stress symptoms. BioMed Research International. 2018. DOI: 10.1155/2018/9814358. Article ID 9814358. pp. 10

[19] NIH. National Institute of Diabetes and Digestive and Kidney Diseases. Overweight and Obesity Statistics. August 2017. Available from: niddk.nih.gov

[20] American College of Obstetricians and Gynecologists. Obesity in adolescents. Committee Opinion No. 714. Obstetrics & Gynecology. 2017;**130**:e1 27–40

[21] Neumark-Sztainer D, Wall M, Guo J, Story M, Haines J, Eisenberg M. Obesity, disordered eating, and eating disorders in a longitudinal study of adolescents: How do dieters fare 5 years later? Journal of the American Dietetic Association. 2006;**106**(4):559-568

[22] da Luz FQ, Hay P, Touyz S, Sainsbury A. Obesity with co-morbid eating disorders: Associated health risks and treatment approaches. Nutrients. 2018;**10**(7):829. DOI: 10.3390/nu10070829

[23] Maslow AH. Motivation and Personality. New York, N.Y: Harper; 1954. ISBN: 978-0-66-041987-5

[24] Brewerton TD. Eating disorders, trauma, and comorbidity: Focus on PTSD. Eating Disorders. 2007;**15**(4):285-304. DOI: 10.1080/10640260701454311

[25] Arcelus JL, Mitchell AJ, Wales J, Nielsen S. Mortality rates in patients with anorexia nervosa and other eating disorders. A meta-analysis of 36 studies. Archives of General Psychiatry. 2011;**68**(7):724-731. DOI: 10.1001/archgenpsychiatry.2011.74

[26] Marzola E, Nasser JA, Hashim SA, et al. Nutritional rehabilitation in anorexia nervosa: Review of the literature and implications for treatment. BMC Psychiatry. 2013;**13**:290. DOI: 10.1186/1471-244X-13-290

[27] Goebel-Fabbri AE, Fikkan J, Franko DL, Pearson K, Anderson BJ, Weinger K. Insulin restriction and associated morbidity and mortality in women with type 1 diabetes. Diabetes Care. 2008;**31**(3):415-419

[28] Troscianko ET. How does metabolic rate really change after anorexia? Part 1. What is the relationship between energy intake, body weight, and metabolic rate in recovery from anorexia? Available from: www.psychologytoday.com-intl-blog-hunger-artist 201603 h. [Accessed: 30 March 2016]

[29] Roots P, Hawker J, Gowers S. The use of target weights in the inpatient treatment of adolescent anorexia nervosa. European Eating Disorders Review. 2006;**14**:323-328. DOI: 10.1002/erv.723

[30] Bouquegneau A, Dubois BE, Krzesinski J, Delanaye P. Anorexia nervosa and the kidney. American Journal of Kidney Disease. 2012;**60**(2):299-307. DOI: 10.1053/j.ajkd.2012.03.019

[31] Hao R, Guo H. Anorexia, undernutrition, weight loss, sarcopenia, and cachexia of aging. European Review of Aging and Physical Activity. 2012;**9**:119-127. DOI: 10.1007/s11556-012-0103-7

[32] Bang L, Rø Ø, Endestad T. Normal gray matter volumes in women recovered from anorexia nervosa: A voxel-based morphometry study. BMC Psychiatry. 2016;**16**:144. DOI: 10.1186/s12888-016-0856-z

[33] Fassino S, Pierò A, Tomba E, et al. Factors associated with dropout from treatment for eating disorders: A comprehensive literature review. BMC Psychiatry. 2009;**9**:67. DOI: 10.1186/1471-244X-9-67

[34] Steinhausen HC, Seidel R, Winkler MC. Evaluation of treatment and intermediate and long-term outcome of adolescent eating disorder. Psychological Medicine. 2000;**30**: 1089-1098

[35] Deep AL, Lilenfeld LR, Plotnicov KH, Pollice C, Kaye WH. Sexual abuse in eating disorder subtypes and control women: The role of co-morbid substance dependence in bulimia nervosa. The International Journal of Eating Disorders. 1999;**25**: 1-10

[36] Mitchell KS, Mazzeo SE, Schlesinger MR, Brewerton TD, Smith BN. Comorbidity of partial and sub-threshold PTSD among men and women with eating disorders in the National Comorbidity Survey Replication Study. The International Journal of Eating Disorders. 2012;**45**(3): 307-315. DOI: 10.1002/eat.20965

[37] Ross CC. Eating Disorders, Trauma, and PTSD. National Eating Disorders Association. 2017. Available from: https://www.nationaleatingdisorders.org/blog/eating-disorders-trauma-ptsd-recovery

[38] Natenshon AH. Reclaiming the lost self in the treatment of bulimia nervosa: A neurobiological approach to recovery that integrates mind, brain, and body. In: Himmerich H, Jáuregui Lobera I, editors. Anorexia and Bulimia Nervosa. Croatia: IntechOpen; 2019. DOI: 10.5772/intechopen.83844. Available from: https://www.intechopen.com/books/anorexia-and-bulimia-nervosa/reclaiming-the-lost-self-in-the-treatment-of-bulimia-nervosa-a-neurobiological-approach-to-recovery-that-integrates-mind-brain-and-body

[39] Everly GS Jr, Benson H. Disorders of arousal and the relaxation response: Speculations on the nature and treatment of stress-related diseases. International Journal of Psychosomatics. 1989;**36**(1-4):15-21

[40] Quintal JS. Trauma resolution treatment; rhizomatics and the processes of change. In: Proceedings of the Selah Freedom: Bringing Light into the Darkness of Sex Trafficking. Conference; 8-9 November (2018) Winnetka, Illinois. 2018

[41] National Task Force on the Prevention and Treatment of Obesity. Dieting and the development of eating disorders in overweight and obese adults. Archives of Internal Medicine. 2000;**160**(17):2581-2589. DOI: 10.1001/archinte.160.17.2581

[42] Colledge F, Cody R, Pühse U, et al. Responses of fitness center employees to cases of suspected eating disorders or excessive exercise. Journal of Eating Disorders. 2020;**8**:8. DOI: 10.1186/s40337-020-0284-9

Chapter 11

Warming in Anorexia Nervosa: A Review

Emilio Gutiérrez and Olaia Carrera

Abstract

Anorexia nervosa (AN) is a severe psychiatric condition primarily affecting young women, and AN has the highest mortality rate among psychiatric disorders. AN continues to be a disorder refractory to psychological or pharmacological treatment. An innovative approach arises from research in rats simultaneously placed on a restricted feeding schedule and given free access to an activity wheel. The detrimental effects of combining diet and exercise in rats can be reversed by a manipulation of ambient temperature (AT). Warming animals exposed to these experimental arrangements reverses running activity, preserves food intake, and enables rats to recover from acute weight loss. This represents a strong preclinical evidence that provides a rationale for a translational approach for the treatment of AN. However, heat application to AN patients was already a recommendation made by William Gull in his seminal paper on AN disorder. A historical perspective of supplying heat to AN patients reviews the circumstances and foundation of this practice. The manipulation of AT in activity-based anorexia (ABA) rats has ended with a period of neglect of AT that parallels the complete neglect of the role of AT in the human AN disorder, either as a risk factor, as a modulating factor in the course of the disorder, or in terms of its utility in the treatment of AN.

Keywords: heat treatment, translational research, ambient temperature, animal research, hyperactivity

1. Introduction

A recent publication analysing the top 100 most cited works on AN reported that only 12 of these papers dealt with treatment, leading the authors to conclude that much work is required to translate 'progress in other areas into effective therapeutic strategies' ([1], p. 13). In contrast to the dearth of literature on treatment, the category encompassing the largest number of papers, 35, addressed the mechanisms underlying the disorder, i.e. 'papers examining diverse theories on AN aetiology and/or maintenance, including family linkage analyses, genetic and heritability studies, biological theories, personality, as well as psychosocial and cultural factors' ([1], p. 10). Moreover, the enterprise of translating theory into effective therapeutic strategies appears to be more challenging than expected. For example, only about 10% of the 4500-word paper, 'Building a model of the aetiology of eating disorders by translating experimental neuroscience into clinical practice' [2], is dedicated to the implications for treatment.

As stated elsewhere [3, 4] given the astonishing contemporary panorama of an absence of psychopharmacological treatments for AN, research with animal analogous models of the human disorder may be helpful in generating new hypotheses for improving AN treatment. A recent example of treatment translation is the reported anxiolytic effect of warmth in anorexia nervosa [5]. In this study postprandial anxiety was significantly reduced in patients resting immediately after lunch for half an hour in a room at 32°C. Bearing in mind the high level of premeal anxiety characteristic of AN patients [6], the significant decrease in postprandial anxiety in warmed AN patients was considerably greater than that achieved by conventional treatments in patients with comparable levels of premeal anxiety such as exposure and response prevention [7].

Interestingly, recent research has underscored the paramount importance of ambient temperature (AT) in the development and more importantly on the reversal of exhaustive running activity, severe weight loss, and self-starvation in rats simultaneously placed on a restricted feeding schedule and given free access to an activity wheel [8–12]. Although self-starvation in rats exposed to this experimental arrangement was first described in the mid-1960s of the twentieth century [13], the term activity-based anorexia (ABA) quickly became dominant describing both the experimental procedure and its resulting behavioural outcome [14]. ABA stands as the best animal model reproducing the main signs of AN (overactivity, extreme weight loss, restricted eating, hypothermia, disturbed sleep, alterations in hypothalamic-pituitary-adrenal/gonadal axis, alterations in diverse appetite-regulating hormones, and severe reductions in grey and white brain matter volume).

Supplying rats exposed to ABA with heat (AT raised to 32°C) reversed excessive activity, improved food intake, and allowed body weight recovery in animals. This reversion was particularly noteworthy as three circumstances concurred in these animals: (a) the increase in AT was delayed until rats had lost 20% of body weight, a point where the spontaneous recovery of rats is unattainable by the animals themselves; (b) animals continued being exposed to the 1.5 h/day restricted food schedule and unrestricted access to the activity wheel; and (c) increased AT allowed for nearly 100% recovery in warmed rats, but there was no single recovery for animals maintained at room temperature (21°C), and a 100% of animals had to be removed to prevent death. This experimental effect of AT has been demonstrated in both male and female animals [10–12].

A more conclusive outcome regarding food intake and body weight was reported in a study [12] where sedentary rats housed at 21°C were food deprived (1.5 h/day) during the first phase of the study that lasted a week. During Phase 2, the animals continued to be submitted to the same restricted feeding schedule for two additional weeks, but AT was increased to 32°C for half of the animals, whereas the other half was maintained at 21°C.

During Phase 2, on average all the animals increased food intake in comparison with Phase 1, but animals maintained at 21°C ate on average 21.5% more than animals housed at 32°C. However, in terms of body weight, only the warmed animals gained a significantly greater amount of weight, and by the end of the experiment, both groups had a similar body weight.

Thus, according to the results, in terms of body weight gain, a warmer environment was more effective than overall food consumption as the buffering effect of higher AT on heat dissipation helped the body weight gain in warmed rats.

In line with this effect of AT on body weight, the same beneficial effect of warming would be expected in AN patients during weight restoration programmes. Moreover, the rate of body weight would be preserved even under a lower caloric supplementation provided that the standard AT of hospital wards was raised. Thus, we should bear in mind the difficulties patients have in gaining weight despite the elevated caloric intake during conventional nutritional rehabilitation programmes [15] and that roughly a third of ingested calories cannot be processed by patients and are dissipated through elevated diet-induced thermogenesis [16, 17] that further heightens the anxiety of AN patients [18]. Recent data indicate that heat is crucial for reducing anxiety following meals when patients remain in a warmer environment at 32° [5].

Unfortunately, the manipulation of AT in ABA rats has been overlooked [19] which deprived us from recognizing the pivotal role of AT in the fate of rats exposed to ABA. Likewise, AN research has also been susceptible to a conspicuous neglect concerning the role of AT in the human disorder, either as a risk factor, as a modulating factor in the course of the disorder, or last but not least its potential in the treatment of AN.

A historical review of the literature reveals that the suggestion of keeping patients warm is not new, since supplying AN patients with heat was first recommended by William Gull [20]. Undoubtedly, the practice of supplying patients with heat was justified by the evidence accrued by a Swiss physiologist, Charles Chossat (1796–1875), [21] with starved animals.

2. First report of heat for the treatment of AN patients: back to the nineteenth century

Although applying heat to AN patients was first prescribed by William Gull (1816–1890) in 1874, this recommendation has been overlooked for over 140 years. On Friday, October 24, 1873, William Gull first reported the use of an external heat supply to AN patients in his seminal presentation on AN to the Clinical Society of London which was published the following year in the Transactions of the Clinical Society of London [20]: 'I have observed that in the extreme emaciation, when the pulse and respiration are slow, the temperature is below the normal standard. This fact together with the observation made by Chossat on the effect of starvation on animals, and their inability to digest food in the state of inanition, without the aid of external heat, has direct clinical bearings—it being often necessary to supply external heat as well as food to patients. The best means of applying heat is to place an india-rubber tube, having a diameter of 2 inches and a length of 3 or 4 feet, filled with a hot water along the spine of the patient, as suggested by Dr. Newington, of Ticehurst' (p. 24).

Gull's recommendation was based on the early preclinical animal starvation studies performed by Chossat who discovered the healing effects of heat on starved animals. Charles Chossat, a physiologist, physician, and politician from Geneva [22], performed detailed observations on the consequences of starvation in different species. Chossat's main work, Recherches expérimentales sur l'inanition [21], advanced many of the findings now established by experimental physiology on the effects of starvation on the contribution to weight loss by the different organs and tissues in animals starved to death. Thus, Ancel Keys and his colleagues in the Minnesota Starvation Experiment found the quantitative experimental studies of Chossat 'were surprisingly elaborate for the time' ([23], p. 198). Furthermore, in Chapter 9, entitled 'Morphology of Some Organs and Tissues', the authors pay tribute to the work of Chossat in the section 'The History of an Error' referring to the erroneous assertion in the physiology textbooks regarding the absence of cardiac atrophy as a result of undernutrition and starvation in spite of the different findings of Chossat [21] regarding heart atrophy in starved animals.

In the 47-page fourth chapter of Recherches expérimentales sur l'inanition, entitled 'Du réchauffement artificiel', Chossat describes the results of 13 experiments on the warming-up of 26 different animals (17 turtledoves, 7 pigeons, 1 hen, and 1 guinea pig), after being starved close to death. The effects of heat on starved animals shocked Chossat himself: 'I confess that this was not without the vivid satisfaction that I saw an animal arrived in a way by the starvation to the last term of the insensitivity, the prostration and the cooling, to revive somehow, and to retake very quickly a big degree of force muscular and of sensitivity, and it without food, without drink, and without other help than the application of the artificial heat' ([21], p. 595, translated from the original in French).

The first animal to be successfully revived was a turtledove with 35% weight loss and a 23°C body temperature (19° below baseline temperature). As a result of rewarming, Chossat observed that 'The appetite comes back at the animal's inanities that one resuscitates by the artificial warming-up; because one sees them leaving the steams and going to tickle everything that they can meet' ([21], p. 604).

However, Chossat found that the recovery of appetite was not necessarily equal to the recovery of the digestive faculties of the animals, as they could not digest food when artificial rewarming was suspended: 'The digestion takes place, on the contrary, while continuing the artificial warming-up during one sufficient time' ([21], p. 605).

Furthermore, Chossat described the purposeful thermoregulatory behaviour of the animals which actively sought the warm walls of the heater: 'I noticed that as the animals took their strength and their temperature, that they preferred to remain perched more and more on the edge of their steams, a position that they often preserved during several consecutive hours, receiving hardly a small amount of heat. It also happened to them to leave the steams and, when they had gotten more or less cold, often one saw them bringing closer to the stove and to warm themselves against its walls' ([21], p. 615).

Was this the first example of translation from lab findings to human treatment?

According to William Gull's reference to Chossat's work, there is uncertainty as to whether the idea of applying heat to patients in advanced malnutrition was developed in Ticehurst in direct relation to Chossat's studies or whether it was William Gull himself who associated the work of Chossat to the use of a heating device. In any case, regardless of who had established the connection with the work of Chossat, there is no doubt that supplying heat to patients represents the first example of translation of basic scientific findings in a laboratory setting into potential treatments for AN patients.

2.1 Ticehurst Asylum, the Newington's, and William Gull: the first extrapolation of applied heat from animals to humans

Gull's description of warming AN patients in advanced starvation was based on a device employed at the Ticehurst Asylum, which was widely acclaimed in political and medical circles as one of the most successful and highly reputable private asylums in England [24, 25], and Gull was the consultant who completed the required medical certification of some of the wealthy clientele who were admitted to Ticehurst [24]. Ticehurst Asylum was licenced as a private madhouse in 1792, and Samuel Newington (1739–1811), an apothecary and surgeon, was the first Newington in charge of the asylum erected in the grounds of his home, The Vineyard. Five generations of doctors from the Newington family, a 'long established' Ticehurst family since the fifteenth century, owned and managed Ticehurst.

How this heat application method was adopted in Ticehurst Asylum is uncertain, but the inventions of the Newingtons to facilitate the feeding of patients refusing voluntary feeding were inaugurated by Charles Newington (1781–1852), who published the description of 'An instrument invented for administering food and medicine to maniacs by the mouth during a closed state of the teeth' [26]. According to Charles Newington's obituary as printed in a local chronicle, he was a very ingenious man, and 'Amongst his numerous inventions, was that of an instrument for feeding those who were bent on self-destruction by starvation. This, in its present modified form, is still used, and has never been known to fail' ([27], p. 55). Following the tradition inaugurated by Charles Newington, his grandson Theodore Newington published a description of an instrument developed while he served as an assistant medical officer at the Bethlem Royal Hospital. The instrument, a nasal tube, allowed feeding patients refusing eating without 'the necessity of having to open the mouth, which, with patients with good teeth and strong jaws, is sometimes exceedingly difficult' ([28], p. 83).

The relationship between William Gull and Ticehurst probably commenced after 1871 with his appointment as a consultant physician [29], a period when the asylum was run by Charles Newington's grandchildren, Dr. Herbert Francis Hayes Newington (1847–1917) and his cousin Dr. Alexander Samuel Lysaght Newington (1846–1914, Theodore Newington's brother). By 1873, Sir William Gull had been awarded the title of Baronet for his successful treatment of the Prince of Wales for a bout of typhoid fever. As an influential physician, Gull medically certified wealthy clientele admitted to Ticehurst, and his visit to Ticehurst Asylum in May 1876 was documented with his confirmation of the diagnosis of general paralysis by Hayes Newington [24].

Another unresolved question concerns the paternity of the idea of applying heat to patients. Undoubtedly, William Gull, lecturer in physiology and comparative anatomy at Guy's Hospital from 1846 to 1856 [30], was familiar with the work of Chossat and in particular his work Recherches expérimentales sur l'inanition [21] which was awarded with the Montyon Prix in experimental physiology in 1841 by the Académie des Sciences de Paris.

Furthermore, the successive members of the Newington family running Ticehurst had completed their academic training in prestigious universities including Oxford and Cambridge. The work of Chossat had extensive diffusion in England both in academic circles and even among laypeople. For example, as soon as Chossat's work was published, it was included in 1844 in the 16th volume of *The Edinburgh Medical and Surgical Journal* whose mission was 'exhibiting a concise view of the latest and most important discoveries in medicine, surgery, and pharmacy' [31]. In the same year, the Analytical and Critical Reviews section of June–April 1844 of the *British and Foreign Medical Review; or Quarterly Journal of Practical Medicine and Surgery* [32] included a harsh critical commentary on Chossat's work criticizing the suffering inflicted on the animals. Thus, almost 30 years before Gull's speech before the Clinical Society of London, a direct link had already been explicitly established between Chossat's 'ingenious experiment of placing animals, whose death seemed impending, under the influence of artificial heat' and the application of heat to people suffering starvation: 'This is evidently a point of much practical importance; and the neglect of sufficient artificial calorification, or the too early suspension of it, has doubtless been a frequent cause of the want of success of the means taken to recover inanitiated persons' ([32], p. 354).

Furthermore, the studies performed by Chossat were readily available even to laypeople in England and were extensively commented in the first scientific dissemination book for the general public written by George H. Lewes (1817–1878): *The Physiology of Common Life* [33]. Written the same year as *On the Origin of Species* by Charles Darwin (1809–1892), Lewes' book was first serialized in *The Cornhill Magazine* [34]. Chapter VII of Volume I, entitled 'Why we are warm, and how we keep so' ([34], pp. 281–315), includes a detailed description of Chossat's starvation experiments that Lewes concluded 'are well known and the results are accessible in almost every text-book' ([34], p. 352). Chossat work was once again reported in *The Cornhill Magazine* [35], mostly read by laypeople in England. The 1861 Russian translation of *The Physiology of Common Life* made a profound impression on the adolescent Ivan Pavlov, who as an elderly man could still quote long sections from it [36].

However, regardless of whether it was Gull or one of the Newingtons who was acquainted with the work of Chossat, the question remains as to why the application of heat was not maintained as a standard strategy and vanished as a treatment for AN patients. Gull's lecture was widely echoed in publications. On November 1, 1873, 1 week after his speech before the Clinical Society of London, the discussion by the attending physicians was included in the Report of the Societies' section in *The British Medical Journal* [37]. The report in *The British Medical Journal* also appeared across the Atlantic in what was to be the last edition of *The Half-Yearly Abstract of the Medical Sciences* published in Philadelphia in 1873 [38].

Although there were several references to the relevance of warming for the treatment of AN patients in the years following Gull's 1874 paper, the interest appears to have waned by the turn of the century. One of the last mentions appeared in the editorial of *The Lancet* issued a week after what happened to be Gull's last publication, a case note of a patient with AN stating 'The cure consists of three things—rest, warmth, and the regular and frequent introduction of food, in utter disregard of the anorexia of the patient' ([39], p. 584).

As far as we are aware, despite the clinical bearing mentioned by Gull, we have found no justification for abandoning his specific recommendation, either founded on its verified clinical uselessness or due to a theoretical reasoning that would render it obsolete or any other reason for it falling into disuse. A plausible explanation is that the initiation of forced feeding displaced the use of heat. As mentioned elsewhere [40], during a 63-day time span following Gull's last publication in 1988, a total of eleven articles appeared commenting Gull's last paper, of which four mentioned force feeding as the optimal strategy: 'forcible administration of nourishment so very simple a process that there need be no hesitation in resorting to it when necessary; these are at once safe and effective, and by their means nutrition can not only be carried on for an indefinite length' ([41], p. 597). Forced feeding had already been voiced by two doctors (Dr. Williams and Dr. Edis) during the discussion that followed Gull speech before the Clinical Society of London on October 24, 1873, but there was no mention on the employment of heat or to Chossat in the minutes of the meeting reported in *The British Medical Journal* [37].

One of the last mentions of the use of heat in the nineteenth century appeared in the first documented necropsy of a patient who died of self-starvation, which noted that all efforts were made to maintain her warm even by wrapping the patient with bandages [42].

In the twentieth century, references to warming AN patients were scarce. Dejerine and Gauckler refer to warming in their treatise *The Psychoneuroses and Their Treatment by Psychotherapy* when they stated 'It may happen that, among certain patients who are extremely weak, one is obliged to seek for aid from ordinary medical therapy; one may thus to give injections of serum, or hypodermics of caffeine, or camphor oil, to warm the patient by artificial means' ([43], p. 321). In 1931, a clinical report [44] informed a treatment of a series of 20 cases of functional anorexia treated at Ruthin Castle, a private hospital (1923–1950) for the investigation and treatment of obscure medical diseases [45], in which patients were kept in bed in a warm room (although the recommended room temperature was unusually low, 60°F, for today's standards). Likewise, in the same decade, two German psychiatrists [46] mentioned in their report on the treatment of a 17-year-old girl the use of heating pads and an electric blanket for heating patients. Later, the use of electric blankets was considered by psychoanalysts not on face value but as a regressive substitute of the umbilical cord: 'Our patient who lay in bed curled up 'attached' to the wall via the electric cord of a heater resting on her abdomen' ([47], p. 395). Furthermore, this blurring of warming is evident in the only figure that appears in Selvini-Palazzolli's book, *Self-Starvation: From the Intrapsychic to the Transpersonal Approach to Anorexia Nervosa* [48]. On page 65 there is an illustration of the analysis of a dream (the ugly yellow dog's dream). In the picture drawn by the adolescent, she appears sitting on the floor covering her mouth while her mother looks from behind a hole in the wall. The girl's back rests on the radiator of the wall, an aspect that is not mentioned at all in the psychoanalytic interpretation.

In relation to the historical journey regarding the use of heat as an adjunctive treatment for AN patients, it is worth noting two spontaneous improvements due to febrile conditions reported by Lasègue [49] and Weizsäcker [50].

Since then, as far as we are aware, we have had to wait until the end of the twentieth century to see the reintroduction of the use of heat in three cases treated with three different strategies of heat application: continuous exposure to a warm environment, wearing a thermal waistcoat, and sauna baths in an infrared cabin [51]. Besides putting an end to the long period of persistent disregard for the role of AT in AN, this paper demands a place for ABA research in AN treatment development.

3. Uncovering the neglected role of ambient temperature in anorexia nervosa

With the exception of research on the effect of season of birth on the subsequent development of anorexia nervosa, AT has been neglected by researchers [52]. However, the first reference to the probable relationship of AN and AT appeared in an editorial in *The Lancet* on March 24, 1888 with a commentary on the paper published by W. Gull on AN that appeared the preceding week in the journal: 'Most of the cases seem to occur in the colder months of the year, and possibly this may be more than a coincidence' ([53], p. 584).

There is growing evidence that AT merits more attention in future research given its paramount importance with respect to several relevant signs of AN such as hyperactivity, body weight, and amenorrhea. Furthermore, there is indirect evidence that the world incidence of the disorder is bound not only to culture but to latitude too [54].

The relevance of AT on the body weight and physical activity of AN patients was first revealed in a study in which adolescent patients with AN showed significantly higher physical activity during the colder months of the year, October to April, than in the warmer months, April to October [55]. In contrast, patients from the warm group were less underweight than those of the cold group. The relationship between AT and physical activity was confirmed by analysing a subset of eight patients with a temperature difference of 6°C on two consecutive days during the monitoring of the patients' physical activity. The physical activity of these patients was significantly higher on colder days, confirming the modulating role of environmental temperature over physical activity beyond the eventual regulatory function of anxiety and negative effect or relevant dimensions of eating psychopathology as body dissatisfaction and drive for thinness. This within subject analysis discarded that the association between AT and activity was mediated by other climatic aspects associated with AT, such as day length or seasonality. It is remarkable that the greater activity of ANR patients during the winter months contrasts with that reported at temperate latitudes for normal body weight people where physical activity decreases in the colder months of the year [56].

Related to the finding of lower body weight and BMI in AN patients during the colder months of the year, a retrospective study covering admissions during a 3-year period (2007–2010) of an adolescent inpatient eating disorders unit revealed that AT was a modulating factor in body mass index (BMI) at hospital admission [52]. The study revealed that AN restrictive (ANR) subtype patients differ from AN binge/purging (ANB/P) subtype patients with respect to the body weight fluctuation pattern throughout the year. The study revealed that differences between both diagnostic subtypes only occurred during the cold semester, revealing that the differences were due to the inverted annual pattern of body weight fluctuation in both groups of patients. Thus, while annual fluctuations in the weight of ANB/P patients were similar to those of the general population, i.e. having a higher BMI during the colder months of the year and a lower one during the warmer months [57], the pattern for ANR patients was the opposite.

Bearing in mind the above, it is hardly surprising that, in comparison to the warm semester, ANR patients admitted to hospital during the colder season had a longer hospital stay, a finding which has been inconsistently replicated in two different German samples [58, 59]. Moreover, due to their lower body weight during the cold semester, ANR patients had longer hospital stays than ANBP patients [52]. Moreover, other researchers have provided strong evidence of the effects of AT on menses recovery in AN patients. During the warmer months of the year, probability of menses recovery was twice as high as in autumn or winter, despite the fact that body weight of the patients were 2 kg less in the warm season than in the cold season, which was directly associated to lower energy expenditure associated with thermoregulation in the spring and summer months [60].

A possible explanation for this pattern of higher activity and lower body weight in AN patients was advanced [19] as a dramatic example of the energy balance equation in which AN patients are locked up. Given their restrictive eating pattern, the lower the AT, the greater the weight loss and consequently the greater the increase in physical activity as a potential surrogate thermoregulation mechanism. However, as ABA research has shown, resorting to increased motor activity raises the body temperature in the short run, but the mobilization of fat reserves to maintain activity which supposes a reduction in body insulation. Moreover, deficient insulation resulting from reduced subcutaneous fat in AN reduces protection against environmental hazards as Arthur Crisp pointed out that 'Fat has general biological purposes as a reserve of energy and a contributor to body temperature regulation, both as a component of resting metabolic rate and, subcutaneously as insulation' ([61], p. 481). Thus, all other things being equal, given the stable restrictive energy intake of ANR patients, a colder environment would impose a greater demand for the maintenance of body temperature. In this scenario, increased physical activity would perform a thermoregulatory function rather than being driven exclusively by psychological factors such as excessive preoccupation with body weight and shape [62].

Besides the aforementioned influence of AT on the hyperactivity and body weight of AN patients, there is also an underreported active search for heat by AN patients. For example, this was the case with the conspicuous absence of reports in the literature of sauna baths as a weight-losing strategy among AN patients [63]. This complete absence of reports contrasted with spontaneous mentions of the use of sauna baths AN patients in their chats on the Internet [64]. It has been suggested that among the possibilities underlying the absence of reports of the use of saunas, there was a possibility that regular sauna bathing may either act in preventing predisposed adolescents from developing the 'full-blown' syndrome or accelerating recovery from AN [63]. Hence, it may be more than mere coincidence that in Finland, where saunas are a substantial part of Finnish culture, the 5-year clinical recovery rates for DSM-IV anorexia nervosa were as high as 68.4% in patients undetected by the health-care system [65].

Furthermore, there is evidence that the world incidence of the disorder could be bound not only to cultural influences but to climate and latitude too [54]. This seems to be the case according to the results gathered by means of a bibliometric perspective where the worldwide distribution of scientific publications was deemed to be an indirect indicator of the incidence and prevalence of the disorder at different latitudes. Two subsequent studies [66, 67] have reported that the distribution of references for anorexia nervosa have remained considerably stable over the last 25 years, associated to higher but not extreme latitudes and to climates with regular seasons with no severe temperature variations across seasons. Thus, references to AN condense into a 40–55° latitude range in the Northern Hemisphere which closely parallels with the vast majority of epidemiological studies undertaken on populations living in this latitude range in the Northern Hemisphere [68].

4. Conclusion: listening to Hippocrates (460–377 BCE)

One of the most important treatises in the *Hippocratic Corpus* entitled *On Airs, Waters and Places* wisely begins with 'Whoever wishes to pursue properly the science of medicine must proceed thus. First, he ought to consider what effects each season of the year can produce; for the seasons are not at all alike, but differ widely both in themselves and at their changes' ([69], p. 71). Without any reasonable doubt, AT has been systematically overlooked in AN research, which has hindered a better understanding of the use of heat in the treatment of AN.

Acknowledgements

The preparation of manuscript and research reported was supported by the research budget of the Unidad Venres Clinicos (University of Santiago de Compostela). The funding sources had no involvement either in the writing of the manuscript or in the decision to submit the paper for publication.

Conflict of interest

The authors declare no conflict of interest.

Author details

Emilio Gutiérrez[1,2*] and Olaia Carrera[2]

1 Department of Clinical Psychology and Psychobiology, College of Psychology, University of Santiago, Santiago de Compostela, Spain

2 Venres Clínicos Unit, College of Psychology, University of Santiago, Santiago de Compostela, Spain

*Address all correspondence to: emilio.gutierrez@usc.es

IntechOpen

© 2020 The Author(s). Licensee IntechOpen. This chapter is distributed under the terms of the Creative Commons Attribution License (http://creativecommons.org/licenses/by/3.0), which permits unrestricted use, distribution, and reproduction in any medium, provided the original work is properly cited.

References

[1] Lipsman N, Woodside DB, Lozano AM. Trends in anorexia nervosa research: An analysis of the top 100 most cited works. European Eating Disorders Review. 2014;**22**:9-14. DOI: 10.1002/erv.2270

[2] Southgate L, Tchanturia K, Treasure J. Building a model of the aetiology of eating disorders by translating experimental neuroscience into clinical practice. Journal of Mental Health. 2005;**14**:553-566. DOI: 10.1080/09638230500347541

[3] Gutierrez E. A rat in the labyrinth of anorexia nervosa: Contributions of the activity-based anorexia rodent model to the understanding of anorexia nervosa. The International Journal of Eating Disorders. 2013;**46**:289-301. DOI: 10.1002/eat.22095

[4] Gutierrez E, Carrera O. Psychotherapy in anorexia nervosa: What does the absence of evidence mean? World Journal of Translational Medicine. 2014;**3**:150-157. DOI: 10.5528/wjtm.v3.i3.150

[5] Zandian M, Holmstedt E, Larsson A, Bergh C, Brodin U, Södersten P. Anxiolytic effect of warmth in anorexia nervosa. Acta Psychiatrica Scandinavica. 2017;**135**:266-267. DOI: 10.1111/acps.12691

[6] Steinglass JE, Sysko R, Mayer L, Berner LA, Schebendach J, Wang Y, et al. Pre-meal anxiety and food intake in anorexia nervosa. Appetite. 2010;**55**:214-218. DOI: 10.1016/j.appet.2010.05.090

[7] Steinglass JE, Albano AM, Simpson HB, Wang Y, Zou J, Attia E, et al. Confronting fear using exposure and response prevention for anorexia nervosa: A randomized controlled pilot study. International Journal of Eating Disorders. 2014;**47**:174-180. DOI: 10.1002/eat.22214

[8] Morrow NS, Schall M, Grijalva CV, Geiselman PJ, Garrick T, Nuccion S, et al. Body temperature and wheel running predict survival times in rats exposed to activity-stress. Physiology & Behavior. 1997;**2**:815-825. DOI: 10.1016/s0031-9384(97)00243-6

[9] Gutierrez E, Baysari M, Carrera O, Whitford T, Boakes R. High ambient temperature reduces rate of body-weight loss produced by increased activity. The Quarterly Journal of Experimental Psychology. 2006;**59**:1196-1211. DOI: 10.1080/17470210500417688

[10] Gutiérrez E, Cerrato M, Carrera O, Vázquez R. Heat reversal of activity-based anorexia: Implications for the treatment of anorexia nervosa. The International Journal of Eating Disorders. 2008;**4**:594-601. DOI: 10.1002/eat.20535

[11] Gutiérrez E, Churruca I, Zárate J, Carrera O, Portillo MP, Cerrato M, et al. High ambient temperature reverses hypothalamic MC4 receptor overexpression in an animal model of anorexia nervosa. Psychoneuroendocrinology. 2009;**34**:420-429. DOI: 10.1016/j.psyneuen.2008.10.003

[12] Cerrato M, Carrera O, Vázquez R, Echevarria E, Gutiérrez E. Heat makes a difference in activity-based anorexia: A translational approach to treatment development in anorexia nervosa. The International Journal of Eating Disorders. 2012;**45**:26-35. DOI: 10.1002/eat.20884

[13] Routtenberg A, Kuznesof AA. Self-starvation of rats living in activity wheels on a restricted feeding schedule. Journal of Comparative and Physiological Psychology.

1967;**64**:414-421. DOI: 10.1037/h0025205

[14] Epling WF, Pierce WD, Stefan LA. Schedule-induced self-starvation. In: Bradshaw CM, Szabadi E, Lowe CF, editors. Quantification of Steady-State Operant Behaviour. Amsterdam: Elsevier/North Holland Biomedical Press; 1981. pp. 393-396

[15] Kaye WH, Gwirtsman HE, Obarzanek E, George T, Jimerson DC, Ebert MH. Caloric intake necessary for weight maintenance in anorexia nervosa: Nonbulimics require greater caloric intake than bulimics. The American Journal of Clinical Nutrition. 1986;**44**:435-443. DOI: 10.1093/ajcn/44.4.435

[16] Moukaddem M, Boulier A, Apfelbaum M, Rigaud D. Increase in diet-induced thermogenesis at the start of refeeding in severely malnourished anorexia nervosa patients. The American Journal of Clinical Nutrition. 1997;**66**:133-140. DOI: 10.1093/ajcn/66.1.133

[17] Russell J, Baur L, Beumont P, Byrnes S, Zipfel S. Refeeding of anorexics: Wasteful not wilful. The Lancet. 1998;**352**:1445-1461. DOI: 10.1016/S0140-6736(05)61269-X

[18] Rigaud D, Verges B, Colas-Linhart N, Petiet A, Moukkaddem M, Van Wymelbeke V, et al. Hormonal and psychological factors linked to the increased thermic effect of food in malnourished fasting anorexia nervosa. The Journal of Clinical Endocrinology and Metabolism. 2007;**92**:1623. DOI: 10.1210/jc.2006-1319

[19] Gutierrez E, Vazquez R, Boakes R. Activity-based anorexia: Ambient temperature has been a neglected factor. Psychonomic Bulletin & Review. 2002;**9**:239-249. DOI: 10.3758/BF03196278

[20] Gull W. Anorexia nervosa (apepsia hysterica, anorexia hysterica). Transactions of the Clinical Society of London. 1874;**7**:22-28

[21] Chossat C. Recherches expérimentales sur l'inanition. Sciences Mathématiques et Psysiques. 1843;**8**:438-640

[22] Dreifuss JJ. Charles Chossat (1796-1875), physiologiste, médecin et homme politique genevois. Gesnerus. 1988;**45**:239-261. DOI: 10.5169/seals-521234

[23] Keys A, Brozek J, Henschel A, Mickelsen O, Taylor HL. The Biology of Human Starvation (2 vols.). Minneapolis: University of Minnesota Press; 1950. 1385 p. DOI: 10.5749/j.ctv9b2tqv

[24] MacKenzie C. Psychiatry for the Rich. A history of Ticehurst Private Asylum, 1792-1917. London: Routledge; 1992. 248 p

[25] Turner TH. A diagnostic analysis of the casebooks of Ticehurst house asylum, 1845-1890. Psychological Medicine. Monograph Supplement. 1992;**21**:1-70. DOI: 10.1017/S0264180100001016

[26] Newington C. An instrument invented for administering food and medicine to maniacs by the mouth during a closed state of the teeth. The Lancet. 1826;**10**:845-846. DOI: 10.1016/S0140-6736(02)95796-X

[27] Lower MA. The Worthies of Sussex. Geo. P. Bacon: Lewes; 1865

[28] Newington T. Feeding by the nose. The Lancet. 1879;**113**:83. DOI: 10.1016/S0140-6736(02)46035-7

[29] Silverman JA. Sir William Gull (1819-1890). Limner of anorexia nervosa and myxoedema. An historical

essay and encomium. Eat Weight Disord-ST. 1997;**2**:111-116. DOI: 10.1007/BF03339960

[30] Pearce JMS. Sir William Withey Gull (1816-1890). European Neurology. 2006;**55**:53-56. DOI: 10.1159/000091430

[31] Chossat C. Experimental researches on inanition. The Edinburgh Medical and Surgical Journal: Exhibiting a Concise View of the Latest and Most Important Discoveries in Medicine, Surgery, and Pharmacy. 1844;**61**:155-162

[32] Chossat C. Experimental researches on inanition; the memoir to which the prize for experimental physiology was adjudged by the academy of sciences in 1841. British and Foreign Medical Review: Or Quarterly Journal of Practical Medicine and Surgery. 1844;**XVII**:344-356

[33] Lewes GH. Physiology of Common Life(2 vols.). Edinburgh: William Blackwood; 1859. 485 p. DOI: 10.1037/12157-000

[34] Smith RE. George Henry Lewes and His "Physiology of Common Life", 1859. Proceedings of the Royal Society of Medicine. 1960;**53**:569-574

[35] Anstie FE. Over-eating and under-eating. Cornhill Magazine. 1863;**8**:35-47

[36] Boakes RA. From Darwin to Behaviourism: Psychology and the Animal Mind. Cambridge, UK: Cambridge University Press; 1984. 296 p. DOI: 10.1002/1520-6696 (198610)22:4<373::AID-JHBS2300220413>3.0.CO;2-Y

[37] Gull W. Anorexia Hysterica (Apepsia Hysterica). British Medical Journal. 1873;**2**:527-528

[38] Gull SG. Hysterical anorexia. The Half-Yearly Abstract of the Medical Sciences: Being a Digest and Continental Medicine, and of the Progress of Medicine and the Collateral Sciences. 1873;**LVIII**:41-44

[39] Gull W. Anorexia nervosa. The Lancet. 1988;**131**:516-517. DOI: 10.1016/S0140-6736(00)48519-3

[40] Silverman JA. Anorexia nervosa in 1888. The Lancet. 1988;**331**:928-930. DOI: 10.1016/S0140-6736(88)91726-6

[41] Adam J. Sir William Gull on Anorexia Nervosa. The Lancet. 1888;**131**:597. DOI: 10.1016/S0140-6736(00)48655-1

[42] Marshall CF. A fatal case of anorexia nervosa. The Lancet. 1895;**145**:149-150. DOI: 10.1016/S0140-6736(01)90912-2

[43] Dejerine J, Gauckler E. The Psychoneuroses and Their Treatment by Psychotherapy. J B Lippincott Company: Philadelphia, PA, US; 1913. 395 p. DOI: 10.1037/14543-000

[44] Allison RS, Belf MD, Davies RP. The treatment of functional anorexia. The Lancet. 1931;**217**:902-907. DOI: 10.1016/S0140-6736(00)30246-X

[45] Allison RS. Ruthin Castle: A private hospital for the investigation and treatment of obscure medical diseases (1923-1950). Ulster Medical Journal. 1977;**46**:22-31

[46] Grote LR, Meng H. Medical and psychotherapeutic treatment of endogenic magersucht. In: Kaufman MR, Heiman M, editors. Evolution of Psychosomatic Concepts. New York: International University Press; 1964. pp. 167-180

[47] Meyer BC, Weinroth LA. Observations on psychological aspects of anorexia nervosa; report of a case. Psychosomatic Medicine. 1957;**19**: 389-398. DOI: 10.1097/00006842-195709000-00006

[48] Selvini Palazzoli M. L'anoressia mentale. Dalla terapia individuale alla terapia familiare. Feltrinelli, Milano, 1963 (Trad. Self-Starvation. From the Intrapsychic to the Transpersonal Approach to Anorexia Nervosa). London: Human Context Books, Chaucer Publishing; 1974. p. 65

[49] Lasègue C. De l'anorexie hystérique. Archives Generales de Medecine. 1873;**21**:385-403

[50] Weizsäcker V. Dreams in endogenic magersucht. In: Kaufman MR, Heiman M, editors. Evolution of Psychosomatic Concepts. New York: International University Press; 1964. pp. 181-197

[51] Gutierrez E, Vazquez R. Heat in the treatment of anorexia nervosa patients. Eating and Weight Disorders. 2001;**6**:49-52. DOI: 10.1007/BF03339752

[52] Fraga A, Caggianesse V, Carrera O, Graell M, Morande G, Gutiérrez E. Seasonal BMI differences between Restrictive and purging anorexia nervosa subtypes. The International Journal of Eating Disorders. 2015;**48**:35-41. DOI: 10.1002/eat.22357

[53] Editorial: Sir William Gull on Anorexia Nervosa. The Lancet. 1888;**131**:583-584. DOI: 10.1016/S0140-6736(00)48620-4

[54] Gutierrez E, Carrera O, Vazquez R, Birmingham CL. Climate might be considered as a risk factor for anorexia nervosa? A hypothesis worth another look. Eating Behaviors. 2013;**14**:278-280. DOI: 10.1016/j.eatbeh.2013.05.006

[55] Carrera O, Adan RAH, Gutierrez E, Danner UN, Hoek HW, van Elburg AA, et al. Anorexia nerviosa: Hyperactivity in anorexia nervosa: Warming up not just burning-off calories. PLoS ONE. 2012;**17**:e41851. DOI: 10.1371/journal.pone.0041851

[56] Buchowski MS, Choi L, Majchrzak KM, Acra S, Matthews CE, Chen KY. Seasonal changes in amount and patterns of physical activity in women. Journal of Physical Activity & Health. 2009;**6**:252-261. DOI: 10.1123/jpah.6.2.252

[57] Dzien A, Dzien-Bischinger C. Seasonal fluctuation in body mass index. Clinical Nutrition. 2003;**22**:425-428. DOI: 10.1016/S0261-5614(03)00051-7

[58] Born C, de la Fontaine L, Winter B, et al. First results of a refeeding program in a psychiatric intensive care unit for patients with extreme anorexia nervosa. BMC Psychiatry. 2015;**15**:57. DOI: 10.1186/s12888-015-0436-7

[59] Kolar DR, Bühren K, Herpertz-Dahlmann B, Becker K, Egberts K, Ehrlich S, et al. Seasonal variation of BMI at admission in German adolescents with anorexia nervosa. PLoS ONE. 2018;**13**(9):e0203844. DOI: 10.1371/journal.pone.0203844

[60] Favaro A, Santonastaso P. Seasonality and the prediction of weight at resumption of menses in anorexia nervosa. Fertility and Sterility. 2008;**91**:1395-1397. DOI: 10.1192/bjp.180.6.480

[61] Crisp AH. A tale of corruption. British Journal of Psychiatry. 2002;**180**:480-482. DOI: 10.1192/bjp.180.6.480

[62] Gutiérrez E, Carrera O. Anorexia nervosa and body-image disturbance. Lancet Psychiatry. 2016;**3**:e9-e10. DOI: 10.1016/S2215-0366(15)00581-7

[63] Gutierrez E, Vazquez R, Beumont PJV. Do people with anorexia nervosa use sauna baths? A reconsideration of heat-treatment in Anorexia Nervosa. Eating Behaviors. 2002;**3**:133-142. DOI: 10.1016/S1471-0153(01)00051-4

[64] Vähäsoini A, Vazquez R, Birmingham CL, Gutierrez E. Unreported sauna use in anorexia nervosa: Evidence from the world-wide-web. Eating and Weight Disorders. 2004;**9**:50-55. DOI: 10.1007/BF03325045

[65] Keski-Rahkonen A, Hoek HW, Susser ES, et al. Epidemiology and course of anorexia nervosa in the community. The American Journal of Psychiatry. 2007;**164**:1259-1265. DOI: 10.1176/appi.ajp.2007.06081388

[66] Vazquez R, Carrera O, Birmingham L, Gutierrez E. Exploring the association between anorexia nervosa and geographical latitude. Eating and Weight Disorders. 2006;**11**:e1-e8. DOI: 10.1007/BF03327745

[67] Gutierrez E, Carrera O, Vázquez R, Puime A, Fraga A, Claver E. The association of anorexia nervosa and climate revisited: A bibliometric perspective. International Journal of Emergency Mental Health and Human Resilience. 2017;**19**:1-7

[68] Hoek HW. Review of the worldwide epidemiology of eating disorders. Current Opinion in Psychiatry. 2016;**29**:336-339. DOI: 10.1097/YCO.0000000000000282

[69] Jones WHS. Air, Waters and Places. Hippocrates Collected Works I. Cambridge, Massachusetts: Harvard University Press; 1923. 432 p. DOI: 10.4159/DLCL.hippocrates_cos-airs_waters_places.1923

Chapter 12

A Software-Assisted Qualitative Study on the Use of Music in People with Anorexia Nervosa

Briana Applewhite, Aishwarya Krishna Priya, Valentina Cardi and Hubertus Himmerich

Abstract

Anorexia nervosa (AN) is an eating disorder associated with a high mortality and an often chronic and disabling course. Thus, novel treatment options should be explored. We performed two focus groups with a total of six people with AN on their use of music and their thoughts about music as an additional therapeutic option. Interviews were transcribed and analyzed in-depth using the NVivo 12 software package. The most prevalent theme throughout the focus groups involved positive expressions, emotions and memories related to music. This theme occurred in ~25% of the data. The importance of music was the second most common theme. Negative feelings and memories associated with music accounted for only ~10% of all references. All six patients expressed that they see benefit in using music therapy as an adjunct to their current treatment. Our analysis shows that people with AN connect music mainly with positive emotions and memories. Therapists might think about applying music more frequently during their sessions with AN patients and consider adding music therapy to their overall treatment concept. However, the results also suggest that music can influence mood not only positively but negatively as well. Quantitative research in bigger patient samples and randomized clinical trials will be necessary to verify these results.

Keywords: music, music therapy, eating disorders, anorexia nervosa, qualitative research, NVivo software

1. Introduction

Anorexia nervosa (AN) is one of the eating and feeding disorders. This group is characterized by a persistently disturbed eating behavior, which leads to changes in food intake, impaired physical health and psychosocial problems. According to the Diagnostic and Statistical Manual of mental disorders (DSM)-5, people with AN show a restrictive eating behavior, a body weight that is significantly too low for age, sex, and developmental trajectory, fear of gaining weight and a disturbance in the perception of one's own body (body image disturbance) [1]. AN occurs in approximately 0.5% of the population, with women being affected about 10 times more often [2]. The risk of death in patients with AN is five times higher compared to people of the same age and gender [3]. The course of AN is often chronic and can lead to a permanent disability.

IntechOpen

The eating and feeding disorders cluster further includes bulimia nervosa (BN), binge eating disorder (BED), avoidant/restrictive food intake disorder (ARFID), pica and rumination disorder.

BN occurs in about 2% of the population with a male to female ratio of about 1:10 [2]. The main criteria for diagnosing BN are recurrent binge eating, compensatory behaviors and excessive concerns with body shape and weight [1]. BED is the most common eating disorder. It is about twice as common (approx. 4% of the population) as the BN, with the proportion of women in patients with BED being around 60% [2]. It is mainly characterized by binge eating without the use of compensation strategies [1]. ARFID is hallmarked by a restrictive eating pattern that leads to malnutrition; pica means the consumption of non-food; and rumination disorder features choking up and chewing food again. Within those eating disorders, clinical features may change over time, with some patients with AN changing to BN or BED. Therefore, we are dealing with a spectrum of eating disorders rather than well-defined disease entities [4].

According to the National Institute for Health and Care Excellence (NICE) [5], the main pillars of therapy for eating disorders such as AN are psychological therapy, diet counseling as well as weight and physical health monitoring. Additional therapies can be family therapy, occupational and art therapy. Despite the availability of these therapies, a recent study that examined acutely ill AN patients over 20 years showed that despite existing therapies, only about 30% recovered after about 10 years and only 60% after 20 years [6]. Thus, there is a demand for additional treatments, and music therapy could be such an additional approach.

In a recently conducted systematic review on the effects of music in people with or at risk for eating disorders, researchers found that the use of music as an adjunct treatment was beneficial in certain cases [7]. The review encompassed 16 studies and 3792 participants using music in an experimental or observational study. Important studies cited in this review found that listening to classical piano improved food consumption with inpatients with AN [8] and that a "vodcast" of visual images and soothing music favorably influenced eating behaviors in patients with AN [9].

Apart from music therapy, the role music as such plays in daily life is expansive. Essentially, all cultures produce and use music in some way. Whether that is listening to a favorite song or dancing at a wedding, music seems to have an expansive power of triggering an emotional response. It is used as a source of healing and can be used as of source of comfort for many. The value of music on a person's life is dependent on the context with which they hear it, how much they engage with it and the feeling that it evokes when listening to it [10]. Music can have transformative effects on stress levels and the autonomic nervous system. For instance, studies have shown that listening to slow and smooth music reduces blood pressure and regulates breathing, in comparison to fast paced music which can lead to increased blood pressure [11]. Music has also been shown to influence neurotransmission such as the amount of dopamine release [12].

We sought to conduct a software-assisted qualitative analysis of two in-depth interviews performed during focus groups with people with AN to find out how they use music in daily life, how they talk about music, and what they think about the therapeutic application of music. We used this qualitative approach, because we wanted to identify and conceptualize aspects of the use of music which are important for them [13–16].

2. Methods

Study participants: Six female patients between 22 and 49 years with AN were recruited at the inpatient eating disorders service at the Bethlem Royal Hospital and the outpatient eating disorders service at the Maudsley Hospital. Both hospitals are managed by the South London and Maudsley NHS Foundation trust (SLaM), London. Patients gave written informed content to participate in the focus groups. They also agreed that the focus group would be recorded and transcribed, the content analyzed, the results of this analysis harnessed for further service development and publication. They also agreed that their recorded and transcribed statements may be cited, potentially verbatim, in an anonymized way.

Study Design: Each patient took part in one of the two focus groups. The focus groups were advertised within both the inpatient and outpatient eating disorders units with posters including the information about the topic and the focus group's research purpose. In preparation of the group, a questionnaire was devised containing 15 questions on listening to music, making music and music as a therapeutic strategy in order to guide the in-depth interviews (see Appendix). The focus groups were recorded, transcribed and subjected to thematic and content analysis [13–16].

Procedure: For evaluation of the transcribed focus groups, we used the NVivo 12 software. NVivo is a qualitative data analysis computer software package for qualitative research on text-based information. It organizes and analyzes non-numerical or unstructured data and allows users to classify, sort and arrange information [17]. Using NVivo, themes were extracted, a word cloud developed, the most frequently used words, and the distribution of coded themes and references analyzed.

3. Results

Following the transcription of both focus groups from audio recordings, a list of 14 themes were extracted from the data collected. Using Nvivo 12 software, the themes derived from both focus groups highlight the effects music has on the participants lives, the emotions experienced while listening to music, as well as the sentiments expressed about music therapy and its uses when treating their AN. The themes generated are as follows: Benefit of Music Therapy, Frequency (of music listening), Genre Listened To, How Music Makes You Feel, Importance of Music, Interest In Music Therapy, Music Dislikes, Music Making, Music Preference, Negative Emotion Elicited, Negative Memory Association, Neutral Emotion Elicited, Positive Emotion Elicited, and Positive Memory Association. **Table 1** illustrates the codebook of the analysis along with the description of the theme, file number and number of references within the data.

A word cloud of the two interviews was developed of the 1000 most frequently used words throughout both focus groups to illustrate which words/phrases appeared most frequently throughout data collection. Words most frequently used are indicated by the larger text size. These include 'music,' 'think,' 'listen,' and 'feel,' suggesting that music elicits a thoughtful emotive reaction within individual participants (**Figure 1**). Music accounts for the most frequently used word amongst participants with a count of 378, while' think' had a count of 327 and 'feel' a count of 145 (**Table 2**).

The individual themes coded with the greatest number of text segments by participants include Music Preference, Positive Emotion Elicited, Positive Memory Association, Importance of Music and How Music Makes You Feel (**Figure 2**).

The themes were grouped into six main segments based on the content outlined by the participant in their responses: Music Therapy, Preference, Positives, Negatives, Neutrals, and Beliefs. The Positives grouping accounted for 25.1% of coded segments, while Preference and Beliefs accounted for 30.9 and 22.2%, respectively (**Table 3**).

Themes	Description	Files	References
Benefit of music therapy	What are the benefits one associates with music therapy?	2	9
Frequency	How often does one listen to music?	2	13
Genre listened to	What type of music one listens to?	2	10
How music makes you feel	What feelings does one experience because of music?	1	22
Importance of music	What value does music have on one's life?	2	24
Interest in music therapy	Is there an interest in the therapeutic uses of music therapy as well as attending a music therapy session?	2	9
Music dislikes	What music does one dislike?	2	14
Music making	Playing an instrument, singing, recording, composition etc.	2	6
Music preference	What does one prefer to listen to? (i.e. favorite artists, song, recording etc.)	2	21
Negative emotion elicited	Is there a negative emotion associated with music?	2	12
Negative memory association	Is there a negative memory associated with music?	2	9
Neutral emotion elicited	Is there an indifference/ impartiality to music?	2	6
Positive emotion elicited	Is there a positive emotion associated with music?	2	28
Positive memory association	Is there a positive memory associated with music?	2	24

Table 1.
Codebook with themes, their description, their appearance in only one or both focus groups and their frequency (extracted from NVivo 12).

Throughout both focus groups, the most commonly shared themes represented positive associations with music, in the form of Positive Memory Associations (28 references) and Positive Emotion Elicited (24 references). A commonality that participants shared throughout the focus group discussions were the positive emotions that music makes them feel. One patient described music as "(it) can be a comfort; it can be something to move you up... (it's) obviously something that's a release of emotions...and it definitely cheers me up and makes me more determined and motivated". This was a popular sentiment amongst and between the two focus groups, with one patient stating "(music) makes me feel good, content even."

The importance of music was also a common theme for participants accounting for 24 references within the data. Patients discussed the uses of music within their day to day life and through their recovery process. One patient stated "(music) gives you space to kind of like describe stuff that you can't necessarily put into words yourself," and serves as an "incentive" or "motivator" throughout their recovery process.

The most commonly discussed themes fall under the Preference grouping with a total of 64 references throughout both focus groups. Accounting for 30.9% of the coded references, patients discussed their music preferences in great detail (**Table 3**). Patients listed the genres they listened to and how often they listened, if they participated in making music, and their music dislikes. Music preference

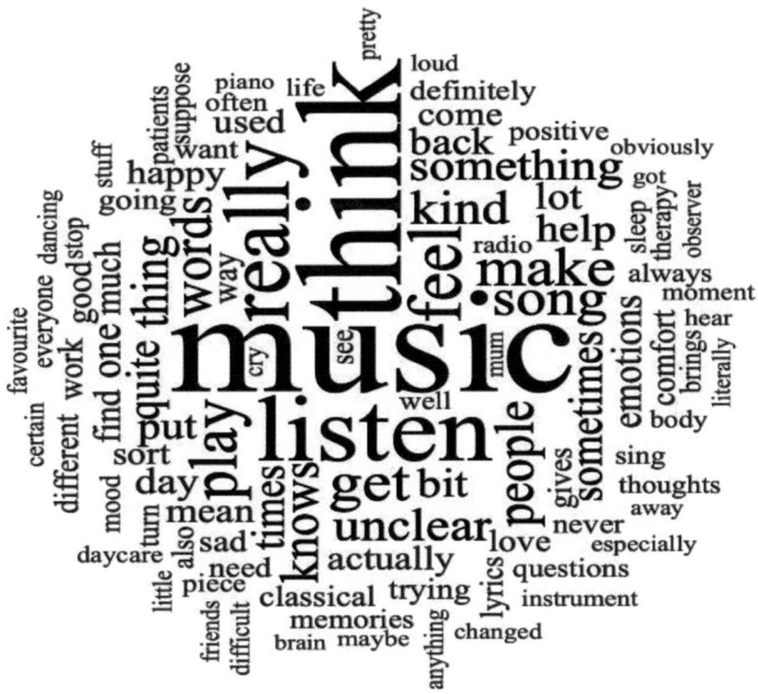

Figure 1.
Word cloud illustrating which words or phrases appeared most frequently throughout both focus groups.

Frequency rank	Word	Length	Count	Weighted percentage	Similar Words
1	Music	5	378	3.52%	Music, Musical, Music's
2	Think	5	327	3.04%	Think, Thinking
3	Listen	6	226	2.10%	Listen, Listening, Listens
4	Really	6	187	1.74%	Really
5	Feel	4	145	1.35%	Feel, Feeling, Feelings, Feels
6	Play	4	126	1.17%	Play, Played, Playful, Playing, Plays
7	Get	3	118	1.10%	Get, Gets, Getting
8	Make	4	115	1.07%	Make, Makes, Making
9	Song	4	106	0.99%	Song, Songs
10	Words	5	100	0.93%	Word, Words

Table 2.
Top 10 most frequently used words including weighted percentages.

accounted for 21 references within both focus groups where patients stated "classical" "pop" "soul" "literally anything" as the genre of choice as well as how they consume the music they listen to ("headphones," "iPod," "CD," "radio").

Neutral themes, defined as an indifference or impartiality to music, represented the smallest percent of coded references (3% of the coded data) (**Table 3**). However, Negative Emotion Elicited and Negative Memory Association accounted for 10.1% of all coded references (**Table 3**). Patients described music as channeling an emotion based on a certain song as well as having a negative memory linked to a

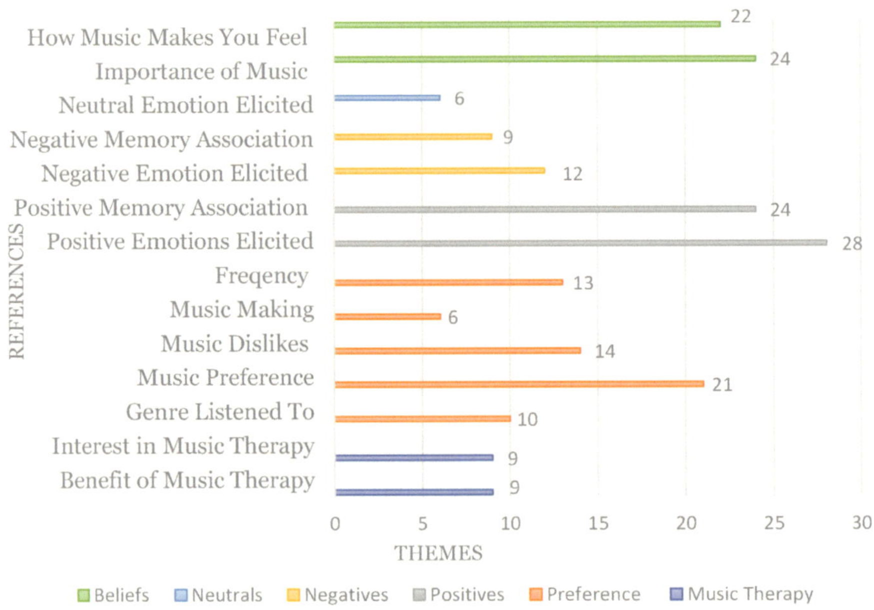

Figure 2.
Distribution of the frequency of themes coded from both focus group.

Coded theme group	Number of coded references	Percentages of all coded references
Music therapy	18	8.7
Preference	64	30.9
Positives	52	25.1
Negatives	21	10.1
Neutrals	6	3
Beliefs	46	22.2

Table 3.
Coded references by group.

piece of music. One patient describes a particularly sad event in their life that was tied to an artist, saying, "that would be with Frank Sinatra's song, that was played at my Granddad's funeral. So, again if I feel like I need to cry and let it all out... Ten out of ten it would make those tears fall." Music seems to elicit an emotive reaction based on the participants life experience.

Music Therapy was discussed totaling 18 references throughout both focus groups (**Figure 2**). Patients were asked for their thoughts on music therapy, if music therapy can be helpful through their recovery process, as well as if they would be interested in attending a music therapy session. None of the patients had any experience with music therapy but all six of the patients unanimously agreed that they would be interested in attending a music therapy session.

There were nine references during the focus groups about the benefits of music therapy. One patient stated "I know it's brilliant. And I know it could help me sort through a lot of issues," while another stated its uses in a group setting with others undergoing treatment for their eating disorder, saying "...a lot of girls I was in daycare with, music was definitely a thing that we did a lot. So, I think that sort of being able to mingle with other people through the recovery process too, I think would be really, really helpful." Overall, patients all seemed to have a strong connection with music, specifically throughout their recovery process and viewed music as an important tool for healing throughout their lives.

4. Discussion

In this study, we conducted a software-assisted qualitative study exploring people with AN's attitudes toward music, music therapy, and the uses of music throughout their life, treatment and recovery. The results of the study point to a promising potential for the varied uses of music throughout the recovery process for eating disorders. Patients were questioned in focus groups concerning the uses of music in their day to day life and as a therapeutic strategy. Responses were analyzed with NVivo 12 qualitative software for recurring themes throughout the discussions.

The most prevalent theme throughout the focus groups involved positive expressions and positive memory associations related to music. This theme occurred in ~25% of the data and totaled 52/207 of all of the coded themes (**Table 3**). This suggests patients have pleasant feelings about music and associate good things that have happened in their lives along with musical experiences. The importance of music was the second most common theme accounting for 24 references throughout the focus groups (**Figure 2**). Patients described the effect music had on their day to day life, with regulating emotions and providing an outlet of peace through their recovery process, suggesting that it was the study participants' opinion that music could be used to improve their mental state throughout their recovery.

Negative feelings and negative memories associated with music accounted for only ~10% of all of the references from both focus groups (**Table 3**). Patients discussed how music they dislike can make them feel low in mood and also described negative memories linked to a certain genre or song. This suggests music can influence mood not only positively but negatively as well.

The final main result concerns the potential uses of music as a therapeutic adjunct to their treatment. When asked about music therapy, 6/6 patients stated they were interested in attending a music therapy session; in addition, all patients expressed that they see benefit in using music therapy as an adjunct to their current treatment for their eating disorder. This suggests music could be helpful for patients in the treatment of AN.

In previous studies on the use of music in eating disorder treatment, researchers found that patients with AN managed to eat more when listening to classical piano music and had a significant reduction in postprandial anxiety when participating and music therapy; listening to a violin concerto by Mozart induced the recall of autobiographical memories in patients with BN and reduced body width estimation [7–9, 18–20]. These previous findings align with the results of our current research as patients described that when listening to their favorite music, they generally feel happier and more positive. In addition, patients expressed their interest in attending music therapy citing the potential benefits it could have in their own life specifically with their treatment of their AN.

In other studies, however, negative symptoms presented when patients watched music videos. More specifically, researchers found that watching music videos was associated with an increase in body dissatisfaction [21], and sexually objectifying videos were associated with increased perception of body size in young women with suffering from low self-esteem [22]. In our study, we found that patients who listened to music outside their usual preference or that they did not like, as a result, had negative emotional reactions (i.e. crying, dissociation). This aligns with the previous findings suggesting that while music not only can produce positive side effects, it can also produce negatives as well [7].

Our study has several limitations. The number of participants (N = 6) was small. All study participants suffered from AN. Due to the small sample size, we could not differentiate between the subtypes of AN (restricting vs. binge eating/purging), length of illness duration and their stage of recovery. Our sample was ethnically homogeneous with only white Caucasian participants, and all patients were female. Thus, the results are not generalizable to other ethnic groups or males. From our perspective, the lack of generalizability is a main problem of research in the area of music therapy for people with eating disorders, and specifically AN. Even though there is plenty of case studies (for a comprehensive review and further literature see [23]), randomized controlled trials (RCT) are scarce [7].

AN is one of several eating disorders. As we have explained in the introduction, eating disorders are not distinct entities, but should rather be seen as symptom clusters within a spectrum of serious problems related to body image disturbance, disordered eating and their physical and psychosocial consequences. Therefore, it might be worth investigating, whether our findings can be reproduced and confirmed in people with BN, BED, ARFID or other eating disorders.

Taken together, our analysis shows that people with AN connect music mainly with positive emotions and memories. Therefore, music may be used more frequently and more extensively in psychological therapies as a tool to modulate emotions. As patients would welcome music therapy as an adjunct treatment option during inpatient or outpatient treatment, therapist might think about including music therapy into their overall treatment concept. However, quantitative research in bigger patient samples and RCTs will be necessary to verify these results.

5. Conclusions

Based on the current study and previous publications on music and music therapy in people with AN, the following preliminary conclusions can be drawn:

- Music elicits mainly positive emotions and memories in people with AN.
- Music is an integral and important part of life.
- Music can help with recovery, overcome anxieties and improve eating.
- People with AN would like to be offered music therapy as an adjunct to their usual treatment.
- Music may be used as a tool to provoke emotions during psychotherapy.
- Music may also elicit negative feelings and memories.
- Watching sexually objectifying music videos can increase body dissatisfaction and the perception of body size in vulnerable people.

Acknowledgements

The MSc Mental Health Studies Programme, Institute of Psychiatry, Psychology and Neuroscience, King's College London funded the publication costs of this book chapter. Hubertus Himmerich has received salary support from the National Institute for Health Research (NIHR) Biomedical Research Centre (BRC) at South London and Maudsley NHS Foundation Trust (SLaM) and King's College London.

Conflict of interest

The authors declare no conflict of interest.

Thanks

The authors thank all six patients who took part in the focus group. They would also like to express their gratitude to Caroline Norton and to Zoe Vazquez-Sanchez for supporting the focus groups in the Maudsley and the Bethlem Royal Hospital.

Appendix: questionnaire for the focus groups

Listening to music:

- How do you find listening to music?
- What impact does listening to your favorite music have on your body and brain?
- How often do you listen to music?
- What type of music do you prefer to listen to?
    - Genre, style
    - Instrumental, vocals, both
    - Stimulating, relaxing
- How do you prefer to listen to music?
    - Recordings, live music
    - TV, radio, DVD, CD, MP3
- How often do you listen to something that is not your usual preference?
- How does listening to music relate to your emotions?
- Can you name of experience where music made you feel happy or sad?
- Is there a time in your life that you connect a certain situation with a specific song?
- How does it make you feel, if you have to listen to music you do not like?

Making music:

- Have you played, or do you play an instrument or sing?
  - Singing alone/in a choir
  - Play instrument alone/in a band/in an orchestra

Music as a therapeutic strategy:

- How could listening to music be helpful to cope with difficult emotions or problems in your life?
- Do you feel that there could be an effect of music in your life?
- Do you have any experience with music therapy?
- Would you attend a music therapy session?

Author details

Briana Applewhite[1†], Aishwarya Krishna Priya[1†], Valentina Cardi[1] and Hubertus Himmerich[1,2*]

1 Department of Psychological Medicine, Institute of Psychiatry, Psychology and Neuroscience, King's College, London, UK

2 South London and Maudsley NHS Foundation Trust, London, UK

*Address all correspondence to: hubertus.himmerich@kcl.ac.uk

† Both authors contributed equally to the manuscript of this chapter.

IntechOpen

© 2020 The Author(s). Licensee IntechOpen. This chapter is distributed under the terms of the Creative Commons Attribution License (http://creativecommons.org/licenses/by/3.0), which permits unrestricted use, distribution, and reproduction in any medium, provided the original work is properly cited.

References

[1] American Psychiatric Association. Diagnostic and Statistical Manual of Mental Disorders (DSM-5). 5th ed. Washington: American Psychiatric Publishing; 2013

[2] Keski-Rahkonen A, Mustelin L. Epidemiology of eating disorders in Europe: Prevalence, incidence, comorbidity, course, consequences, and risk factors. Current Opinion in Psychiatry. 2016;**29**:340-345. DOI: 10.1097/YCO.0000000000000278

[3] Himmerich H, Hotopf M, Shetty H, Schmidt U, Treasure J, Hayes RD, et al. Psychiatric comorbidity as a risk factor for mortality in people with anorexia nervosa. European Archives of Psychiatry and Clinical Neuroscience. 2019;**269**:351-359. DOI: 10.1007/s00406-018-0937-8

[4] Himmerich H, Treasure J. Psychopharmacological advances in eating disorders. Expert Review of Clinical Pharmacology. 2018;**11**:95-108. DOI: 10.1080/17512433.2018

[5] National Institute for Health and Care Excellence (NICE): Eating Disorders: Recognition and Treatment. 2017. Available from: https://www.nice.org.uk/guidance/ng69

[6] Eddy KT, Tabri N, Thomas JJ, Murray HB, Keshaviah A, Hastings E, et al. Recovery from anorexia nervosa and bulimia nervosa at 22-year follow-up. The Journal of Clinical Psychiatry. 2017;**78**:184-189. DOI: 10.4088/JCP.15m10393

[7] Testa F, Arunachalam S, Heiderscheit A, Himmerich H. A systematic review of scientific studies on the effects of music in people with or at risk for eating disorders. Psychiatria Danubina. 2020. Accepted

[8] Cardi V, Lounes N, Kan C, Treasure J. Meal support using mobile technology in anorexia nervosa. Contextual differences between inpatient and outpatient settings. Appetite. 2013;**60**:33-39. DOI: 10.1016/j.appet.2012.10.004

[9] Cardi V, Esposito M, Clarke A, Schifano S, Treasure J. The impact of induced positive mood on symptomatic behaviour in eating disorders. An experimental, AB/BA crossover design testing a multimodal presentation during a test-meal. Appetite. 2015;**87**:192-198. DOI: 10.1016/j.appet.2014.12.224

[10] North AC, Hargreaves DJ, Hargreaves JJ. Uses of music in everyday life. Music Perception. 2004;**22**:41-77. DOI: 10.1525/mp.2004.22.1.41

[11] Linnemann A, Strahler J, Nater UM. Assessing the effects of music listening on psychobiological stress in daily life. Journal of Visualized Experiments. 2017;**120**. DOI: 10.3791/54920

[12] Salimpoor VN, Benovoy M, Larcher K, Dagher A, Zatorre RJ. Anatomically distinct dopamine release during anticipation and experience of peak emotion to music. Nature Neuroscience. 2011;**14**:257-262. DOI: 10.1038/nn.2726

[13] Moser A, Korstjens I. Series: Practical guidance to qualitative research. Part 3: Sampling, data collection and analysis. The European Journal of General Practice. 2018;**24**:9-18. DOI: 10.1080/13814788.2017.1375091

[14] Braun V, Clarke V. Using thematic analysis in psychology. Qualitative Research in Psychology. 2006;**3**:77-101. DOI: 10.1191/1478088706qp063oa

[15] Elo S, Kääriäinen M, Kanste O, Pölkki T, Utriainen K, Kyngäs H. Qualitative content analysis: A focus on trustworthiness. SAGE Open. 2014;**1**: 1-10. DOI: 10.1177/2158244014522633

[16] Fitzpatrick R, Boulton M. Qualitative methods for assessing health care. Quality in Health Care. 1994;**3**: 107-113. DOI: 10.1136/qshc.3.2.107

[17] Richards T. An intellectual history of NUD*IST and NVivo. International Journal of Social Research Methodology. 2002;**5**:199-214. DOI: 10.1080/13645570210146267

[18] Bibb J, Castle D, Newton R. The role of music therapy in reducing post meal related anxiety for patients with anorexia nervosa. Journal of Eating Disorders. 2015;**3**:50. DOI: 10.1186/s40337-015-0088-5

[19] Bibb J, Castle D, Skewes McFerran K. Reducing anxiety through music therapy at an outpatient eating disorder recovery service. Journal of Creativity in Mental Health. 2019;**14**:306-314. DOI: 10.1080/15401383.2019.1595804

[20] Kulbartz-Klatt Y, Florin I, Pook M. Bulimia nervosa: Mood changes do have an impact on body width estimation. The British Journal of Clinical Psychology. 1999;**38**:279-287. DOI: 10.1348/014466599162854

[21] Tiggemann M, Pickering A. Role of television in adolescent women's body dissatisfaction and drive for thinness. The International Journal of Eating Disorders. 1996;**20**:199-203. DOI: 10.1002/(SICI)1098-108X(199609)20:2<199::AID-EAT11>3.0.CO;2-Z

[22] Mischner IHS, van Schie HT, Wigboldus DHJ, van Baaren RB, Engels RCME. Thinking big: The effect of sexually objectifying music videos on bodily self-perception in young women. Body Image. 2013;**10**:26-34. DOI: 10.1016/j.bodyim.2012.08.004

[23] Heiderscheit A. Creative Arts Therapies and Clients with Eating Disorders. London/Philadelphia: Jessica Kingsley Publishers; 2016

Chapter 13

Evidence-Based and Novel Psychological Therapies for People with Anorexia Nervosa

Anna Carr, Kate Tchanturia, Emmanuelle Dufour, Mary Cowan and Hubertus Himmerich

Abstract

Anorexia nervosa (AN) is a serious and often highly persistent psychiatric disorder, whereby sufferers struggle to maintain a healthy weight. Its complexity creates challenges regarding treatment, however psychological therapy is recommended by the National Institute for Heath and Care Excellence (NICE). There are four major evidence-based psychotherapies recommended for treating adults – enhanced cognitive behavioural therapy (CBT-E), the Maudsley model of anorexia nervosa treatment for adults (MANTRA), specialist supportive clinical management (SSCM) and focal psychodynamic therapy (FPT)—and three main psychotherapies recommended for treating adolescents with anorexia-family therapy for anorexia nervosa (FT-AN), enhanced cognitive behavioural therapy (CBT-E) and adolescent focused therapy for anorexia nervosa (AFP-AN). Additionally, several novel adjunct treatments are under examination, two of which—cognitive remediation therapy (CRT) and cognitive remediation and emotion skills training (CREST)—are also discussed in this chapter. Other relevant areas regarding psychological treatment include: combinations of medication or occupational therapy and psychotherapy, treating individuals with comorbidities, the challenges of studying psychological treatment for anorexia and future directions of psychotherapies for anorexia, and are also discussed.

Keywords: anorexia nervosa, predisposing factors, precipitating factors, perpetuating factors, treatment, psychological therapy, psychotherapy

1. Introduction

Anorexia Nervosa (AN) is a serious and often highly persistent psychiatric disorder, whereby sufferers struggle to maintain a healthy weight. According to the Diagnostic and Statistical Manual of Mental Disorders, 5th edition (DSM-5), the diagnostic criteria for AN are as follows:

a. the restricting of energy intake to a level lower than required in order to maintain a healthy body weight resulting in significantly low body weight relevant to a person's age, gender, development stage and physical health

b. an extreme fear of weight gain or fatness, or continued attempts to interfere with weight gain

c. disturbances to one's view of their body, e.g., the body being an unusually high basis for self-evaluation or an inability to recognise the seriousness of the low body weight [1].

It should be noted, here, the significant changes to the diagnostic criteria presented in the DSM-5 compared to the previous edition. These are revised guidelines for determining weight loss severity, revised weight loss criterion (specifying the significance of weight in relation to differences in individuals' age, gender, developmental stage or physical health), the omission of amenorrhoea and the absence of the need for the explicit verbalisation of fear of weight gain, so long as behaviours intentionally inhibiting weight gain are evident [1, 2]. Consistent with the DSM-5, AN can be divided into two subtypes, restricting and binge-eating/purging. A sufferer with restricting subtype predominantly uses dieting, fasting and/or excessive exercise to achieve a low body weight, with the absence of any recurrent binging or purging behaviours in the 3 months before diagnosis. Binging and purging behaviours include self-induced vomiting and/or laxative, diuretic or enema abuse. The binge-eating/purging subtype is characterised by repeated displays of such behaviours in the 3 months before diagnosis [1].

Anorexia can affect any individual, irrelevant of their age, gender, race or ethnicity, however it has been found to be most common in adolescent and young females [3]. Whilst some research has found a higher prevalence of AN in white adults, these findings are quite inconsistent, with others indicating no significant differences in rates of AN for different ethnicities [4]. Anorexia is highly comorbid, with significant numbers of sufferers reporting diagnoses of other psychiatric illnesses such as substance use disorders, personality disorders, anxiety disorders, mood disorders, obsessive–compulsive disorders and autism spectrum disorders [3, 5, 6], as well as an increased suicide risk [7]. Additionally, many negative physical consequences and health complications are associated with anorexia, including cardiovascular, gastrointestinal, endocrine and metabolic, pulmonary and dermatologic complications. Almost all of the body's organ systems can be negatively impacted as a result of malnutrition or other behaviours associated with AN (e.g., purging), and despite varying outcomes, anorexia is often extremely persistent, has a relatively high risk of relapse, and the highest mortality rate among psychiatric disorders [7].

2. Predisposing, precipitating and perpetuating factors of AN

A functional analysis of anorexia by Slade [8] describes "antecedent events", divided into "general setting conditions" and "specific psychosocial stimuli", that cause changes in an individual's behaviour/biological adaptation, the consequences of which lead to anorexia. Setting conditions such as low self-esteem, issues during development or perfectionistic tendencies, combine with specific psychosocial stimuli such as comments from others about weight or learnt dieting behaviour and trigger initial food restricting behaviour, indicating the first step towards an eating disorder. Changes in behaviour/biological adaptation are shown in response to these events, specifically restricting food intake and weight loss, and endocrine disturbances that may result in amenorrhoea in females, either due to the effects of low weight or due to a stress induced functional disorder. Slade then describes "consequences" of these behaviours in the form of positive reinforcers, feelings of control, success etc., and negative reinforcers, avoiding weight gain, or changes in body shape. These limited "antecedent events," "specific psychosocial stimuli" and "consequences" discussed by Slade are now commonly referred to as predisposing, precipitating and perpetuating factors and cover a wide range of potential contributory factors to the development, onset and maintenance of anorexia.

It is now widely accepted that anorexia is developed, triggered and maintained by a combination of many different biological, psychological and social factors [9] with various models theorising the involvement of different core factors to different extents [10, 11]. Separating factors into those that predispose a person to anorexia and those that perpetuate the illness is crucial for identifying which are relevant for preventative strategies (i.e., predisposing or risk factors) and which are relevant to treatment and interventions (perpetuating or maintaining factors) [12]. It is also important to note that there is some overlap between factors as they converge and combine to increase risk of anorexia, for example some predisposing factors may also act as perpetuating factors. Additionally, some factors do not work independently and may be closely linked or impact upon each other, for example a social factor might serve to reinforce an existing psychological factor [11]. **Table 1** gives a summary of the predisposing, precipitating and perpetuating factors for anorexia and demonstrates how they can be categorised into psychological, biological and socio-cultural factors.

Many theories and models of anorexia nervosa consider there to be a vital role for psychological factors in predisposing an individual to the disorder, such as personality and cognitive variables [13]. Literature frequently discusses personality characteristics that are thought to be common among individuals with anorexia including: traits associated with anxiety and depression, obsessive–compulsive traits such as rigidity and concern with detail, perfectionism, being high achieving, socially withdrawn, sensitive and introverted. These characteristics combine with other risk factors and increase an individual's vulnerability to the illness [14, 15]. In addition to personality characteristics, combinations of experiences and events lead to the creation of various distorted cognitions, creating vulnerability in an individual for developing anorexia, for example beliefs about the importance of thinness and the need to feel in control, or a cognitive bias towards food, eating, weight or body shape information processing. Fairburn et al.'s [16] cognitive behavioural theory focuses on the need for control as a central feature of anorexia and suggests that a combination of existing feelings of ineffectiveness, perfectionistic tendencies and low self-esteem underpin this need for control. Other predisposing cognitive factors for anorexia include difficulties switching between tasks (set shifting) and a preference for 'detail-focused' thinking rather than 'bigger picture' thinking (poor central coherence) [9]. Biological models highlight a number of genetic predispositions and neurobiological factors involved in the development of anorexia [14], such as malfunctions of particular neurotransmitters that may increase risk of anorexia by altering appetite regulation and increasing locomotor activity levels, or specific inherited genes that may be responsible for altered mechanisms involved in energy metabolism or appetite and feeding regulation. For a full review see [17]. Sociocultural influences might also predispose an individual to anorexia, for example insecure attachment types as a child or stressful or traumatic life events can result in interpersonal issues and emotional avoidance, common in those with anorexia [14, 18, 19].

With existing predisposing factors in place, the onset of the illness may be triggered by one or more precipitating factors [14] such as periods of isolation or self-doubt, interpersonal conflict, existing loss or trauma, culture among particular occupations, e.g., ballet dancers, models or athletes, disrupted family dynamics and peer influence, for example dieting behaviour, teasing or body dissatisfaction. Additionally, biological factors like pregnancy [20–22] or weight loss [23] may influence eating disorder symptomology, psychopathology or behaviours.

	Predisposing factors	Precipitating factors	Perpetuating factors
Psychological factors	• Personality traits (e.g., anxiousness, concern with detail, perfectionism, high achieving) • Distorted cognitions, e.g., regarding need for control • Cognitive bias towards food, eating, weight etc. • Cognitive inflexibility	• Direct reinforcement that restricting food intake = control • Salient eating behaviours in the family shifting need for control to focus on food • Threat to self-control • Negative psychological states, e.g., isolation, self-doubt • Developmental crisis, e.g., fearing puberty/independence	• Association of self-control with self-worth • High standards and perfectionism applied to restriction of food intake • Effects of starvation threaten self-control and strengthen value of controlling food, e.g., preoccupation with food, poor concentration • Emotions less salient/numbed – belief that anorexia can manage adverse emotional states • Mood intolerance • Anxiety • Personality traits, e.g., perfectionism, high achieving, fear of making mistakes • Low self-esteem • Distorted cognitive beliefs, e.g., about benefits of anorexia • Impaired cognitive functioning, e.g., weak central coherence, poor set-shifting ability
Biological factors	• Inherited malfunctions to neurotransmitters involved in appetite regulation or locomotor activity levels • Genetic predisposition for altered energy metabolism or appetite and feeding regulation • Pre-natal stress exposure	• Weight loss • Pregnancy	• Altered physiological processes cause cognitive and psychological disturbances • Changes to hormone levels and digestive system due to malnourishment • Changes to serotonin/dopamine systems
Social factors	• Learnt beliefs/adopted values about importance of weight/shape • Insecure attachment types • Stressful/traumatic life events, e.g., abuse, disrupted family dynamics	• Interpersonal conflict • Loss or trauma • Occupational cultures, e.g., ballet dancers, models, athletes • Disrupted family dynamics • Peer influence, e.g., dieting, teasing, body dissatisfaction	• Difficult family dynamics/family conflicts • Concern from close others/enabling behaviours • Lack of family coping strategies • Societal ideals for thinness • Extreme concern/overvalued importance of weight/shape • Comments from others boosts confidence/gives attention • Body dissatisfaction

Table 1.
Summary of predisposing, precipitating and perpetuating factors in AN.

It has been suggested that the most useful models for understanding the illness in terms of advancing treatment are maintenance models, focusing more specifically on factors that maintain the illness rather than those involved in the development of it [19, 24], though there is often a lot of overlap with some factors acting not only as perpetuating factors but also precipitating or predisposing ones. Many models of AN discuss psychological factors that perpetuate anorexia, either internally (self-perpetuating factors) or externally. Fairburn et al.'s [16] cognitive behavioural theory proposes a number of psychological maintaining factors. Fairburn et al. posit that achieving successful dietary restriction creates a sense of self-control in an individual, in turn improving their self-worth until restriction becomes an indication of both self-control and self-worth. This may be exacerbated by a highly perfectionist individual applying their high standards to restriction in the form of strict dietary rules. A second maintaining factor suggested in the theory is the direct effect of starvation on cognition. Intense feelings of hunger, exaggerated feelings of fullness, poorer concentration and preoccupation with food may cause an individual to feel their self-control is threatened or failing and strengthen the value that controlling food holds on the individual's self-control and self-worth. Finally, Fairburn et al. suggest extreme concerns about weight or shape is involved in perpetuating the illness, whereby an individual evaluates their self-worth highly on their weight and shape. This may be exacerbated by body checking behaviours, particularly when an individual is in an aroused and anxious state, which serves to enhance the individual's perceived imperfections regarding their body shape, encouraging further restricting and creating a vicious cycle. As a consequence of starvation, many of the aforementioned maintaining factors are worsened, facilitating the formation of vicious cycles that allow these maintaining factors and the illness to persist [15]. Further psychological, biological and social perpetuating factors are listed in **Table 1**.

3. History of treatment for AN

Historically, treatment for AN relied heavily on antipsychotic medication up until the second half of the 1990s when the shift towards a more complex approach to treatment began, taking into account an individual's biological and developmental factors and involving individual psychotherapy [25]. Advancements were made following this shift such as the introduction of cognitive and behavioural treatments. For example, an operant conditioning technique used from the mid-1960s involved the delivery of positive (e.g., more freedom) or negative reinforcers (e.g., bed rest) in response to desired behaviour (e.g., completing a meal). Despite being deemed effective at the time, questions surrounding its durability and wider impact (not just on weight), along with concerns about its coercive and controlling nature and lack of regard for other maintaining factors of the illness, dispute the claim of its superiority to other existing approaches for intervention [26].

A number of the cognitive techniques used at the time resemble a more basic and general version of cognitive therapy still used in present times [27], originating from the work of Bruch [28]. Bruch argued that psychotherapy to treat anorexia should be aimed at addressing the distorted thinking patterns and flawed core beliefs/assumptions that the sufferer holds, acquired as a result of their experiences during development. This might be accomplished using cognitive techniques such as *decentering* (adopting a less egocentric perspective for example by asking oneself 'do I notice this as much in others as I do in myself?') or *decatastrophising* (encouraging patients to imagine right through to the end of a feared situation to gauge the realistic likelihood of an event occurring and how bad it will be, rather than assuming the worst and catastrophising immediately) [29]. After further refining of Bruch's (1973) ideas, a cognitive-behavioural approach to treatment for AN based on Beck's cognitive model of depression was developed by Garner and Bemis [16, 29, 30], which involved a mixture of cognitive techniques like those mentioned, along with behavioural techniques such as "scheduling pleasant events" (to help establish other reinforcers for pleasure other than those driving the eating disorder) and "behavioural rehearsal" (e.g., role playing scary events to they can be better coped with) [30]. Other research around this time emphasised the importance of therapy that addresses the need for control [8]. Garner et al.'s [31] model of cognitive-behavioural therapy for anorexia became the leading approach of its time and involved addressing core maintaining mechanisms such as low weight, the use of weight and shape as means of achieving self-control/self-worth and body checking, as well as other issues such as low self-esteem, poor emotion recognition and expression, disruptions in the family and interpersonal difficulties [16]. Following this, and with more recent research and models highlighting the importance of other maintaining factors for the illness, cognitive-behavioural therapy (CBT) for anorexia was further adapted and developed to become more focused on the central mechanisms involved in the maintenance of the disorder, with the suggestion that other issues only be targeted by treatment if they are preventative of change [16, 32], allowing a more person-centred treatment [9].

Family therapy for the treatment of eating disorders was introduced in the 1970s following changes to the accepted general beliefs and assumptions of the role family processes play in the development and maintenance of anorexia [25, 33]. For example, Minuchin et al.'s [34] psychosomatic family model argues that family processes involving rigidity, over-involvement and conflict avoidance, along with existing psychological vulnerability in the individual, underpin the development of anorexia, and therapy should therefore involve the family to work towards changing the family dynamic. Until this time, families were generally considered to hinder treatment and so patients were treated in isolation from their parents [35]. Other associations between eating disorders and family dynamics have since been examined suggesting specific areas where families have an impact, such as attachment, parenting style, communication orientation or family conflict [18, 36, 37], though more recent models hold in mind that no blame should be attributed to the family, rather treatment works with the family [33].

By the end of the twentieth century AN was rarely treated with medication alone, instead using a multifaceted approach involving both medication and psychological intervention to better suit the individual [25].

4. Evidence-based psychological treatment for AN

The current recommended treatment for AN is guided by The National Institute for Health Care and Excellence (NICE) guidelines and aims to improve care for sufferers of anorexia by providing details of what are considered to be the most effective interventions for AN in both adults, children and young people, and allowing for an individualized and integrated approach to be adopted. According to the guidelines, treatment for anorexia should involve one or more psychological therapy, along with additional support including psychoeducation about the illness, monitoring of mental and physical health including weight and risk factors, family/carer involvement and a multidisciplinary team approach from health-care professionals. The recommended psychological interventions differ for adults and children and young people as indicated below [38]. See **Table 2** for a brief summary of the psychological therapies for AN in adults and adolescents.

Psychological treatments	Evidence from clinical studies	Evidence from RCTs	Recommended in NICE guidelines
Established treatments			
Psychological treatments for AN in adults			
Eating-disorder-focused cognitive behavioural therapy (CBT-ED)	+	+	☑
Maudsley Anorexia Nervosa Treatment for Adults (MANTRA)	+	+	☑
Specialist supportive clinical management (SSCM)	+	+	☑
Eating-disorder-focused focal psychodynamic therapy (FPT)	+	+	☑
Psychological treatments for AN in children and young people			
Anorexia-nervosa-focused family therapy (FT-AN)	+	+	☑
Eating-disorder-focused cognitive behavioural therapy (CBT-ED)	−/+	−/+	☑
Adolescent-focused psychotherapy for anorexia nervosa (AFP-AN)	−/+	N/A	☑
Novel treatments			
Psychological treatments for AN in adults			
Cognitive Remediation Therapy (CRT)	+	−/+	☐
Cognitive Remediation and Emotion Skills Training (CREST)	−/+	N/A	☐

Abbreviations: Not tested (N/A), negative study results (−), positive study result (+), inconsistent or limited results (−/+), recommended in the NICE guidelines (☑), not mentioned in the NICE guidelines (☐).

Table 2.
Psychological therapies for AN in adults and adolescents: Evidence from clinical studies (including feasibility studies and non-randomised trials) and randomised controlled trials (RCTs) and whether they are recommended by the NICE guidelines.

4.1 Psychotherapies for AN in adults

The NICE guidelines recommend four major evidence-based psychological interventions for the treatment of AN in adults. These are: individual eating-disorder-focused cognitive behavioural therapy (CBT-ED), Maudsley Anorexia Nervosa Treatment for Adults (MANTRA), specialist supportive clinical management (SSCM) and eating-disorder-focused focal psychodynamic therapy (FPT). The guidelines recommend beginning with the first three mentioned therapies and, if found to be unsuitable or ineffective, then considering FPT [38].

4.1.1 Eating-disorder-focused cognitive behavioural therapy (CBT-ED)

CBT-ED is delivered on an individual basis, consisting of 20–40 sessions over 20 weeks, depending on the version used. An enhanced version of CBT is most commonly used (CBT-E) which originated from CBT for bulimia nervosa (CBT-BN), though as a "transdiagnostic" treatment can be used to treat a broad range of eating disorders including anorexia. It has two versions, a focused version which is shorter and just involves the core treatment, and a broad version which addresses further maintaining mechanisms, such as perfectionism, low self-esteem or interpersonal difficulties, in addition to the core treatment. CBT-E aims to alter faulty cognitions by focusing on behavioural changes and monitoring the effects and implications of behaviours that reinforce the eating disorder [38, 39].

CBT-E is delivered in four main stages, the first of which aims to encourage the patient to engage with treatment, identify the processes that are maintaining the individual's illness, provide psychoeducation and introduce two essential elements of the therapy: weighing and regular eating. Stage two is a chance for the patient and therapist to review progress so far and plan for stage three, the main body of treatment. This main stage is tailored to the individual and targets the patient's own maintaining processes. These processes generally fall under six core headings: the over-evaluation of shape and weight, the over-evaluation of control over eating, dietary restraint, dietary restriction, being underweight and event- or mood-triggered changes in eating. If the patient has additional factors that are creating a barrier to change, e.g., high perfectionism, core low self-esteem or pronounced interpersonal problems, the broad form of therapy might be used and these additional maintaining mechanisms are addressed more specifically. Mood intolerance was originally included as an additional mechanism to be addressed in the broad form of therapy however is now included in the core treatment. Finally, stage four is in place to ensure changes are maintained following treatment ending and to minimise the risk of relapse [40].

A review of treatments for adults with anorexia concludes that there is a moderate evidence base for CBT-E for adults, with evidence suggesting that it produces a moderate and lasting beneficial effect. This is an improvement on the older version of CBT which was found to have weak evidence base and only a slight beneficial effect [9]. Another review found a large effect of CBT-E on EDE-Q (Eating Disorder Examination Questionnaire—indicating eating disorder psychopathology) outcomes specifically for AN [41]. Generally, studies show that CBT-E produces good outcomes regarding increases in BMI and decreases in eating disorder psychopathology and conclude that it is an effective and viable treatment option for anorexia. However, there does not yet appear to be any consistent convincing evidence to suggest it is superior to comparable psychotherapies [42–50]. There is some evidence to suggest that CBT-E may be feasible to deliver in a group setting for patients with eating disorders, including those with anorexia, without losing the desired positive outcomes regarding weight gain and reduction in eating disorder psychopathology [51], however sample sizes are small and so this requires further examining.

Despite its apparent success in the treatment of other eating disorders such as bulimia or binge eating disorder, and theoretical suitability for treating anorexia, there is less evidence to support its success in those with anorexia [49, 52]. It has been suggested that a combination of the malnourished brain, as a result of extremely low weight, and the ego-syntonic nature of anorexia makes motivation to engage with treatment low and the challenging of distorted cognitions even more difficult and distressing for the individual [52, 53].

4.1.2 Maudsley anorexia nervosa treatment for adults (MANTRA)

MANTRA is a flexible treatment based around a patient workbook and delivered over 10–20 sessions depending on the complexity of the patient's problems [38]. It is based on Schmidt and Treasure's [24] cognitive-interpersonal maintenance model and aims to target the maintaining factors of anorexia, for example unhelpful thinking styles, including rigidity, perfectionism and obsessive–compulsive traits, faulty cognition and beliefs, e.g., the benefits of AN, emotion avoidance and responses from others that do not support recovery such as criticism or enabling of behaviours [15, 54]. MANTRA is taught in modules that address various aspects of the patient's life and recovery, for example nutrition, identity, cognitive styles or interpersonal relationships. It can be individualised once the core module of case formulation is complete by emphasising the optional modules to a greater or lesser extent depending on how ready or motivated the individual is, and by tailoring the therapy to match an individual's clinical symptoms, personality and neuropsychological traits. It is specifically designed for anorexia treatment and is tailored to suit the common temperamental traits associated with the illness, delivered using elements of motivational interviewing and CBT [9, 55].

In a number of RCTs comparing treatment for anorexia, MANTRA was found to have positive outcomes regarding BMI and eating disorder psychopathology though was not statistically significantly different in comparison with CBT-E or SSCM. However, MANTRA was more favourably rated by patients and resulted in increasing weight even in severely unwell patients [44, 54, 55]. A review of evidence from RCTs comparing treatments for anorexia concluded that MANTRA has a moderate evidence base which shows that it produces a moderate and lasting beneficial effect [9].

4.1.3 Specialist supportive clinical management (SSCM)

SSCM was developed as a standardised outpatient treatment to help support individuals with anorexia through education, advice, therapeutic guidance and reassurance [56, 57]. It is delivered in an outpatient setting as weekly sessions for 20 or more weeks depending on the severity of the individual's illness. The treatment aims to support the patient in gradually normalising their eating behaviour and gaining weight through physical health monitoring, clinical management and therapeutic content. This includes psychoeducation, nutritional advice and support in setting goals and understanding the link between their symptoms and abnormal eating behaviour [9, 38].

Evidence from RCTs suggests SSCM to be at least comparable to CBT and IPT regarding improved outcomes and global anorexia rating [56, 58]. Compared to MANTRA, SSCM seems to perform equally well overall, however in the treatment of particularly severely ill patients SSCM is slightly less successful in producing longer-term weight gain than MANTRA. There is the suggestion that SSCM might produce quicker responses to treatment and be best used for patients with less severe cases of anorexia who have higher motivation for treatment [54, 55, 58]. Still, other findings show no significant differences in outcome regarding BMI, eating disorder psychopathology or general psychopathology between SSCM, MANTRA and CBT-E [44]. Despite some mixed findings, a review of evidence from RCTs comparing treatments for anorexia concluded that SSCM has a moderate evidence based that demonstrates its moderate beneficial effect [9].

4.1.4 Eating-disorder-focused focal psychodynamic therapy (FPT)

Designed as an outpatient treatment, FPT is a person-centred treatment whereby an individualised hypothesis is created regarding how the person experiences their own symptoms. The patient's relevant central psychodynamic features are identified by the therapist using a standardised interview tool. Treatment is then delivered in three rough phases, the first of which centres around building a good therapeutic relationship, self-esteem, pro-AN beliefs and the ego-syntonic nature of anorexia. The second phase is focused on the link between interpersonal relationships and eating disorder behaviours, and the third attends to the transfer from treatment to real life and preparing the patient for the end of treatment [9, 43, 59].

Although being an effective treatment in terms of weight gain, when compared to other specialist psychological treatments (family therapy and cognitive analytical therapy), FPT does not appear to be superior [60]. Additionally, FPT has shown no greater success than CBT-E and TAU regarding weight gain or reduction in anorexic psychopathology after treatment, though at 12-month follow up has shown significantly higher recovery rates than TAU as measured by global outcome (a combination of BMI and eating disorder psychopathology) [43].

One review of treatment for anorexia conclude there is a moderate evidence base for the treatment, and a moderate and lasting beneficial treatment effect of FPT for adults with anorexia [9]. There is the suggestion from existing eating disorder literature that due to the interpersonal element in psychodynamic interventions, they may need a longer timeframe for their positive effects to be exhibited [58]. In light of this, and due to a large part of FPT being focused on interpersonal relationships, there is the possibility that its strength lies in better long-term results [43].

4.2 Psychological treatment for AN in children and young people

For treating anorexia in children and young people, the NICE guidelines recommend one of the following: anorexia-nervosa-focused family therapy (FT-AN), CBT-ED or adolescent-focused psychotherapy for anorexia nervosa (AFP-AN). It is recommended that FT-AN is considered first, with CBT-ED or AFP-AN being considered if FT-AN is unacceptable, ill-advised or ineffective for the individual [38].

4.2.1 Anorexia-nervosa-focused family therapy (FT-AN)

FT-AN (or family-based therapy; FBT) is typically delivered in 10–20 sessions over 6 months to a year and is structured in three rough phases. FBT has a behavioural focus, whereby the family is encouraged to take some control and support the patient with weight restoration, making healthy diet decisions and gaining autonomy around eating. Despite an emphasis on the role that an individual's family has in their recovery, care should be taken to ensure no blame is attributed to either the patient or their family. The family should be encouraged to temporarily be part of helping the individual to manage their eating. The first phase of treatment is centred on the forming of therapeutic relationships between the therapist, patient and family members, weight restoration and a return to a more physically healthy state. The next phase involves supporting the patient to gradually acquire some autonomy that is appropriate for their age and development, for example portioning their own meals under the supervision of a parent or carer. Finally, phase three aims to identify any anticipated developmental challenges for the young person and how to manage them and establish plans following termination of treatment or in case of relapse [38, 61]. Family therapy is thought to be particularly useful for treating adolescents with the illness as it is during this time that individuals are going through critical development times that are often taking place in a home environment among family [62].

Reviews of FBT have summarised studies comparing different formats of FBT, and different types of family therapy to FBT [33, 61], finding no significant differences between the various formats and types. For example, comparing conjoint therapy (for family and patient together) to separate therapy (patient and family seen separately), studies have found no significant differences in outcomes [63, 64]. Additionally, a comparison of FBT of different lengths found no significant differences between short- and long-term FBT at end of treatment and 4-year follow-up [65]. Comparisons of FBT with different types of family therapy, for example systemic family therapy, which is concerned more with the family system and issues surrounding relationships, interactions and dynamics [66], reveal no significant differences in terms of primary outcome, though FBT did produce more rapid weight gain and less incidents of hospitalisation for those assigned to it. Several reviews conclude that no one format for content/delivery of FT-AN has consistently been significantly more successful than another [50, 62, 67].

An expanding pool of evidence exists that supports the use of FBT as the primary intervention for treating children and young people with anorexia [9, 68] however there is still limited evidence to suggest FBT is consistently superior to other psychological treatments or treatment as usual [33]. Despite much of the research on anorexia treatment for adolescents focusing on FT-AN, a lack of high-quality studies comparing FT-AN to individual treatments means it cannot reliably be deemed superior [69]. Other reviews have concluded that FBT is no more successful in addressing anorexic psychopathology than other psychotherapies [70] and highlight the issue that it is not necessarily successful for all adolescents, for example for families with single or separated parents, or where the young person has high levels of obsessive–compulsive traits [61, 71].

4.2.2 Eating-disorder-focused cognitive behavioural therapy (CBT-ED)

Although designed as a treatment for adults, CBT-E for eating disorders can be adapted to be suitable for treating young people several ways. For example, many young people live at home in a family unit where they might become dependent on a parent or carer, therefore treatment should be delivered in such a way that encourages and facilitates the young person to take some responsibility and develop independence so that a return to normal adolescent development can be made following treatment. Due to the family involvement that is common and expected among young people living at home, care should also be taken to ensure the best use of the family's involvement, without the patient perceiving this as over-involvement and threating their autonomy. Motivation for treatment is often quite low in younger patients making it important to incorporate strategies to engage the patient with the therapy. The therapy itself is delivered in largely the same way for children and adolescents as it is for adults, though minor adaptations may be made to ensure it is suitable and meets the additional needs of young people [72].

Studies show some promise from CBT-E regarding weight gain and reduced eating disorder and general psychopathology among adolescents with anorexia which lasted at follow up [73–75], and suggest that CBT-E may be even more successful in adolescents than adults [76]. Despite this, one study review concluded that there is a weak to moderate evidence base for CBT for young people with eating disorders, with inconsistent results regarding effects of treatment for CBT and only slightly beneficial effects for CBT-E [9].

4.2.3 Adolescent-focused psychotherapy for anorexia nervosa (AFP-AN)

AFP-AN (previously named ego-oriented individual therapy before being manualised) [77] is delivered primarily through up to around 40 individual sessions with the individual, with an additional 8–12 sessions involving the patient's family or carer(s) to support the individual work. Treatment begins more intensively, with regular sessions aiming to allow the therapist to establish a strong therapeutic relationship with the patient, as well as build the patient's motivation for behaviour change. The aim of AFP-AN is to facilitate independence and self-efficacy around eating behaviour through sessions focusing on the link between the person's eating disorder and their self-image, emotion processing and regulation, and interpersonal processes. This helps the individual develop an understanding of how their self-concept perpetuates the illness and how they use their anorexia as a coping strategy. Unlike CBT, however, AFP is more concerned with employing strategies to challenge underlying psychological or developmental deficits rather than issues directly associated with food, weight or shape, for example. AFP supports the individual to manage fears surrounding weight gain and find alternative ways to cope with stress or adverse emotions, as well as providing psychoeducation about the consequences of malnourishment and the importance of nutrition and weight gain. As treatment is in its final stage, the emphasis is on applying the skills and knowledge acquired from treatment in real life situations [38, 71, 77, 78].

AFP was found to match FBT in terms of treatment completion and outcome in a clinical trial comparing the two [78]. However, at follow-up AFP was found to be statistically inferior to FBT regarding outcome, suggested to be due to fewer instances of full-remission threshold being met following treatment, as well as higher relapse rates, in individuals who completed AFP. One trial also found that AFP was less successful in treating patients with severe eating disorder psychopathology than FBT [79].

4.3 Conclusion

Though there appears to be some success for psychotherapies, still it is proving difficult to achieve consistently good outcomes with the treatments that are currently available for anorexia, particularly in adults [44]. Additionally, there is a consensus that despite a growing evidence-base for treatments for anorexia and a preference for psychotherapy as treatment, there still remains no established leading treatment [9, 80]. A number of treatment reviews conclude that among a variety of psychotherapies, including the aforementioned treatments recommended by the NICE guidelines, there is no convincing evidence to suggest one consistently superior intervention for treating adults, children or adolescents with anorexia nervosa [44, 50, 69, 81]. This is largely due to the difficulty of trialling treatments for anorexia because of difficulty recruiting participants, high rates of patient drop-out or non-adherence to treatment and withdrawal from clinicians as a result of risk not being stabilised [50]. Still, psychotherapies that include the family seem to be more promising and tentatively deemed most appropriate and preferred in the treatment of children and adolescents with anorexia [81].

5. Novel adjunct psychological treatments for AN

In addition to the aforementioned NICE recommended treatments, a number of novel adjunct treatments are being used and explored, generally in addition to other more established intensive psychotherapies [82]. The two adjunct psychological interventions are relatively new, though a growing evidence base for them is emerging. **Table 2** gives a brief indication of the current climate regarding the literature for the two following treatments.

5.1 Cognitive remediation therapy (CRT)

CRT was originally developed to be used for the rehabilitation of individuals with various neuropsychological issues, however has since been adapted to address the common problem of cognitive inflexibility (i.e., poor set shifting—inability to move flexibly between different tasks or stimuli—and weak central coherence—inability to process information as a whole leading to a focus on details) among individuals with anorexia. The therapy aims to encourage switching between tasks, multitasking and bigger picture thinking to break inflexible thinking patterns and habits through the practice of simple tasks and mental exercises. After practicing these tasks, patients are encouraged to reflect on what cognitive style they have used to complete the task, explore how this may be helpful or unhelpful in day-to-day life and learn new strategies to help make small positive behavioural changes. CRT can be delivered either on a 1:1 basis typically over 10 45-min sessions, or as a briefer format in a group setting over 5 or 6 sessions. It can be used with adults or children and adolescents and is suitable even for patients with very low BMI, unlike most talking therapies, allowing them to engage in psychological work early on in treatment [83–85].

Based on evidence from randomised treatment trials, CRT reduces drop-out rates, with a 10–20% drop-out rate reported across these studies, suggesting that CRT can be a useful step to begin patient engagement with psychological interventions. In addition to low drop-out rates, qualitative feedback about CRT from both patients and therapists is very positive [86–88]. There is evidence from several RCTs that CRT improves performance and subjective evaluation of cognitive processes. This general improvement in cognition supports better general functioning [84, 85]. Available research across the lifespan suggests CRT can be used as an adjunct therapy to engage patients, improve cognitive processes and prepare grounds for further psychological work. However, CRT is not a stand-alone treatment for eating disorders, does not directly target weight change and, as such, is not included in the NICE guidelines.

5.2 Cognitive remediation and emotion skills training (CREST)

CREST is an intervention developed to address problems with identifying, managing and expressing emotions among individuals with anorexia nervosa. Like CRT, it is an intervention that can be offered early on in treatment when patients may not be able to use more complex psychological therapies. CREST is generally delivered over 8–10 sessions. Typically, if a patient has previously had CRT, they are offered eight individual sessions of CREST. If patients have not had any experience of CRT, they will first have two sessions focused on thinking styles, followed by eight sessions involving the psychoeducation and experiential elements of CREST [89].

The main evidence for CREST comes from qualitative and quantitative evaluation of the case series in individual (8–10 sessions) and group format (5–6 sessions). Whilst the majority of studies available examine the efficacy of CREST for adults, showing some promise, more recently there have been some studies published investigating CREST for adolescents with anorexia and findings suggest that is may also be suitable for this patient group [90]. At the present time, the efficacy of CREST in individual and group formats is still being examined. Detailed studies using qualitative data and self-report questionnaires offer positive feedback and show promise; however, more studies with RCT methodology are required to endorse this.

6. Discussion

The current chapter has given a brief introduction to the diagnosis of anorexia nervosa and a short history of its treatment. It has then described the current evidence-based psychological treatments for anorexia, as recommended by the NICE guidelines, and presented a summary of the literature regarding the efficacy of these treatments. In addition to the standard treatment for anorexia, a number of more recently developed adjunct therapies are under examination. Two of these are described and again a summary of the literature investigating their efficacy is presented.

An alternative to psychotherapy alone for anorexia nervosa is to treat using combinations of treatment types and approaches. The following presents some of the current combinations under examination in the treatment of anorexia. Adapting treatment approach may be particularly important for treating individuals with comorbid diagnoses, which is discussed in this section, as well as some of the difficulties conducting studies that explore psychotherapy for anorexia, limitations of this chapter and future directions of the literature.

6.1 Combinations of medications and psychological therapy

One recognised potential treatment alternative to psychotherapy alone is the use of oxytocin, a hormone and neuropeptide that is involved in the modulation of a number of functions including eating behaviour and food consumption, emotional reactivity, stress and anxiety, trust and social interactions and bond formation [82, 91]. Evidence from reviews of the literature suggest that the oxytocin system becomes disrupted in individuals with anorexia, affecting oxytocin levels in response to stimulation or after a meal, among other things, that may return to "normal" following recovery [92]. If this is the case, there is the potential for oxytocin administration to be beneficial for treating anorexia. On the contrary, findings from RCTs show no significant weight gain following oxytocin administration in people with anorexia, however do propose that it may reduce the stress response in anticipation of food [91, 93]. Alternatively, oxytocin might impact some of the maintaining factors of anorexia, such as attachment and interpersonal issues or aspects of social cognition, e.g., emotion recognition [94–96]. With the suggestion that difficulties with emotional processing contribute to less effectivity from cognitive therapy [97], the addition of oxytocin to such psychotherapies may be beneficial, however findings on this remain inconclusive [94, 98, 99].

D-cycloserine is another drug that is suggested to show some promise in augmenting psychological treatment for anorexia [100]. For example, d-cycloserine is suggested to enhance CBT, by contributing to the consolidation of therapeutic learning from the treatment, and exposure therapy, by strengthening the mechanisms involved in fear extinction [101]. However, the results of one trial did not support this, finding that administering d-cycloserine to individuals with anorexia led to no significant differences in outcome measures following four exposure-therapy based training meals, though it was noted that the lack of effect may be due to the small sample size used [102]. On the other hand, a later RCT found that the administration of d-cycloserine with exposure therapy for individuals with anorexia led to significantly greater increases in BMI following treatment compared to placebo [103]. Still, there is certainly a need for a better understanding of the effect of combinations of medications and psychotherapies and it is clear that many more trials are required to investigate the impact of drugs such as oxytocin and d-cycloserine on treatment for anorexia [103, 104].

6.2 Combinations of occupational therapy (OT) and psychological therapy

Psychological treatment for anorexia nervosa should be part of a whole therapeutic programme including diet counselling, as well as weight and physical health monitoring, but may additionally offer occupational therapy (OT) and art therapy, typically led by occupational therapists [105]. OT is a profession which enables engagement and performance [106]. It is a patient-centred health profession concerned with promoting health and well-being through occupation by enabling people to participate in activities they want to do, need to do and are expected to do [107]. Occupational therapists use psychotherapeutic skills and approaches and reflect on their relationship with the patients and families. They use approaches from psychodynamic therapy and DBT such as transference and countertransference. Occupational therapists use similar frames of reference to psychologists but through an activity-orientated approach in order to maximise the person's level of psychosocial functioning [108]. Eating disorders influence people's lives and the way they engage in meaningful occupations and OT can explore the meaning of new occupations which can emerge from the eating disorder. Through specific OT assessments using the Model of Human Occupation [109], OT can examine people's motivation, routine, habits, roles and skills in a range of areas such as self-care, leisure and productivity in order to promote a more adaptive occupational participation in daily activities. OT provides a unique opportunity to implement individual and group work provided in eating disorders services supporting plans made for the patients within the multidisciplinary team. OT works with the person within their social and physical environments using meaningful activities, which often support CBT and psychological changes in different areas of life. Providing occupationally focused interventions means that most goals can be addressed using everyday activities. Through OT interventions, people can learn to transfer their experience and skills from intervention to daily life. OT teams can receive psychotherapeutic supervision and are involved in handovers, meetings and ward rounds to feed information back to the multidisciplinary team, and thus contribute to or even lead the psychotherapeutic process by bringing a unique perspective of function to the team. Its contribution can be beneficial regarding improvements to self-awareness, self-esteem and greater independence [110]. For some patients, additional physiotherapy including strength training does also seem to be beneficial [111].

6.3 Psychological treatment for people with comorbidities

Autism spectrum disorder (ASD) is significantly overrepresented among individuals with eating disorders and a relatively common comorbidity of anorexia [112, 113]. Evidence suggests that this comorbidity is associated with more severe presentation, poorer illness outcomes and can hinder engagement with usual treatment, negatively impacting treatment outcome. This is perhaps due to some overlap in traits, e.g., poor flexibility, weak central coherence, emotional difficulties and poor introspection potentially exacerbating the maintaining factors of AN, such as rules and rigidity, which may be applied to food restriction or exercise, for example [6, 112, 114, 115]. There is the suggestion that cognitive remediation may be beneficial in the treatment of individuals high in traits like weak central coherence and poor flexibility, common to both ASD and AN [116]. As discussed, CRT and CREST are of interest in eating disorder literature and have attracted some attention regarding their use with individuals with both ASD and anorexia. Small trials and case studies indicate some potential and suitability for CRT and CREST in the treatment of AN, though further investigating is required regarding the efficacy of psychological treatment for anorexia in those with and without ASD traits, with the potential of adapting treatments to be more appropriate for use with individuals with both AN and ASD [115, 117, 118].

Also of a high comorbidity with anorexia are personality disorders (PD), with estimates of over 50% of individuals with eating disorders having comorbid diagnoses of PDs, most commonly borderline personality disorder (BPD), avoidant personality disorder (APD) and obsessive–compulsive personality disorder

(OCPD) [119]. There is the suggestion that a comorbid diagnosis of a PD with anorexia may lead to adverse implications regarding more chronic illness course, lower levels of functioning, higher rates of treatment termination and less positive outcomes. Such implications may be due to various influences of PD traits including increased self-harm/suicide risk, a lack of trust in the therapist interfering with therapy engagement, poor insight into own illness and exacerbated maintaining factors of anorexia like dysregulated emotion control [114, 119–121]. In light of this there appears to be a need for adapting the therapy approach used to better suit these individuals and their co-occurring symptoms [122], for example using adapted versions of alternative psychotherapies such as dialectical behavioural therapy (DBT) to treat individuals with comorbid diagnoses of anorexia and BPD [123, 124]. Likewise, similar dysfunctions in brain circuitry suggested to underlie both obsessive–compulsive personality traits and impairments to cognitive flexibility may explain some of the overlap in diagnoses of anorexia and OCPD and obsessive–compulsive disorder (OCD). Perhaps, then, therapies that target these cognitive maintaining factors of anorexia, such as CRT or CREST, could be most appropriate for treating individuals with comorbid diagnoses of OCPD or OCD and AN, though this merits further examination [125].

6.4 Difficulties conducting studies exploring psychotherapy for anorexia

Several factors make exploring the efficacy of psychotherapy for anorexia nervosa particularly difficult, leaving almost all treatment trials in the field inherently methodologically limited before they have even begun [50]. For example, the severity of the illness makes recruiting participants challenging and participant that are recruited are almost always female only samples, with very few studies investigating the efficacy of treatments for males or minority groups with anorexia [50, 126]. This leaves an absence of knowledge regarding the way males respond to treatment and the impact of culture, race, gender and sexuality on treatment, creating a large gap in the literature regarding the efficacy of treatments for males and minority groups with anorexia [81]. Additionally, drop-out rates are particularly high leading to small or incomplete data sets, or a lack of follow-up data. These issues create problems regarding cost, statistical power, interpretation and comparison of results, and potentially undermine research results, biasing estimates of treatment effects [50, 126]. One suggested explanation for the high drop-out rates is the role of personality. With PDs having relatively high comorbidity with anorexia, issues forming and maintaining interpersonal therapeutic relationships may be exacerbated due to the nature of the PD, making continued engagement in therapy difficult [119].

Despite the growing evidence base for psychotherapies for anorexia, another major issue that persists is the absence of untreated comparison groups or control groups altogether [69]. Due to the severity of the physical effects of anorexia, as well as its high mortality rate and often chronic course of development, it is unethical for patient groups to remain untreated or on waiting lists as a control group as part of a study. For this reason, it is only possible to evaluate the superiority of a treatment when compared to an alternative active treatment, often referred to as "treatment as usual" (TAU), rather than its real efficacy when compared to no treatment. However, this creates further methodological issues as TAU varies from study to study and so does not provide a common comparison group, meaning findings supporting a treatment's superiority, or inferiority, to another still cannot be reliably compared [50, 69]. Likewise, with recovery rates varying due to different definitions of recovery, varying outcome measures and inconsistent follow-up lengths between studies, the problem of reliably comparing treatments for anorexia is exacerbated [82]. Poor clarity of the "criteria" for recovery and measures of recovery being based on physical changes, such as weight gain, skews the apparent efficacy of treatment, sometimes ignoring the impact of the participants' initial weights (some perhaps being much lower than others), as well as cognitive and behavioural changes that might indicate recovery leading to outcomes appearing more or less positive [69, 81]. For example, one systematic review found that family-based therapies yielded a very slight superiority regarding impact on weight outcome, but the same was not true for psychological outcomes [127]. Furthermore, a lack of independently replicated studies comparing treatments for anorexia contributes to the lack of reliable estimates of which treatments are most efficacious [69].

6.5 Limitations of chapter

Several limitations of this chapter should be noted. The chapter has summarised some of the literature relevant to psychological therapies for anorexia nervosa however is not a systematic review, therefore does not present *all* of the current research in the field. Additionally, the therapies discussed that make up the main section of the chapter are those recommended by the National Institute for Health and Care Excellence (NICE) who provide recommendations for health and care only in the UK [128]. Therefore these are not necessarily the first choice of treatment for other countries, though it does not go unrecognised that many other countries have developed practices and guidelines for treating eating disorders including anorexia. This is relevant as despite a consensus regarding the importance of psychotherapy in the treatment of anorexia across a number of countries' guidelines, including several European countries, Australia, New Zealand and the US, there still remains some inconsistencies regarding the recommended first-line treatment, optimal intensity of treatment (i.e., inpatient, outpatient or day patient) for different stages of the illness and criteria for hospitalisation. Furthermore, many of the available studies evaluating the various therapies for anorexia come from highly Westernised, English speaking countries such as the UK, US, Australia and some of Europe, with few to none from places such as Africa, South America, Eastern Europe and Asia. This may impact heavily on the efficacy of different treatments and their formats, as well as treatment adherence, due to sociocultural influences such as family ties, cultural beliefs and values, parenting styles and education [81]. Thus, this chapter may be most helpful for colleagues who practice in the UK or for readers who are interested in the psychological treatment of AN in the UK, but our chapter does not provide a comprehensive worldwide view on the topic.

6.6 Future directions

There appears to still be a lot of progression required regarding treatment for anorexia nervosa and what is most effective, though looking to the future there are a number of suggestions under investigation. For example, identifying individuals who may not be suitable for conventional treatments, perhaps those with comorbidities, and adapting treatments in response to this may increase the number of patients that treatments are efficacious for. For example, systemic family therapy may be more beneficial than FBT for individuals with obsessive–compulsive traits [66], and an adapted version of DBT might be a more suitable and effective way of treating individuals with comorbid diagnoses of anorexia and PD [123, 124]. For individuals with a comorbid diagnosis of ASD, specific maintaining factors of AN, such as weak central coherence, poor flexibility and emotional difficulties, are often particularly apparent and problematic. Therefore, for these patients it may that treatments that target these traits, e.g., CRT or CREST, could be most effective [116], particularly if modified to suit these individuals' needs [129]. Perhaps, then, the answer to this could be identifying patient subgroups that might respond particularly well (or not) to one treatment over another and tailoring treatment accordingly [69], though this is yet to be examined fully.

An additional consideration looking forward it that much of the current research is conducted in outpatient settings, omitting those most critically ill (who are most likely to be using inpatient services) from being participants and limiting the ability of researchers to evaluate the impact that different treatment settings have on the efficacy of psychological treatments, how successfully treatments translate to different levels of care and make recommendations regarding the best setting for treatment [50]. More intense treatment contexts such as inpatient or day-patient typically mean that patients live-in or spend up to around 10 h at the treatment location, which is significantly more therapeutic input than the typical 1 h per week of treatment offered to less chronically ill patients who access outpatient treatment [130]. Despite this, research indicates that evidence comparing inpatient and outpatient treatment shows there to be little or no differences regarding outcome between the two treatment settings and the majority of young people suffering with anorexia can be kept safe and managed well as outpatients, with high levels of patient satisfaction and significantly lower costs [131, 132]. Though the severity of some cases might mean that inpatient treatment is necessary to reduce immediate risk, research shows that a short inpatient stay followed by day-patient treatment was no less successful or safe than inpatient treatment [133], and extended hospital admissions might actually have adverse impacts on long-term recovery [134]. Considering such research, further investigation about effective settings for psychological treatment would be beneficial so that better informed decisions can be made regarding efficacy, safety, suitability for various age groups or stages of illness and cost effectiveness of treatment for anorexia in various settings.

Acknowledgements

Kate Tchanturia has received research support from The Health Foundation and the Maudsley Charity. The Health Foundation is an independent charity committed to improving health care for people in the UK. The Maudsley Charity is an independent NHS mental health charity which works in partnership with patients and families, clinical care teams and researchers at the South London and Maudsley NHS Foundation Trust, the Institute of Psychiatry, Psychology and Neuroscience at King's College London, and community organisations, with a common goal of improving mental health, to support innovation, research and service improvement. Hubertus Himmerich has received salary support from the National Institute for Health Research (NIHR) Biomedical Research Centre (BRC) at South London and Maudsley NHS Foundation Trust (SLaM) and King's College London.

Conflict of interest

The authors declare no conflict of interest.

Author details

Anna Carr[1], Kate Tchanturia[1,2], Emmanuelle Dufour[1], Mary Cowan[1] and Hubertus Himmerich[1,2]*

1 South London and Maudsley NHS Foundation Trust, London, UK

2 Department of Psychological Medicine, Institute of Psychiatry, Psychology and Neuroscience, King's College London, London, UK

*Address all correspondence to: hubertus.himmerich@kcl.ac.uk

IntechOpen

© 2020 The Author(s). Licensee IntechOpen. This chapter is distributed under the terms of the Creative Commons Attribution License (http://creativecommons.org/licenses/by/3.0), which permits unrestricted use, distribution, and reproduction in any medium, provided the original work is properly cited. CC BY

References

[1] American Psychiatric Association. Diagnostic and Statistical Manual of Mental Disorders (DSM-5). 5th ed. Washington: American Psychiatric Publishing; 2013

[2] Attia E, Becker AE, Bryant-Waugh R, Hoek HW, Kreipe RE, Marcus MD, et al. Feeding and eating disorders in DSM-5. The American Journal of Psychiatry. 2013;**170**:1237-1239. DOI: 10.1176/appi.ajp.2013.13030326

[3] Keski-Rahkonen A, Mustelin L. Epidemiology of eating disorders in Europe: Prevalence, incidence, comorbidity, course, consequences, and risk factors. Current Opinion in Psychiatry. 2016;**29**:340-345. DOI: 10.1097/YCO.0000000000000278

[4] Cheng ZH, Perko VL, Fuller-Marashi L, Gau JM, Stice E. Ethnic differences in eating disorder prevalence, risk factors, and predictive effects of risk factors among young women. Eating Behaviors. 2019;**32**:23-30. DOI: 10.1016/j.eatbeh.2018.11.004

[5] Himmerich H, Hotopf M, Shetty H, Schmidt U, Treasure J, Hayes RD, et al. Psychiatric comorbidity as a risk factor for mortality in people with anorexia nervosa. European Archives of Psychiatry and Clinical Neuroscience. 2019;**269**:351-359. DOI: 10.1007/s00406-018-0937-8

[6] Westwood H, Tchanturia K. Autism spectrum disorder in anorexia nervosa: An updated literature review. Current Psychiatry Reports. 2017;**19**:1-10. DOI: 10.1007/s11920-017-0791-9

[7] Treasure J, Duarte TA, Schmidt U. Eating disorders. Lancet. 2020;**395**:899-911. DOI: 10.1016/S0140-6736(20)30059-3

[8] Slade P. Towards a functional analysis of anorexia nervosa and bulimia nervosa. British Journal of Clinical Psychology. 1982;**21**:167-179. DOI: 10.1111/j.2044-8260.1982.tb00549.x

[9] Zipfel S, Giel KE, Bulik CM, Hay PH, Schmidt U. Anorexia nervosa: Aetiology, assessment, and treatment. The Lancet Psychiatry. 2015;**2**:1099-1111. DOI: 10.1016/S2215-0366(15)00356-9

[10] Munro C, Randell L, Lawrie SM. An integrative bio-psycho-social theory of anorexia nervosa. Clinical Psychology & Psychotherapy. 2016;**24**:1-21. DOI: 10.1002/cpp.2047

[11] Murray T. Wait not, want not: Factors contributing to the development of anorexia nervosa and bulimia nervosa. The Family Journal. 2003;**11**:276-280. DOI: 10.1177/1066480703252470

[12] Stice E. Risk and maintenance factors for eating pathology: A meta-analytic review. Psychological Bulletin. 2002;**128**:825-848. DOI: 10.1037/0033-2909.128.5.825

[13] Vitousek K, Manke F. Personality variables and disorders in anorexia nervosa and bulimia nervosa. Journal of Abnormal Psychology. 1994;**103**:137-147. DOI: 10.1037//0021-843x.103.1.137

[14] Woerwag-Mehta S, Treasure J. Causes of anorexia nervosa. Psychiatry. 2008;**7**:147-151. DOI: 10.1016/j.mppsy.2008.02.010

[15] Schmidt U. Maudsley model of anorexia nervosa treatment for adults (MANTRA): A cognitive-interpersonal model of illness development and maintenance. In: Wade T, editor. Encyclopedia of Feeding and Eating Disorders. Singapore: Springer; 2015. pp. 1-5. DOI: 10.1007/978-981-287-087-2_95-1

[16] Fairburn CG, Shafran R, Cooper Z. A cognitive behavioural theory of

anorexia nervosa. Behaviour Research and Therapy. 1999;**37**:1-13. DOI: 10.1016/S0005-7967(98)00102-8

[17] Himmerich H, Bentley J, Kan C, Treasure J. Genetic risk factors for eating disorders: An update and insights into pathophysiology. Therapeutic Advances in Psychopharmacology. 2019;**9**:1-20. DOI: 10.1177/2045125318814734

[18] Jewell T, Collyer H, Gardner T, Tchanturia K, Simic M, Fonagy P, et al. Attachment and mentalization and their association with child and adolescent eating pathology: A systematic review. International Journal of Eating Disorders. 2016;**49**:354-373. DOI: 10.1002/eat.22473

[19] Treasure J, Schmidt U. The cognitive-interpersonal maintenance model of anorexia nervosa revisited: A summary of the evidence for cognitive, socio-emotional and interpersonal predisposing and perpetuating factors. Journal of Eating Disorders. 2013;**1**:1-10. DOI: 10.1186/2050-2974-1-13

[20] Micali N, Treasure J, Simonoff E. Eating disorders symptoms in pregnancy: A longitudinal study of women with recent and past eating disorders and obesity. Journal of Psychosomatic Research. 2007;**63**:297-303. DOI: 10.1016/j.jpsychores.2007.05.003

[21] Micali N. Eating disorders and pregnancy. Psychiatry. 2008;**7**:191-193. DOI: 10.1016/j.mppsy.2008.02.003

[22] Tiller J, Treasure J. Eating disorders precipitated by pregnancy. European Eating Disorders Review. 1998;**6**:178-187. DOI: 10.1002/(SICI)1099-0968(199809)6:3<178::AID-ERV231>3.0.CO;2-Y

[23] Brandenburg BMP, Andersen AE. Unintentional onset of anorexia nervosa. Eating and Weight Disorders. 2007;**12**:97-100. DOI: 10.1007/BF03327584

[24] Schmidt U, Treasure J. Anorexia nervosa: Valued and visible. A cognitive-interpersonal maintenance model and its implications of research and practice. British Journal of Clinical Psychology. 2006;**45**:343-366. DOI: 10.1348/014466505x53902

[25] Steinhausen H. The outcome of anorexia nervosa in the 20th century. The American Journal of Psychiatry. 2002;**159**:1284-1293. DOI: 10.1176/appi.ajp.159.8.1284

[26] Bemis KM. The present status of operant conditioning for the treatment of anorexia nervosa. Behavior Modification. 1987;**11**:432-463. DOI: 10.1177/01454455870114003

[27] Grave RD, Ghoch ME, Sartirana M, Calugi S. Cognitive behavioural therapy for anorexia nervosa: An update. Current Psychiatry Reports. 2015;**18**:1-8. DOI: 10.1007/s11920-015-0643-4

[28] Bruch H. Eating Disorders: Obesity, Anorexia Nervosa and the Person Within. New York: Basic Books; 1973

[29] Garner DM, Bemis KM. Cognitive therapy for anorexia nervosa. In: Garner DM, Garfinkel PE, editors. Handbook of Psychotherapy for Anorexia Nervosa and Bulimia. New York: The Guilford Press; 1985. pp. 107-146

[30] Garner DM, Bemis KM. A cognitive-behavioral approach to anorexia nervosa. Cognitive Therapy and Research. 1982;**6**:123-150. DOI: 10.1007/BF01183887

[31] Garner DM, Vitousek KM, Pike KM. Cognitive-behavioral therapy for anorexia nervosa. In: Garner DM, Garfinkel PE, editors. Handbook of Treatment for Eating Disorders.

New York: Guilford Press; 1997. pp. 94-144

[32] Turner H. Classics revisited. Garner and Bemis (1982): "A cognitive-behavioural approach to anorexia nervosa". Advances in Eating Disorders: Theory, Research and Practice. 2014;**2**:300-306. DOI: 10.1080/02619288.2014.875675

[33] Fisher CA, Skocic S, Rutherford KA, Hetrick SE. Family therapy approaches for anorexia nervosa. Cochrane Database of Systematic Reviews. 2019;**5**:1-165. DOI: 10.1002/14651858.CD004780.pub3

[34] Minuchin S, Rosman BL, Baker L. Psychosomatic Families: Anorexia Nervosa in Context. Cambridge: Harvard University Press; 1978. DOI: 10.4159/harvard.9780674418233

[35] Le Grange D, Eisler I. Family interventions in adolescent anorexia nervosa. Child and Adolescent Psychiatric Clinics of North America. 2009;**18**:159-173. DOI: 10.1016/j.chc.2008.07.004

[36] Cerniglia L, Cimino S, Tafà M, Marzilli E, Ballarotto G, Bracaglia F. Family profiles in eating disorders: Family functioning and psychopathology. Psychology Research and Behavior Management. 2017;**10**:305-312. DOI: 10.2147/PRBM.S145463

[37] Miller-Day M, Marks JD. Perceptions of parental communication orientation, perfectionism, and disordered eating behaviors of sons and daughters. Health Communication. 2006;**19**:153-163. DOI: 10.1207/s15327027hc1902_7

[38] National Institute for Health and Care Excellence. Eating Disorder: Recognition and Treatment [Internet]. 2017. Available from https://www.nice.org.uk/guidance/ng69/chapter/Recommendations [Accessed: 10 December 2019]

[39] Fairburn CG, Cooper Z, Shafran R. Enhanced cognitive behaviour therapy for eating disorders ("CBT-E"): An overview. In: Fairburn CG, editor. Cognitive Behavior Therapy and Eating Disorders. New York: Guilford Press; 2008

[40] Fairburn CG, Cooper Z, Shafran R, Bohn K, Hawker DM, Murphy R, et al. Enhanced cognitive behavior therapy for eating disorders: The core protocol. In: Fairburn CG, editor. Cognitive Behavior Therapy and Eating Disorders. New York: Guilford Press; 2008

[41] Dahlenburg SC, Gleaves DH, Hutchinson AD. Treatment outcome research of enhanced cognitive behaviour therapy for eating disorders: A systematic review with narrative and meta-analytic synthesis. Eating Disorders. 2019;**27**:482-502. DOI: 10.1080/10640266.2018.1560240

[42] Calugi S, El Ghoch M, Dalle GR. Intensive enhanced cognitive behavioural therapy for severe and enduring anorexia nervosa: A longitudinal outcome study. Behaviour Research and Therapy. 2017;**89**:41-48. DOI: 10.1016/j.brat.2016.11.006

[43] Zipfel S, Wild B, Groβ G, Friederich HC, Teufel M, Schellberg D, et al. Focal psychodynamic therapy, cognitive behaviour therapy, and optimised treatment as usual in outpatients with anorexia nervosa (ANTOP study): Randomised controlled trial. Lancet. 2014;**383**:127-137. DOI: 10.1016/S0140-6736(13)61746-8

[44] Byrne S, Wade T, Hay P, Touyz S, Fairburn CG, Treasure J, et al. A randomised controlled trial of three psychological treatments for anorexia nervosa. Psychological Medicine.

2017;**47**:2823-2833. DOI: 10.1017/S0033291717001349

[45] Atwood ME, Friedman A. A systematic review of enhanced cognitive behavioral therapy (CBT-E) for eating disorders. International Journal of Eating Disorders. 2020;**53**:311-330. DOI: 10.1002/eat.23206

[46] Agras WS. Cognitive behavior therapy for the eating disorders. Psychiatric Clinics of North America. 2019;**42**:169-179. DOI: 10.1016/j.psc.2019.01.001

[47] Dalle Grave R, El Ghoch M, Sartirana M, Calugi S. Cognitive behavioral therapy for anorexia nervosa: An update. Current Psychiatry Reports. 2016;**18**:1-8. DOI: 10.1007/s11920-015-0643-4

[48] Hay PJ, Claudino AM, Touyz S, Abd EG. Individual psychological therapy in the outpatient treatment of adults with anorexia nervosa. Cochrane Database of Systematic Reviews. 2015;**7**:1-97. DOI: 10.1002/14651858.cd003909.pub2

[49] Galsworthy-Francis L, Allan S. Cognitive behavioural therapy for anorexia nervosa: A systematic review. Clinical Psychology Review. 2014;**34**:54-72. DOI: 10.1016/j.cpr.2013.11.001

[50] Watson HJ, Bulik CM. Update on the treatment of anorexia nervosa: Review of clinical trials, practice guidelines and emerging interventions. Psychological Medicine. 2013;**43**:2477-2500. DOI: 10.1017/S0033291712002620

[51] Wade S, Byrne S, Allen K. Enhanced cognitive behavioral therapy for eating disorders adapted for a group setting. International Journal of Eating Disorders. 2017;**50**:863-872. DOI: 10.1002/eat.22723

[52] Bamford BH, Mountford VA. Cognitive behavioural therapy for individuals with longstanding anorexia nervosa: Adaptations, clinician survival and system issues. European Eating Disorders Review. 2012;**20**:49-59. DOI: 10.1002/erv.1080

[53] Gregertsen EC, Mandy W, Serpell L. The egosyntonic nature of anorexia: An impediment to recovery in anorexia nervosa treatment. Frontiers in Psychology. 2017;**8**:1-9. DOI: 10.3389/fpsyg.2017.02273

[54] Schmidt U, Oldershaw A, Jichi F, Sternheim L, Startup H, McIntosh V, et al. Out-patient psychological therapies for adults with anorexia nervosa: Randomised controlled trial. British Journal of Psychiatry. 2012;**201**:392-399. DOI: 10.1192/bjp.bp.112.112078

[55] Schmidt U, Magill N, Renwick B, Keyes A, Kenyon M, Dejong H, et al. The Maudsley outpatient study of treatments for anorexia nervosa and related conditions (MOSAIC): Comparison of the Maudsley model of anorexia nervosa treatment for adults (MANTRA) with specialist supportive clinical management (SSCM) in outpatients with broadly defined anorexia nervosa: A randomized controlled trial. Journal of Consulting and Clinical Psychology. 2015;**83**:796-807. DOI: 10.1037/ccp0000019

[56] McIntosh VVW, Jordan J, Carter FA, Luty SE, McKenzie JM, Bulik CM, et al. Three psychotherapies for anorexia nervosa: A randomized, controlled trial. American Journal of Psychiatry. 2005;**162**:741-747. DOI: 10.1176/appi.ajp.162.4.741

[57] McIntosh VVW, Jordan J, Luty SE, Carter FA, McKenzie JM, Bulik CM, et al. Specialist supportive clinical management for anorexia nervosa. International Journal of Eating Disorders. 2006;**39**:625-632. DOI: 10.1002/eat.20297

[58] Carter FA, Jordan J, McIntosh VV, Luty SE, McKenzie JM, Framton CM, et al. The long-term efficacy of three psychotherapies for anorexia nervosa: A randomized, controlled trial. International Journal of Eating Disorders. 2011;**44**:647-654. DOI: 10.1002/eat.20879

[59] Wild B, Friederich H-C, Gross G, Teufel M, Herzog W, Giel KE, et al. The ANTOP study: Focal psychodynamic psychotherapy, cognitive-behavioural therapy, and treatment-as-usual in outpatients with anorexia nervosa—A randomised controlled trial. Trials. 2009;**10**:1-7. DOI: 10.1186/1745-6215-10-23

[60] Dare C, Eisler I, Russell G, Treasure J, Dodge L. Psychological therapies for adults with anorexia nervosa. British Journal of Psychiatry. 2001;**178**:216-221. DOI: 10.1192/bjp.178.3.216

[61] Rienecke R. Family-based treatment of eating disorders in adolescents: Current insights. Adolescent Health, Medicine and Therapeutics. 2017;**8**:69-79. DOI: 10.2147/AHMT.S115775

[62] Le Grange D, Lock J. The dearth of psychological treatment studies for anorexia nervosa. International Journal of Eating Disorders. 2005;**37**:79-91. DOI: 10.1002/eat.20085

[63] Eisler I, Dare C, Hodes M, Russell G, Dodge E, Le Grange D. Family therapy for adolescent anorexia nervosa: The results of a controlled comparison of two family interventions. Journal of Child Psychology and Psychiatry. 2000;**41**:727-736. DOI: 10.1111/1469-7610.00660

[64] Le Grange D, Eisler I, Dare C, Russell GF. Evaluation of family treatments in adolescent anorexia nervosa: A pilot study. International Journal of Eating Disorders. 1992;**12**:347-357. DOI: 10.1002/1098-108X(199212)12:4<347::AID-EAT2260120402>3.0.CO;2-W

[65] Lock J, Agras WS, Bryson S, Kraemer HC. A comparison of short- and long-term family therapy for adolescent anorexia nervosa. Journal of the American Academy of Child and Adolescent Psychiatry. 2005;**44**:632-639. DOI: 10.1097/01.chi.0000161647.82775.0a

[66] Agras WS, Lock J, Brandt H, Bryson SW, Dodge E, Halmi KA, et al. Comparison of 2 family therapies for adolescent anorexia nervosa: A randomized parallel trial. JAMA Psychiatry. 2014;**71**:1279-1286. DOI: 10.1001/jamapsychiatry.2014.1025

[67] Keel PK, Haedt A. Evidence-based psychosocial treatments for eating problems and eating disorders. Journal of Clinical Child and Adolescent Psychology. 2008;**37**:39-61. DOI: 10.1080/15374410701817832

[68] Lock J. An update on evidence-based psychological treatments for eating disorders in children and adolescents. Journal of Clinical Child and Adolescent Psychology. 2015;**44**:707-721. DOI: 10.1080/15374416.2014.971458

[69] Zeeck A, Herpertz-Dahlmann B, Friederich H, Brockmeyer T, Resmark G, Hagenah U, et al. Psychotherapeutic treatment for anorexia nervosa: A systematic review and network meta-analysis. Frontiers in Psychiatry. 2018;**9**:1-14. DOI: 10.3389/fpsyt.2018.00158

[70] Lock J, Nicholls D. Toward a greater understanding of the ways family-based treatment addresses the full range of psychopathology of adolescent anorexia nervosa. Frontiers in Psychiatry. 2020;**10**:1-8. DOI: 10.3389/fpsyt.2019.00968

[71] Lock J, Fitzpatrick KK. Advances in psychotherapy for children and adolescents with eating disorders. American Journal of Psychotherapy. 2009;**63**:287-303. DOI: 10.1176/appi.psychotherapy.2009.63.4.287

[72] Cooper Z, Stewart A. CBT-E and the younger patient. In: Fairburn CG, editor. Cognitive Behavior Therapy and Eating Disorders. New York: Guilford Press; 2008. pp. 221-230

[73] Dalle Grave R, Sartirana M, Calugi S. Enhanced cognitive behavioural therapy for adolescents with anorexia nervosa: Outcomes and predictors of change in a real-world setting. International Journal of Eating Disorders. 2019;**52**:1042-1046. DOI: 10.1002/eat.23122

[74] Dalle Grave R, Calugi S, El Ghoch M, Conti M, Fairburn CG. Inpatient cognitive behavior therapy for adolescents with anorexia nervosa: Immediate and long-term effects. Frontiers in Psychiatry. 2014;**5**:1-7. DOI: 10.3389/fpsyt.2014.00014

[75] Dalle Grave R, Calugi S, Doll HA, Fairburn CG. Enhanced cognitive behaviour therapy for adolescents with anorexia nervosa: An alternative to family therapy? Behaviour Research and Therapy. 2013;**51**:R9-R12. DOI: 10.1016/j.brat.2012.09.008

[76] Calugi S, Dalle Grave R, Sartirana M, Fairburn CG. Time to restore body weight in adults and adolescents receiving cognitive behaviour therapy for anorexia nervosa. Journal of Eating Disorders. 2015;**3**:1-6. DOI: 10.1186/s40337-015-0057-z

[77] Fitzpatrick KK, Moye A, Hoste R, Lock J, Le Grange D. Adolescent focused psychotherapy for adolescents with anorexia nervosa. Journal of Contemporary Psychotherapy. 2010;**40**:31-39. DOI: 10.1007/s10879-009-9123-7

[78] Lock J, Le Grange D, Agras WS, Moye A, Bryson SW, Jo B. Randomized clinical trial comparing family-based treatment with adolescent-focused individual therapy for adolescents with anorexia nervosa. Archives of General Psychiatry. 2010;**67**:1025-1032. DOI: 10.1001/archgenpsychiatry.2010.128

[79] Le Grange D, Lock J, Agras WS, Moye A, Bryson SW, Jo B, et al. Moderators and mediators of remission in family-based treatment and adolescent focused therapy for anorexia nervosa. Behaviour Research and Therapy. 2012;**50**:85-92. DOI: 10.1016/j.brat.2011.11.003

[80] Van den Berg E, Houtzager L, de Vos J, Daemen I, Katsaragaki G, Karyotaki E, et al. Meta-analysis on the efficacy of psychological treatments for anorexia nervosa. European Eating Disorders Review. 2019;**27**:331-351. DOI: 10.1002/erv.2683

[81] Alckmin-Carvalho F, Vega JB, Cobelo AW, Fabbri AD, Pinzon VD, Melo MHS. Evidence-based psychotherapy for treatment of anorexia nervosa in children and adolescents: Systematic review. Archives of Clinical Psychiatry. 2018;**45**:41-48. DOI: 10.1590/0101-60830000000154

[82] Brockmeyer T, Friederich HC, Schmidt U. Advances in the treatment of anorexia nervosa: A review of established and emerging interventions. Psychological Medicine. 2018;**48**:1228-1256. DOI: 10.1017/S0033291717002604

[83] Tchanturia K, editor. Cognitive Remediation Therapy (CRT) for Eating and Weight Disorders. Sussex: Routledge; 2015

[84] Tchanturia K, Lounes N, Holttum S. Cognitive remediation in anorexia nervosa and related conditions: A systematic review. European Eating Disorders Review. 2014;**22**:454-462. DOI: 10.1002/erv.2326

[85] Tchanturia K, Giombini L, Leppanen J, Kinnaird E. Evidence for cognitive remediation therapy in young people with anorexia nervosa: Systematic review and meta-analysis of the literature. European Eating Disorders Review. 2017;**25**:227-236. DOI: 10.1002/erv.2522

[86] Tchanturia K, Lloyd S, Lang K. Cognitive remediation therapy for anorexia nervosa: Current evidence and future research directions. International Journal of Eating Disorders. 2013;**46**:492-495. DOI: 10.1002/eat.22106

[87] Whitney J, Easter A, Tchanturia K. Service users' feedback on cognitive training in the treatment of anorexia nervosa: A qualitative study. International Journal of Eating Disorders. 2008;**41**:542-550. DOI: 10.1002/eat.20536

[88] Easter A, Tchanturia K. Therapists' experiences of cognitive remediation therapy for anorexia nervosa: Implications for working with adolescents. Clinical Child Psychology and Psychiatry. 2011;**16**:233-246. DOI: 10.1177/1359104511401185

[89] Tchanturia K, Brown A, Fleming C. Thinking about emotions: CREST group. In: Tchanturia K, editor. Brief Group Psychotherapy for Eating Disorders: Inpatient Protocols. Sussex: Routledge; 2015. pp. 74-106

[90] Giombini L, Nesbitt S, Leppanen J, Cox H, Foxall A, Easter A, et al. Emotions in play: Young people's and clinician's experience of 'thinking about emotions' group. Eating and Weight Disorders. 2019;**24**:605-614. DOI: 10.1007/s40519-019-00646-3

[91] Russell J, Maguire S, Hunt GE, Kesby A, Suraev A, Stuart J, et al. Intranasal oxytocin in the treatment of anorexia nervosa: Randomized controlled trial during refeeding. Psychoneuroendocrinology. 2018;**87**:83-92. DOI: 10.1016/j.psyneuen.2017.10.014

[92] Maguire S, O'Dell A, Touyz L, Russell J. Oxytocin and anorexia nervosa: A review of the emerging literature. European Eating Disorders Review. 2013;**21**:475-478. DOI: 10.1002/erv.2252

[93] Russell J, Maguire S, Kesby A, McGregor I, O'Dell A, Treasure J. Oxytocin as a treatment enhancer in anorexia nervosa. European Psychiatry. 2017;**41**:S37. DOI: 10.1016/j.eurpsy.2017.01.171

[94] Giel K, Zipfel S, Hallschmid M. Oxytocin and eating disorders: A narrative review on emerging findings and perspectives. Current Neuropharmacology. 2018;**16**:1111-1121. DOI: 10.2174/1570159X15666171128143158

[95] Galbiati F, Aulinas A, Eddy K, Miller K, Klibanski A, Plessow F, et al. SAT-441 oxytocin levels are associated with psychopathology in restricting but not binge-purge subtype of anorexia nervosa. Journal of the Endocrine Society. 2019;**3**:S1. DOI: 10.1210/js.2019-SAT-441

[96] Schmelkin C, Plessow F, Thomas JJ, Gray EK, Marengi DA, Pulumo R, et al. Low oxytocin levels are related to alexithymia in anorexia nervosa. International Journal of Eating Disorders. 2017;**50**:1332-1338. DOI: 10.1002/eat.22784

[97] Jänsch C, Harmer C, Cooper MJ. Emotional processing in women with anorexia nervosa and healthy volunteers. Eating Behavior. 2009;**10**:184-191. DOI: 10.1016/j.eatbeh.2009.06.001

[98] Leppanen J, Ng KW, Tchanturia K, Treasure J. Meta-analysis of the effects of intranasal oxytocin on interpretation and expression of emotions.

Neuroscience and Biobehavioral Reviews. 2017;**78**:125-144. DOI: 10.1016/j.neubiorev.2017.04.010

[99] Plessow F, Eddy KT, Lawson EA. The neuropeptide hormone oxytocin in eating disorders. Current Psychiatry Reports. 2018;**20**:1-11. DOI: 10.1007/s11920-018-0957-0

[100] Schade S, Paulus W. D-cycloserine in neuropsychiatric diseases: A systematic review. International Journal of Neuropsychopharmacology. 2016;**19**:1-7. DOI: 10.1093/ijnp/pyv102

[101] Otto MW, Kredlow MA, Smits JAJ, Hofmann SG, Tolin DF, de Kleine RA, et al. Enhancement of psychosocial treatment with d-cycloserine: Models, moderators, and future directions. Biological Psychiatry. 2016;**80**:274-283. DOI: 10.1016/j.biopsych.2015.09.007

[102] Steinglass J, Sysko R, Schebendach J, Broft A, Strober M, Walsh BT. The application of exposure therapy and d-cycloserine to the treatment of anorexia nervosa: A preliminary trial. Journal of Psychiatric Practice. 2007;**13**:238-245. DOI: 10.1097/01.pra.0000281484.89075.a8

[103] Levinson CA, Rodebaugh TL, Fewell L, Kass AE, Riley EN, Stark L, et al. D-Cycloserine facilitation of exposure therapy improves weight regain in patients with anorexia nervosa: A randomized controlled trial. Journal of Clinical Psychiatry. 2015;**76**:787-793. DOI: 10.4088/JCP.14m09299

[104] Ori R, Amos T, Bergman H, Soares-Weiser K, Ipser JC, Stein DJ. Augmentation of cognitive and behavioural therapies (CBT) with d-cycloserine for anxiety and related disorders. Cochrane Database of Systematic Reviews. 2015;**5**:1-131. DOI: 10.1002/14651858.CD007803.pub2

[105] Hughes K, Halford SJ, Cowan M, Himmerich H, Tchanturia K. Evaluation of a step-up treatment programme for individuals inscribed with a psychiatric diagnosis of eating disorder. Clinical Psychology Forum. 2019;**324**:23-36

[106] Turner A, Alsop A. Unique core skills: Exploring occupational therapists' hidden assets. British Journal of Occupational Therapy. 2015;**78**:739-749. DOI: 10.1177/0308022615601443

[107] World Federation of Occupational Therapists. About Occupational Therapy [Internet]. 2020. Available from: https://wfot.org/about/about-occupational-therapy. [Accessed: 03 April 2020]

[108] Giles GM, Allen ME. Occupational therapy in the rehabilitation of the patient with anorexia nervosa. Occupational Therapy in Mental Health. 1986;**6**:47-66. DOI: 10.1300/J004v06n01_04

[109] Taylor RR. Kielhofner's Model of Human Occupation: Theory and Application. 5th ed. Philadelphia: Lippincott Williams & Wilkins; 2017

[110] Harris P. Facilitating change in anorexia nervosa: The role of occupational therapy. British Journal of Occupational Therapy. 1992;**55**(9):334-339. DOI: 10.1177/030802269205500903

[111] Hughes K, Woodgate D, Halford SJ, Cowan M, Himmerich H. The therapeutic effect of physical activity in a day-hospital patient with anorexia nervosa. Psychiatria Danubina. 2019;**31**:201-203. DOI: 10.24869/psyd.2019.201

[112] Kinnaird E, Norton C, Tchanturia K. Clinicians' views on working with anorexia nervosa and autism spectrum disorder comorbidity: A qualitative study. BMC Psychiatry. 2017;**17**:1-8. DOI: 10.1186/s12888-017-1455-3

[113] Huke V, Turk J, Saeidi S, Kent A, Morgan JF. Autism spectrum disorders in eating disorder populations: A systematic review. European Eating Disorders Review. 2013;**21**:345-351. DOI: 10.1002/erv.2244

[114] Kelly C, Davies M. A review of anorexia nervosa, its relationship to autism and borderline personality disorder, and implications for patient related outcomes. Journal of Psychiatry and Psychiatric Disorders. 2019;**3**:207-215. DOI: 10.26502/jppd.2572-519X0075

[115] Adamson J, Leppanen J, Murin M, Tchanturia K. Effectiveness of emotional skills training for patients with anorexia nervosa with autistic symptoms in group and individual format. European Eating Disorders Review. 2018;**26**:367-375. DOI: 10.1002/erv.2594

[116] Treasure J. Coherence and other autistic spectrum traits and eating disorders: Building from mechanism to treatment. The Birgit Olsson lecture. Nordic Journal of Psychiatry. 2013;**67**:38-42. DOI: 10.3109/08039488.2012.674554

[117] Dandil Y, Baillie C, Tchanturia K. Cognitive remediation therapy as a feasible treatment for a young person with anorexia nervosa and autism spectrum disorder comorbidity: A case study. Clinical Case Studies. 2020;**19**:115-132. DOI: 10.1177/1534650119890425

[118] Kinnaird E, Norton C, Stewart C, Tchanturia K. Same behaviours, different reasons: What do patients with co-occurring anorexia and autism want from treatment? International Review of Psychiatry. 2019;**31**:308-317. DOI: 10.1080/09540261.2018.1531831

[119] Martinussen M, Friborg O, Schmierer P, Kaiser S, Øvergård KT, Neunhoeffer A-L, et al. The comorbidity of personality disorder in eating disorders: A meta-analysis. Eating and Weight Disorders – Studies on Anorexia, Bulimia and Obesity. 2017;**22**:201-209. DOI: 10.1007/s40519-016-0345-x

[120] Link TM, Beermann U, Mestel R, Gander M. Treatment outcome in female in-patients with anorexia nervosa and comorbid personality disorders prevalence—Therapy drop out and weight gain. Psychotherapy, Psychosomatic, Psychological Medicine. 2017;**67**:420-430. DOI: 10.1055/s-0043-103271

[121] Skodol AE, Oldham JM, Hyler SE, Kellman HD, Doidge N, Davies M. Comorbidity of DSM-III-R eating disorders and personality disorders. International Journal of Eating Disorders. 1993;**14**:403-416. DOI: 10.1002/1098-108x(199312)14:4<403::aid-eat2260140403>3.0.co;2-x

[122] Miller AE, Racine SE, Klonksy ED. Symptoms of anorexia nervosa and bulimia nervosa have differential relationships to borderline personality disorder symptoms. Eating Disorders. 2019;**15**:1-14. DOI: 10.1080/10640266.2019.1642034

[123] Navarro-Haro MV, Botella C, Guillen V, Moliner R, Marco H, Jorquera M, et al. Dialectical behaviour therapy in the treatment of borderline personality disorder and eating disorders comorbidity: A pilot study in a naturalistic setting. Cognitive Therapy and Research. 2018;**42**:636-649. DOI: 10.1007/s10608-018-9906-9

[124] Bankoff SM, Karpel MG, Forbes HE, Pantalone DW. A systematic review of dialectical behaviour therapy for the treatment of eating disorders. Eating Disorders. 2012;**20**:196-215. DOI: 10.1080/10640266.2012.668478

[125] Friederich HC, Herzog W. Cognitive-behavioural flexibility in anorexia nervosa. In: Adan RAH, Kaye WH, editors.

Behavioral Neurobiology of Eating Disorders. Heidelberg/Berlin: Springer; 2010. pp. 111-123

[126] Downs KJ, Blow AJ. A substantive and methodological review of family-based treatment for eating disorders: The last 25 years of research. Journal of Family Therapy. 2013;**35**:3-28. DOI: 10.1111/j.1467-6427.2011.00566.x

[127] Murray SB, Quintana DS, Loeb KL, Griffiths S, Le Grange D. Treatment outcomes for anorexia nervosa: A systematic review and meta-analysis of randomized controlled trials. Psychological Medicine. 2018;**49**:535-544. DOI: 10.1017/S0033291718002088

[128] National Institute for Health and Care Excellence. NICE Guidelines [Internet]. 2020. Available from: https://www.nice.org.uk/about/what-we-do/our-programmes/nice-guidance/nice-guidelines [Accessed: 19 March 2020]

[129] Tchanturia K, Larsson E, Brown A. Benefits from group cognitive remediation therapy in anorexia nervosa: Case series. Neuropsychiatry. 2016;**30**:42-49. DOI: 10.1007/s40211-016-0177-y

[130] Friedman K, Ramirez AL, Murray SB, Anderson LK, Cusack A, Boutelle KN, et al. A narrative review of outcome studies for residential and partial hospital-based treatment of eating disorders. European Eating Disorders Review. 2016;**24**:263-276. DOI: 10.1002/erv.2449

[131] Gowers SG, Clark AF, Roberts C, Byford S, Barrett B, Griffiths A, et al. A randomised controlled multicentre trial of treatments for adolescent anorexia nervosa including assessment of cost-effectiveness and patient acceptability. Health Technology Assessment. 2010;**14**:1-98. DOI: 10.3310/hta14150

[132] Madden S, Hay P, Touyz S. Systematic review of evidence for different treatment settings in anorexia nervosa. World Journal of Psychiatry. 2015;**5**:147-153. DOI: 10.5498/wjp.v5.i1.147

[133] Herpertz-Dahlmann B, Schwarte R, Krei M, Warnke A, Wewetzer C, Pfeiffer E, et al. Day-patient treatment after short inpatient care versus continued inpatient treatment in adolescents with anorexia nervosa (ANDI): A multicentre, randomised, open-label, non-inferiority trial. The Lancet. 2014;**383**:1222-1229. DOI: 10.1016/S0140-6736(13)62411-3

[134] Gowers SG, An JW, Shore A, Hossain F, Elvins R. Impact of hospitalisation on the outcome of adolescent anorexia nervosa. British Journal of Psychiatry. 2000;**176**:138-141. DOI: 10.1192/bjp.176.2.138

Section 4

Prevention and Treatment of Obesity - Difficulties and Novel Ideas

Chapter 14

Anti-Obesity Medical Devices

Hassan M. Heshmati

Abstract

Obesity is a major health problem worldwide responsible for increased morbidity/mortality and high cost for the society. Management of obesity requires multidisciplinary approaches including diet, food supplement, exercise, behavior change, drug, medical device, gut microbiome manipulation, and surgery. Anti-obesity medical devices are an option for subjects who have not responded to more conservative medical treatments but want an alternative to surgery. Compared to bariatric surgery, they have the advantage of being less invasive, easier to perform, and reversible. In the United States of America (USA), based on the expected weight loss, the Center for Devices and Radiological Health (CDRH) of the Food and Drug Administration (FDA) categorizes anti-obesity medical devices as weight-loss devices or weight-management devices. The weight-loss devices include gastric band devices, gastric space-occupying devices, and gastric emptying devices. The weight-management devices include oral removable palatal space-occupying devices and ingested transient gastric space-occupying devices. The effectiveness, safety, and cost of anti-obesity medical devices vary considerably by the type of medical device. Their use should always be combined with lifestyle changes. Considering the large market size of obesity treatment, anti-obesity medical devices can play a major role in the management of obesity.

Keywords: medical devices, obesity, weight loss, weight management

1. Introduction

Obesity is excess body weight for a given height, defined by a body mass index (BMI) ≥ 30 kg/m^2. In some Asian countries (e.g., Japan), the threshold to define obesity is lower (25 kg/m^2). Obesity is a major health problem worldwide associated with increased morbidity/mortality and high cost for the society. The prevalence of obesity has doubled in more than 70 countries since 1980. The number of adult subjects with obesity is around 700 million worldwide. Nearly 4 million subjects die each year from the consequences of obesity. The annual cost of obesity is more than $2 trillion [1–3].

Management of obesity requires multidisciplinary approaches including diet, food supplement, exercise, behavior change, drug, medical device, gut microbiome manipulation, and surgery [1, 4–9]. The annual obesity treatment market is around $6 billion. In the USA, among subjects with obesity, only 2% receive drug therapy and less than 1% who are eligible for bariatric surgery benefits from it. The reasons for these undertreatment rates are mainly related to adverse effects/complications and cost of drugs and bariatric surgery.

Medical devices available 100 years ago were limited to stethoscope, original medical X-ray imaging device, and electrocardiograph [10]. Over the past several

IntechOpen

decades, the number of medical devices has increased exponentially. Anti-obesity medical devices are positioned to bridge the gap between more conservative treatments (e.g., lifestyle) and more aggressive interventions (e.g., bariatric surgery). Compared to bariatric surgery, they have the advantage of being less invasive, easier to perform, and reversible. Anti-obesity medical devices are available upon prescription or as over-the-counter products.

2. Heterogeneity of anti-obesity medical devices

Anti-obesity medical devices represent a heterogeneous family of devices in terms of presentation, usage/administration, mechanism of action, effectiveness, safety, regulation, availability, and cost [8, 11–14]. The devices can be as different as an intragastric balloon, a stomach aspiration system, or particles administered orally in capsule.

3. General characteristics of anti-obesity medical devices

Unlike anti-obesity drugs that act chemically through specific receptors, anti-obesity medical devices act rather mechanically. They do not have systemic absorption, specific metabolism, or receptors. Their research and development pattern follow specific models. The terminology used for medical devices differs slightly from that used for drugs (e.g., sham instead of placebo, effectiveness instead of efficacy). With some medical devices, it is not possible to use a sham for ethical and/or technical reasons. Compared to drugs, medical devices have different effectiveness dynamics. Unlike drugs, for some anti-obesity medical devices, there is no compliance issue with the device use since the device is placed in the body for several months and there is no need for repeated administration that might be affected by the subject's discipline. Because there is no systemic absorption, there are no side effects related to the impact of medical devices on different organs through the bloodstream. The regulatory systems ruling anti-obesity medical devices are based on short product life cycles. The marketing and sales of anti-obesity medical devices are based on different models as compared to drugs.

4. Mechanism of action of anti-obesity medical devices

Anti-obesity medical devices can cause weight loss through different mechanisms by acting at different levels.

4.1 Decrease in food intake

Although the primary impact of the anti-obesity medical devices is mechanical, the final effect may be achieved through changes in several factors controlling appetite and food intake, especially the gastrointestinal hormones (e.g., decrease in ghrelin, increase in glucagon-like peptide-1).

4.1.1 Oral cavity

An anti-obesity medical device can decrease the food intake by limiting the bite size in the oral cavity.

4.1.2 Stomach

An anti-obesity medical device can decrease the food intake by reducing the available stomach volume.

4.1.3 Others

Other levels of impact to achieve food intake reduction are possible and have been or will be investigated.

4.2 Decrease in available/absorbed nutrient

4.2.1 Stomach

An anti-obesity medical device can decrease the amount of available nutrient by removing part of the gastric contents.

4.2.2 Intestine

An anti-obesity medical device can decrease the absorbed nutrient by bypassing part of the intestine.

5. Challenges in developing anti-obesity medical devices

The main challenges in the development of anti-obesity medical devices are due to lack of unique regulatory guidance and disparities in time and cost of approval processes in different countries.

6. Regulation and approval/clearance of anti-obesity medical devices

The regulation of anti-obesity medical devices varies by countries or group of countries. There are important differences in the regulatory processes, cost, and time to approval between the USA and Europe [15].

Over-the-counter anti-obesity medical devices may or may not need regulation and approval/clearance depending on the devices and countries.

6.1 USA

In the USA, the regulation of medical devices is centralized since 1976 through the FDA. This centralized process allows a better coordination and enforcement of rules. The CDRH is in charge of approval/clearance of anti-obesity medical devices. There are three regulatory classes of medical devices: Class I (low risk), Class II (moderate risk), and Class III (high risk). Based on the expected weight loss, two categories of anti-obesity medical devices have been defined: weight-loss devices ("more" weight loss) and weight-management devices ("less" weight loss). The approval/clearance is through premarket notification process [510(k)] or premarket approval (PMA) process and is based on safety and effectiveness.

A new guidance using benefit-risk approaches is in preparation by the CDRH taking into account the weight loss (extent and duration), the rate of responders ($\geq$ 5% weight loss), the reduction of comorbidities (e.g., hypertension, dyslipidemia, type 2 diabetes), and the safety [rate and severity of adverse events (AEs)].

6.2 Europe

Since its formation in 1993, the European Union (EU), currently a group of 27 countries (after the recent removal of the United Kingdom), has established rules for the approval of medical devices. Anti-obesity medical devices are regulated under directive 93/42/EC. There are four regulatory classes of medical devices: Class I (low risk), Class IIa (low-moderate risk), Class IIb (moderate-high risk), and Class III (high risk). Each member country has a regulatory entity called Competent Authority (CA). The CA certifies/notifies entities called Notified Bodies (NBs) in each country. The NBs are private, for-profit companies responsible for conformity assessment and CE (Conformité Européenne) mark. There are over 50 NBs in the EU. The NBs contract with the manufacturers to supply the CE mark and the approval is based on safety and performance. Clinical effectiveness is not a requirement. An anti-obesity medical device with a CE mark can be marketed in any EU member country.

In the EU, the approval process is more flexible, faster, and less expensive in comparison to the USA.

6.3 Other countries

Other countries have different regulatory procedures. The approval process has varying degrees of sophistication and challenges. In Japan for example, the application is processed by the Pharmaceutical and Medical Device Agency (PMDA). Although the Japanese market is very attractive for foreign manufacturers, the approval process is complicated, long, and expensive due to multiple factors (e.g., lack of translated documents from Japanese, need to perform specific and costly studies in the Japanese population).

Several countries accept the FDA approval/clearance or the CE mark.

7. Approved/cleared anti-obesity medical devices

Several anti-obesity medical devices have been approved/cleared in the USA, in the EU, and in other countries. Some devices have been approved first in the EU before being approved several years later in the USA. This section focuses on anti-obesity medical devices regulated in the USA.

Below are the anti-obesity medical devices approved/cleared in the USA (**Table 1**). Their use should always be in conjunction with lifestyle recommendations on diet and exercise.

Medical device	Approval date	Indication
Lap-Band®	June 5, 2001	Weight-loss device (BMI ≥ 35 kg/m^2)
Orbera™ Intragastric Balloon System	August 5, 2015	Weight-loss device (BMI 30–40 kg/m^2)
AspireAssist®	June 14, 2016	Weight-loss device (BMI 35–55 kg/m^2)
Obalon Balloon System	September 8, 2016	Weight-loss device (BMI 30–40 kg/m^2)
SmartByte Device	May 18, 2017	Weight-management device (BMI 27–35 kg/m^2)
Plenity™	April 12, 2019	Weight-management device (BMI 25–40 kg/m^2)
TransPyloric Shuttle	April 16, 2019	Weight-loss device (BMI 30–40 kg/m^2)

Table 1.
Approved/cleared anti-obesity medical devices in the USA ranked by approval date.

7.1 Weight-loss devices

7.1.1 Gastric band devices

7.1.1.1 Lap-Band®

Lap-Band® (BioEnterics Corporation) is an adjustable silicone band placed laparoscopically around the proximal stomach immediately below the gastro-esophageal junction and attached to a subcutaneous reservoir (**Figure 1**). The level of pressure is adjusted by varying the amount of fluid that is inserted into the band. The technique is reversible, has low procedural risk, and can be performed in an outpatient setting. Lap-Band® can be revised and/or replaced as needed. The pressure imposed to the proximal stomach causes early satiety and a decrease in food intake with subsequent weight loss [8].

In the pivotal study, 292 subjects (247 females, 45 males, mean BMI = 47.4 kg/m^2) were implanted with Lap-Band® and had follow-up evaluations for 36 months. The primary effectiveness endpoint, assessed in the per protocol population at Month 36, was the excess weight loss. Safety analysis also included an additional seven subjects who previously received a similar device. At Month 36, the excess weight loss was 36.2%, relatively stable over the previous 18 months (the weight loss was 18.0%). AEs were observed in 266 subjects (89.0%). Most AEs were of gastrointestinal origin (mainly nausea/vomiting, gastroesophageal reflux, and abdominal pain, mild in the majority of cases). Serious AEs (SAEs) were observed in 16 subjects (5.4%), mainly port leakage and 2 deaths (unrelated to device).

Overall, Lap-Band® is relatively safe and has a strong effectiveness. The device was approved by the FDA in June 2001. It is indicated for weight loss in severe obesity with BMI ≥ 40 kg/m^2 or obesity with BMI ≥ 35 kg/m^2 in the presence of one or more severe comorbidities, in conjunction with lifestyle recommendations, in subjects who failed to respond to diet, exercise, and behavior change. It is contraindicated in several conditions including pregnancy, non-adult subjects, inflammatory diseases of the gastrointestinal tract, upper gastrointestinal bleeding conditions,

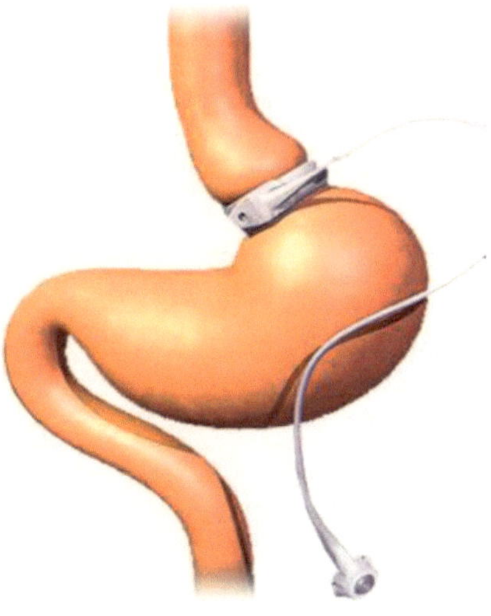

Figure 1.
Lap-Band® (BioEnterics Corporation—Picture downloaded from the internet).

portal hypertension, and severe cardiopulmonary diseases (non-exhaustive list). Complications include proximal gastric enlargement, erosion or migration of the band, and leaks of the band system (non-exhaustive list).

7.1.2 Gastric space-occupying devices

7.1.2.1 Orbera™ Intragastric balloon system

Orbera™ Intragastric Balloon System (Apollo Endosurgery, Inc.) is a balloon made of silicone placed endoscopically in the stomach (**Figure 2**). The balloon is filled with saline mixed with methylene blue (450–700 mL). The methylene blue is a marker for balloon dysfunction. In case of balloon rupture, the methylene blue will be systematically absorbed and change the color of urine to blue. The procedure is minimally invasive and can be performed in an outpatient setting. The balloon is removed endoscopically after 6 months. By occupying gastric volume, Orbera™ Intragastric Balloon System causes early satiety and a decrease in food intake with subsequent weight loss [8, 11, 13, 14].

In the pivotal study, 255 subjects (229 females, 26 males, mean BMI = 35.3 kg/m^2) were randomized into Orbera™ Intragastric Balloon System (n = 125) or control (no intragastric intervention, n = 130) arms for 6 months and 6 months follow-up after Orbera™ Intragastric Balloon System removal. Safety analysis also included an additional 35 run-in, non-randomized subjects who received Orbera™ Intragastric Balloon System. All subjects were given lifestyle recommendations. The co-primary effectiveness endpoints, assessed in the modified intention-to-treat (mITT) population at Month 9, were the excess weight loss in Orbera™ Intragastric Balloon System arm and a significantly greater weight loss in Orbera™ Intragastric Balloon System arm compared to control arm. At Month 9, the excess weight loss was 26.5% in Orbera™ Intragastric Balloon System arm, and the weight losses were 9.1 and 3.4% in Orbera™ Intragastric Balloon System and control arms, respectively. The study did not meet the first co-primary effectiveness endpoint but met the second co-primary effectiveness endpoint. At Month 6, the weight losses were 10.2 and 3.3% in Orbera™ Intragastric Balloon System and control arms, respectively. A total of 810 device-related AEs was observed (mainly nausea/vomiting, gastroesophageal reflux, and abdominal pain, mild or moderate in the majority of cases). Fourteen device- or procedure-related SAEs were observed, mainly device intolerance but no death.

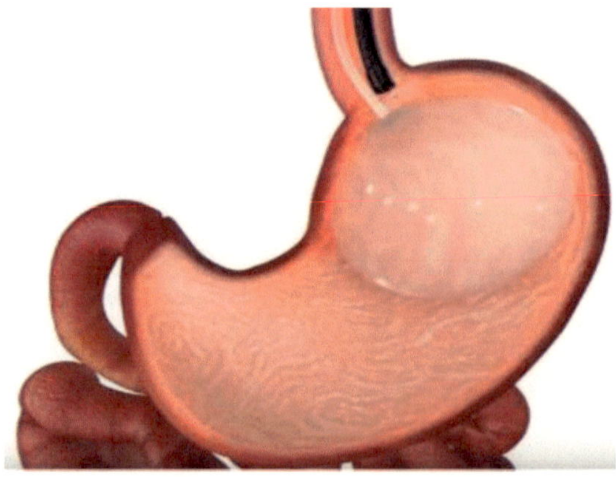

Figure 2.
Orbera™ Intragastric Balloon System (Apollo Endosurgery, Inc.—Picture downloaded from the internet).

Overall, Orbera™ Intragastric Balloon System is relatively safe and has a strong effectiveness. The device was approved by the FDA in August 2015. It is indicated for weight loss in obesity with BMI between 30 and 40 kg/m^2, in conjunction with lifestyle recommendations, in subjects who failed to respond to diet, exercise, and behavior change. It is contraindicated in several conditions including pregnancy, non-adult subjects, prior bariatric surgery, inflammatory diseases of the gastrointestinal tract, upper gastrointestinal bleeding conditions, and liver deficiency (non-exhaustive list). Complications include balloon migration, intestinal obstruction, gastric ulcer, and gastric perforation (non-exhaustive list).

7.1.2.2 Obalon Balloon System

Obalon Balloon System (Obalon Therapeutics, Inc.) is a swallowable balloon made of nylon and polyethylene contained within a gelatin capsule (attached to a thin inflation catheter) that is taken orally. The correct position of the capsule is confirmed with fluoroscopy. The capsule disintegrates in the stomach and releases the balloon. The balloon is filled with air (250 cc of nitrogen and sulfur hexafluoride gas mixture). Up to three balloons can be placed in the same session or sequentially over a 6-month period (**Figure 3**). The procedure is minimally invasive and can be performed in an outpatient setting without endoscopy. The balloon is removed endoscopically after 6 months. By occupying gastric volume, Obalon Balloon System causes early satiety and a decrease in food intake with subsequent weight loss [8, 13, 14].

In the pivotal study, 387 subjects (341 females, 46 males, mean BMI = 35.2 kg/m^2) were randomized into Obalon Balloon System (n = 198) or control (sham capsule, n = 189) arms for 6 months. At Month 6, the eligible control arm subjects were permitted to crossover and receive Obalon Balloon System for 6 months. All subjects were given lifestyle recommendations. The co-primary effectiveness endpoints, assessed in the mITT population at Month 6, were a significantly greater weight loss in Obalon Balloon System arm compared to control arm (super-superiority) and the responder rate at 5% weight loss in Obalon Balloon System arm. Device-related safety analysis also included 138 subjects who switched at Month 6 from control to Obalon Balloon System. At Month 6, the weight losses were 6.6 and 3.4% in Obalon Balloon System and control arms, respectively, and the responder rate at 5% weight loss in Obalon Balloon System arm was 62.1%. The study met both co-primary effectiveness endpoints. Most device-related AEs were of gastrointestinal origin (mainly abdominal pain and nausea/vomiting, mild in the majority of cases), observed in

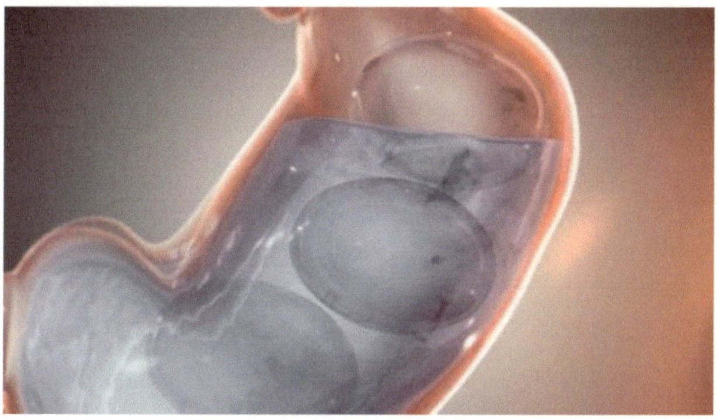

Figure 3.
Obalon Balloon System (Obalon Therapeutics, Inc.—Picture downloaded from the internet).

300 subjects (89.3%). Device- or procedure-related SAEs were observed in one subject (0.3%), a case of peptic ulcer disease.

Overall, Obalon Balloon System is relatively safe and has a modest effectiveness. The device was approved by the FDA in September 2016. It is indicated for weight loss in obesity with BMI between 30 and 40 kg/m^2, in conjunction with lifestyle recommendations, in subjects who failed to respond to diet, exercise, and behavior change. It is contraindicated in several conditions including pregnancy, non-adult subjects, prior bariatric surgery, inflammatory diseases of the gastrointestinal tract, gastric diseases, and eating disorders (non-exhaustive list). Complications include balloon migration, intestinal obstruction, gastric ulcer, and gastric perforation (non-exhaustive list).

7.1.2.3 TransPyloric Shuttle

TransPyloric Shuttle (BAROnova, Inc.) is a device placed endoscopically in the stomach (**Figure 4**). It is not strictly a balloon but functions like a balloon. It has two asymmetrical bulbs made of silicone connected by a flexible catheter. The procedure is minimally invasive and can be performed in an outpatient setting. The shuttle is removed endoscopically after 12 months. By creating intermittent obstruction to gastric outflow that delays gastric emptying, TransPyloric Shuttle causes early satiety and a decrease in food intake with subsequent weight loss [8, 13].

In the pivotal study, 270 subjects (252 females, 18 males, mean BMI = 36.6 kg/m^2) were randomized into TransPyloric Shuttle (n = 181) or control (sham endoscopic procedure, n = 89) arms for 12 months. The TransPyloric Shuttle was successfully placed in 171 subjects. The study also included an additional 32 open-label subjects who received TransPyloric Shuttle. All subjects were given lifestyle recommendations. The co-primary effectiveness endpoints, assessed in the per protocol population at Month 12, were a significantly greater weight loss in TransPyloric Shuttle arm compared to control arm and the responder rate at 5% weight loss in TransPyloric Shuttle arm. At Month 12, the weight losses were 9.5 and 2.8% in TransPyloric Shuttle and control arms, respectively, and the responder rate at 5% weight loss in TransPyloric Shuttle arm was 66.8%. The study met both co-primary effectiveness endpoints. Most device-related AEs were of gastrointestinal origin (mainly nausea/vomiting, abdominal pain, and dyspepsia, mild or moderate in the majority of

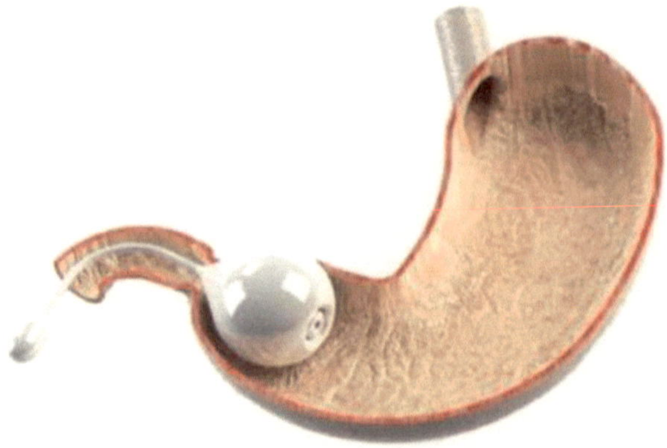

Figure 4.
TransPyloric Shuttle (BAROnova, Inc.—Picture downloaded from the internet).

cases), observed in 200 subjects (98.5%). Device- or procedure-related SAEs were observed in six subjects (3.0%), mainly device impaction but no death.

Overall, TransPyloric Shuttle is relatively safe and has a strong effectiveness. The device was approved by the FDA in April 2019. It is indicated for weight loss in obesity with BMI between 35 and 40 kg/m^2 or obesity with BMI between 30 and < 35 kg/m^2 in the presence of one or more comorbidities, in conjunction with lifestyle recommendations, in subjects who failed to respond to diet, exercise, and behavior change. It is contraindicated in several conditions including pregnancy, non-adult subjects, prior bariatric surgery, inflammatory diseases of the gastrointestinal tract, gastric diseases, and eating disorders (non-exhaustive list). Complications include device impaction and gastric ulcer (non-exhaustive list).

7.1.3 Gastric emptying devices

7.1.3.1 AspireAssist®

AspireAssist® (Aspire Bariatrics, Inc.) is a device attached to a percutaneous endoscopic gastrostomy tube implanted endoscopically (**Figure 5**). It allows the aspiration of gastric contents 20–30 minutes after each major meal (a meal containing more than 200 calories). Thorough chewing of food is required to facilitate aspiration with the 6-mm-diameter tube. The procedure is minimally invasive and can be performed in an outpatient setting. The device is removed when the desired body weight is reached. By allowing the removal of approximately 30% of ingested calories over 5–10 minutes, AspireAssist® causes decreased absorption of gastrointestinal nutrients with subsequent weight loss [8, 11–14].

In the pivotal study, 171 subjects (149 females, 22 males, mean BMI = 41.6 kg/m^2) were randomized into AspireAssist® (n = 111) or control (no intragastric intervention, n = 60) arms for 12 months. All subjects were given lifestyle recommendations. The co-primary effectiveness endpoints, assessed in the mITT population at Month 12, were a significantly greater excess weight loss in AspireAssist® arm compared to control arm (super-superiority) and the responder rate at 25% excess weight loss in AspireAssist® arm. At Month 12, the excess weight losses were 31.5 and 9.8% in AspireAssist® and control arms, respectively, and the responder rate at 25% excess weight loss in AspireAssist® arm was 56.8%. The study met the first co-primary effectiveness endpoint but not the second co-primary effectiveness endpoint. At Month 12, the weight losses were 12.1 and 3.6% in AspireAssist® and

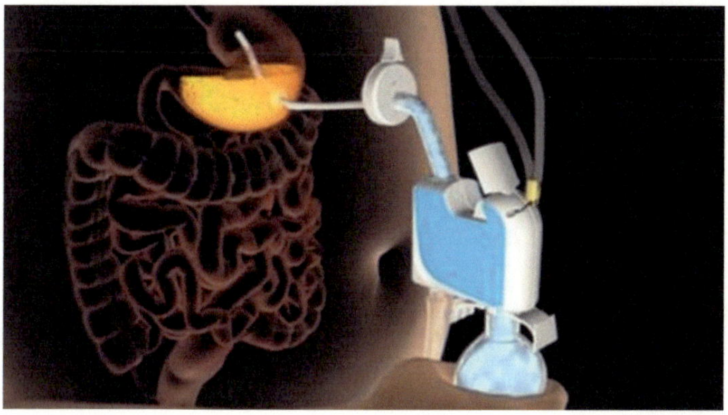

Figure 5.
AspireAssist® (Aspire Bariatrics, Inc.—Picture downloaded from the internet).

control arms, respectively. Device- or procedure-related AEs were observed in 93 subjects (83.8%, mainly peristomal granulation tissue, abdominal pain, and nausea/vomiting, mild in the majority of cases). Device- or procedure-related SAEs were observed in four subjects (3.6%), including peritonitis but no death.

Overall, AspireAssist® is relatively safe and has a strong effectiveness. The device was approved by the FDA in June 2016. It is indicated for weight loss in obesity with BMI between 35 and 55 kg/m^2, in conjunction with lifestyle recommendations, in subjects who failed to respond to non-surgical weight-loss therapy. It is contraindicated in several conditions including pregnancy, non-adult subjects, upper gastrointestinal bleeding conditions, chronic abdominal pain, severe cardiopulmonary diseases, and eating disorders (non-exhaustive list). Complications include skin irritation, infection, and electrolyte abnormalities (non-exhaustive list).

7.2 Weight-management devices

7.2.1 Oral removable palatal space-occupying devices

7.2.1.1 SmartByte Device

SmartByte Device (Scientific Intake) is an oral device occupying space on the upper palate. It includes a temperature-recording sensor to monitor usage (**Figure 6**). It is worn in mouth during meal consumption. The device is renewed every 12 months. By creating limited bite size and slower eating, SmartByte Device causes a decrease in food intake with subsequent weight loss [16].

In the pivotal study, 173 subjects (BMI between 26 and 36 kg/m^2) were randomized into SmartByte Device (n = 102) or control (no oral intervention, n = 71) arms for 4 months. All subjects were given lifestyle recommendations. The primary effectiveness endpoint, assessed in the ITT population at Month 4, was a greater responder rate at 5% weight loss in SmartByte Device arm compared to control arm. At Month 4, the responder rates at 5% weight loss were 20.6 and 5.6% in SmartByte Device and control arms, respectively. The study did not meet the primary effectiveness endpoint. At Month 4, the weight losses were 1.7 and 0.4% in SmartByte Device and control arms, respectively. Device-related AEs were observed in five subjects (4.9%, including two episodes of transient choking on food). No device-related SAEs were observed.

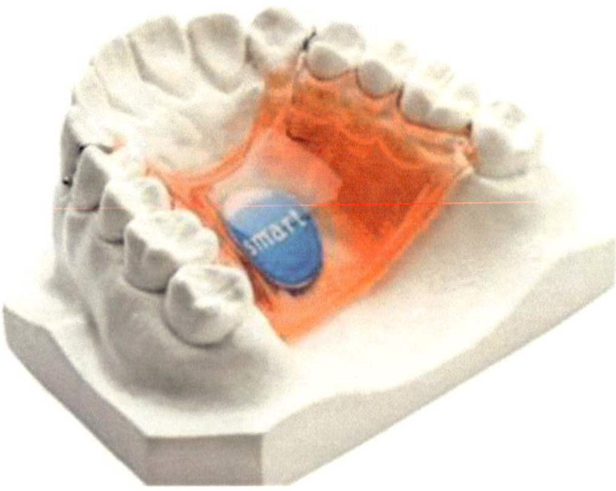

Figure 6.
SmartByte Device (Scientific Intake—Picture downloaded from the internet).

Overall, SmartByte Device is safe and has a weak effectiveness. The device was cleared by the FDA in May 2017. It is indicated to aid in weight management in overweight and obesity with BMI between 27 and 35 kg/m^2, in conjunction with lifestyle recommendations. It is contraindicated in pregnancy and eating disorders. Complications include choking on food and mouth soreness (non-exhaustive list).

7.2.2 Ingested transient gastric space-occupying devices

7.2.2.1 Plenity™

Plenity™ (Gelesis, Inc.) is a superabsorbent hydrogel (cellulose and citric acid, forming a three-dimensional matrix) administered orally in capsules with 500 mL of water (three capsules, 20–30 minutes before lunch and dinner). The hydrogel particles hydrate up to 100 times their initial weight in the stomach and intestine (**Figure** 7). The particles mix with ingested food and create a larger volume with higher elasticity and viscosity. The particles degrade in the colon and are eliminated in the feces. By creating a larger volume with higher elasticity in the stomach and intestine, Plenity™ causes early satiety and a decrease in food intake with subsequent weight loss [17].

In the pivotal study, 436 subjects (245 females, 191 males, mean BMI = 33.8 kg/m^2) were randomized into Plenity™ (n = 223) or control (sham capsule, n = 213) arms for 6 months. All subjects were given lifestyle recommendations. The co-primary effectiveness endpoints, assessed in the ITT population (multiple imputation) at Month 6, were a significantly greater weight loss in Plenity™ arm compared to control arm (super-superiority) and the responder rate at 5% weight loss in Plenity™ arm. At Month 6, the weight losses were 6.4 and 4.4% in Plenity™ and control arms, respectively, and the responder rate at 5% weight loss in Plenity™ arm was 58.6%. The study did not meet the first co-primary effectiveness endpoint but met the second co-primary effectiveness endpoint. Most device-related AEs were of gastrointestinal origin (mainly abdominal distension, diarrhea, infrequent bowel movements, and flatulence, mild in the majority of cases), observed in 84 subjects (37.7%). No device-related SAEs were observed.

Overall, Plenity™ is safe and has a modest effectiveness. The device was cleared by the FDA in April 2019. It is indicated to aid in weight management in overweight and obesity with BMI between 25 and 40 kg/m^2, in conjunction with lifestyle recommendations. It is contraindicated in pregnancy, non-adult subjects, and history of allergic reaction to the components of Plenity™ capsule. No relevant complications have been reported.

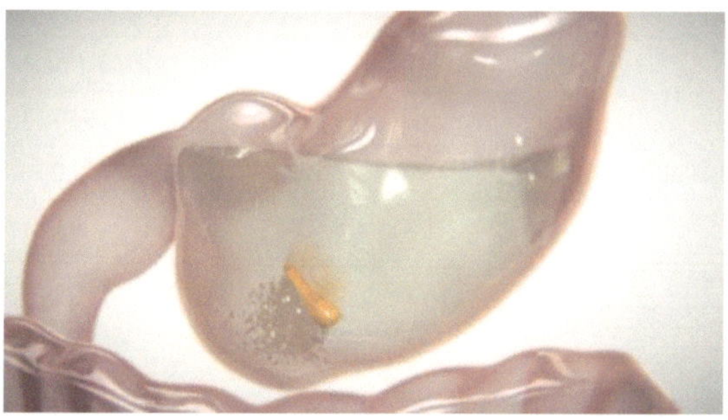

Figure 7.
Plenity™ (Gelesis, Inc.—Picture downloaded from the internet).

Comparative effectiveness of the above anti-obesity medical devices is reported in **Table 2**.

Medical device	Treatment duration	Total body weight loss
Lap-Band®	36 months	18.0%
AspireAssist®	12 months	12.1%
Orbera™ Intragastric Balloon System	6 months	10.2%
TransPyloric Shuttle	12 months	9.5%
Obalon Balloon System	6 months	6.6%
Plenity™	6 months	6.4%
SmartByte Device	4 months	1.7%

Table 2.
Approved/cleared anti-obesity medical devices in the USA ranked by extent of total body weight loss in pivotal studies.

Relevant complications (non-exhaustive list), some being very rare, of the above anti-obesity medical devices are reported in **Table 3**.

Medical device	Treatment duration	Relevant complication
Lap-Band®	36 months	Proximal gastric enlargement, band erosion or migration, system leaks
AspireAssist®	12 months	Skin irritation, infection, electrolyte abnormalities
Orbera™ Intragastric Balloon System	6 months	Balloon migration, intestinal obstruction, gastric ulcer, gastric perforation
TransPyloric Shuttle	12 months	Device impaction, gastric ulcer
Obalon Balloon System	6 months	Balloon migration, intestinal obstruction, gastric ulcer, gastric perforation
Plenity™	6 months	None
SmartByte Device	4 months	Choking on food, mouth soreness

Table 3.
Relevant complications of the approved/cleared anti-obesity medical devices in the USA in pivotal studies.

Cost of the above anti-obesity medical devices is reported in **Table 4**.

Medical device	Average cost (Range)
Lap-Band®	$15,000 ($10,000–$30,000)
AspireAssist®	$10,000 ($7,000–$13,000)
Orbera™ Intragastric Balloon System	$6,000 ($3,000–$9,000)
TransPyloric Shuttle	To be determined
Obalon Balloon System	$8,000 ($6,000–$9,000)
Plenity™	$100/month
SmartByte Device	$500

Table 4.
Cost of the approved/cleared anti-obesity medical devices in the USA.

8. Anti-obesity medical devices withdrawn from the market in the USA

Several anti-obesity medical devices have been withdrawn by the manufacturers from the market in the USA after approval by the FDA (e.g., Maestro Rechargeable System, Realize Adjustable Gastric Band, ReShape Integrated Dual Balloon System, Garren Gastric Bubble).

9. Anti-obesity medical devices under investigation or pending approval

Several anti-obesity medical devices are currently in development in different countries (e.g., Epitomee Device [18]).

EndoBarrier® has obtained a CE mark in the EU but its approval in the USA has been challenged for safety reasons [8, 11–14].

10. Over-the-counter anti-obesity medical devices

A variety of anti-obesity medical devices are available as over-the-counter products (e.g., NozNoz, slow control fork, slipper genie).

11. Conclusions

Anti-obesity medical devices represent a heterogenous family of devices in terms of presentation, usage/administration, mechanism of action, effectiveness, safety, regulation, availability, and cost. They offer an attractive approach in managing obesity. Anti-obesity medical devices are positioned to bridge the gap between more conservative treatments (e.g., lifestyle) and more aggressive interventions (e.g., bariatric surgery). Their use should always be combined with lifestyle changes.

Considering the large market size of obesity treatment and the small percentage of subjects treated with drugs or bariatric surgery, anti-obesity medical devices can play a major role in the management of obesity.

Conflict of interest

The author received honorarium for consultancy from Gelesis, Inc.

Author details

Hassan M. Heshmati
Endocrinology Metabolism Consulting, LLC, Anthem, AZ, USA

*Address all correspondence to: hassanheshmati@yahoo.com

IntechOpen

© 2020 The Author(s). Licensee IntechOpen. This chapter is distributed under the terms of the Creative Commons Attribution License (http://creativecommons.org/licenses/by/3.0), which permits unrestricted use, distribution, and reproduction in any medium, provided the original work is properly cited. CC BY

References

[1] Gadde KM, Martin CK, Berthoud HR, Heymsfield SB. Obesity. Pathophysiology and management. Journal of the American College of Cardiology. 2018;**71**:69-84. DOI: 10.1016/j.jacc.2017.11.011

[2] GBD 2015 Obesity Collaborators, Afshin A, Forouzanfar MH, Reitsma MB, et al. Health effects of overweight and obesity in 195 countries over 25 years. The New England Journal of Medicine. 2017;**377**:13-27. DOI: 10.1056/NEJMoa1614362

[3] Shephard RJ. On determining how much obesity is costing society. The Health & Fitness Journal of Canada. 2019;**12**:80-116. DOI: 10.14288/hfjc.v12i1.276

[4] Freedman MR, King J, Kennedy E. Popular diets: A scientific review. Obesity Research. 2001;**9**(Suppl 1): 1S-40S

[5] Onakpoya IJ, Wider B, Pittler MH, Ernst E. Food supplements for body weight reduction: A systematic review of systematic reviews. Obesity. 2011;**19**: 239-244. DOI: 10.1038/oby.2010.185

[6] Wadden TA, Butryn ML, Hong PS, Tsai AG. Behavioral treatment of obesity in patients encountered in primary care settings. A systematic review. Journal of the American Medical Association. 2014;**312**:1779-1791. DOI: 10.1001/jama.2014.14173

[7] Saxon DR, Iwamoto SJ, Mettenbrink CJ, et al. Antiobesity medication use in 2.2 million adults across eight large health care organizations: 2009-2015. Obesity. 2019;**27**:1975-1981. DOI: 10.1002/oby.22581

[8] Lee PC, Dixon J. Medical devices for the treatment of obesity. Nature Reviews. Gastroenterology & Hepatology. 2017;**14**:553-564. DOI: 10.1038/nrgastro.2017.80

[9] Radvinsky D, Iskandar M, Ferzli G. Bariatric surgery today: The good, the bad, and the ugly. Annals of Laparoscopic and Endoscopic Surgery. 2017;**2**:52. DOI: 10.21037/ales.2017.02.26

[10] Neuman MR, Baura GD, Meldrum S, et al. Advances in medical devices and medical electronics. Proceedings of the IEEE. 2012;**100**:1537-1550. DOI: 10.1109/JPROC.2012.2190684

[11] Chang J, Brethauer S. Medical devices in the treatment of obesity. Endocrinology and Metabolism Clinics of North America. 2016;**45**:657-665. DOI: 10.1016/j.ecl.2016.04.014

[12] Ruban A, Doshi A, Lam E, Teare JP. Medical devices in obesity treatment. Current Diabetes Reports. 2019;**19**:90. DOI: 10.1007/s11892-019-1217-3

[13] Bazerbachi F, Vargas Valls EJ, Abu Dayyeh BK. Recent clinical results of endoscopic bariatric therapies as an obesity intervention. Clinical Endoscopy. 2017;**50**:42-50. DOI: 10.5946/ce.2017.013

[14] Glass J, Chaudhry A, Zeeshan MS, Ramzan Z. New era: Endoscopic treatment options in obesity – A paradigm shift. World Journal of Gastroenterology. 2019;**25**:4567-4579. DOI: 10.3748/wjg.v25.i32.4567

[15] Van Norman GA. Drugs and devices. Comparison of European and U.S. approval processes. JACC: Basic to Translational Science. 2016;**1**:399-412. DOI: 10.1016/j.jacbts.2016.06.003

[16] Ryan DH, Parkin CG, Longley W, Dixon J, Apovian C, Bode B. Efficacy and safety of an oral device to reduce food intake and promote weight loss. Obesity Science & Practice. 2018;**4**: 52-61. DOI: 10.1002/osp4.139

[17] Greenway FL, Aronne LJ, Raben A, et al. A randomized, double-blind, placebo-controlled study of Gelesis100: A novel nonsystemic oral hydrogel for weight loss. Obesity. 2019;**27**:205-216. DOI: 10.1002/oby.22347

[18] Shirin H, Richter V, Matalon S, et al. Safety, tolerability and efficacy of a novel self-use biodegradable device for management of obesity. Obesity Science & Practice. 2019;**5**:376-382. DOI: 10.1002/osp4.343

Chapter 15

Gut Microbiome in Obesity Management

Hassan M. Heshmati

Abstract

Obesity is a worldwide pandemic causing increased morbidity/mortality and high cost for the society. Management of obesity requires multidisciplinary approaches including diet, food supplement, exercise, behavior change, drug, medical device, gut microbiome manipulation, and surgery. Over the past two decades, there has been a growing awareness of the importance of gut microbiome in human health and disease. Profound changes affecting the diversity and the abundance of gut microbiome are associated with several disorders including obesity. A decrease in microbiome diversity and an increase in the ratio of Firmicutes-to-Bacteroidetes phyla have been reported in obese subjects. The gut microbiome can be manipulated to change the host metabolism and manage obesity. Potential interventions include diet (e.g., low calories, low fat, and high fiber), prebiotics (e.g., inulin, lactulose, and resistant starch), probiotics (e.g., yogurt, cheese, and milk), synbiotics (combination of prebiotics and probiotics), bariatric surgery (e.g., Roux-en-Y gastric bypass), and fecal microbiota transplantation (through colonoscopy, esophagogastroduodenoscopy, orogastric tube, or oral capsule). A better understanding of the interactions between different diets and gut microbiome should help the development of new guidelines for the prevention and management of obesity.

Keywords: gut microbiome, obesity, weight management

1. Introduction

Obesity is excess body weight for a given height, defined by a body mass index (BMI) ≥ 30 kg/m^2. In some Asian countries (e.g., Japan), the threshold to define obesity is 25 kg/m^2. The main cause of obesity is an imbalance between energy intake and energy expenditure. Obesity is a worldwide pandemic associated with increased morbidity/mortality and high cost for the society. The prevalence of obesity is increasing exponentially. The number of adult subjects with obesity is around 700 million worldwide. Near 4 million subjects die each year from the consequences of obesity. The annual cost of obesity is more than $2 trillion [1–3].

Management of obesity requires multidisciplinary approaches including diet, food supplement, exercise, behavior change, drug, medical device, gut microbiome manipulation, and surgery [1, 4–9]. The annual obesity treatment market is around $6 billion.

The human intestine harbors a complex and diverse microbial ecosystem referred to as gut microbiome [10–14]. This rich community of microorganisms

IntechOpen

has co-evolved in a symbiotic relationship with humans. Its diversity is influenced by several factors including host genetics, mode of birth, age, gender, pregnancy, BMI, diet, medications, and surgery [12, 15–31]. The understanding of the gut microbiome evolves at a rapid pace, but the practical application of this knowledge is still in its infancy. The gut microbiome is essential for the maintenance of human health. It is involved in protection against pathogens and regulation of immune system and metabolism [32]. Profound changes affecting the diversity and the abundance of gut microbiome (dysbiosis) are associated with several disorders including obesity [33]. The prevention and management of obesity may benefit from manipulation of gut microbiome.

2. Gut microbiome description and composition

Gut microbiome is a complex community of microorganisms living in the digestive tract, mainly in the colon (**Figure 1**). Variable pH and oxygen concentration affect the abundance of gut microbiome across the gastrointestinal tract. Gut microbiome represents up to 60% of the dry mass of feces (biomass around 1.5 kg), has more cells than host somatic cells and at least 100 times more genes than human genome [10–14].

Gut microbiome is established within the few first years of life and contains up to 100 trillion microbes, mainly bacteria (more than 1,000 species) but also fungi, protozoa, archaea, and viruses. The taxonomic ranking of gut microbiome includes species, genera, families, orders, classes, and phyla. Most of the species belong to Actinobacteria, Bacteroidetes, Firmicutes, Proteobacteria, and Verrucomicrobia phyla. The predominant phyla (90%) are Firmicutes (e.g., *Ruminococcus* and *Lactobacillus* genera) and Bacteroidetes (e.g., *Bacteroides* and *Prevotella* genera). Three enterotypes with functional differences have been defined based on variation in the level of genera: Enterotype 1 (*Bacteroides*), Enterotype 2 (*Prevotella*), and Enterotype 3 (*Ruminococcus*).

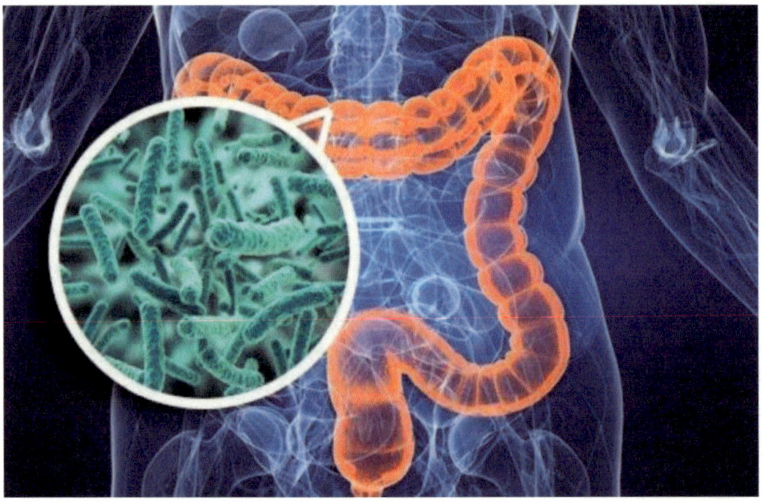

Figure 1.
Gut microbiome is mainly located in the colon (Picture downloaded from the internet).

3. Gut microbiome projects

There are two major gut microbiome projects: European Megagenomics of the Human Intestinal Tract and US Human Microbiome Project [11]. For gut microbiome studies, multiple fecal collections of the same subject are recommended. The assessments are DNA-based methods (16S rDNA sequencing, whole genome shotgun sequencing) (**Figure 2**) [32, 34, 35]. The challenges in the assessments of gut microbiome are due to the diversity and the inter/intra-individual variability caused by different factors such as age and diet.

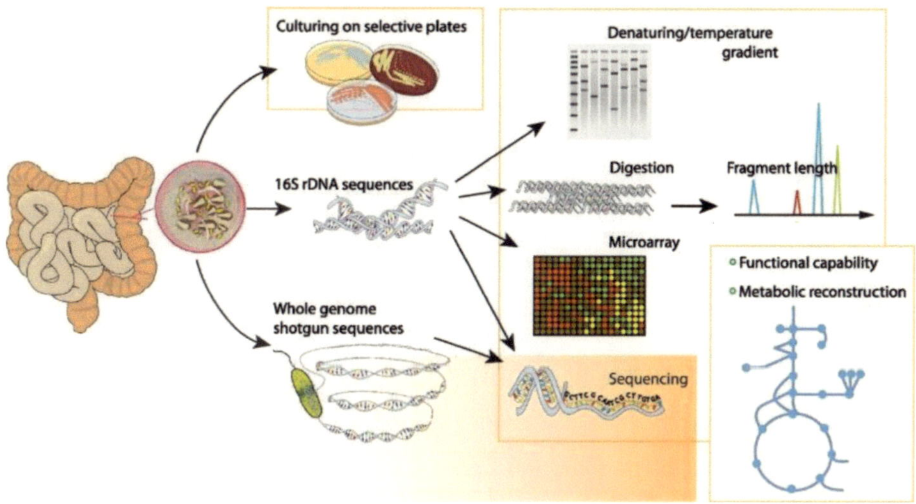

Figure 2.
Assessment of gut microbiome (Picture downloaded from the internet).

4. Gut microbiome metabolism

4.1 Nutrition sources

The sources for nutrition of gut microbiome are ingested dietary components (carbohydrate, protein, lipid) and host-derived components (shed epithelial cells, mucus).

4.2 Metabolites

Several metabolites are produced by gut microbiome. They include short-chain fatty acids (following carbohydrate fermentation), phenolic substances (following protein fermentation), and vitamins (vitamin B, vitamin K).

5. Gut microbiome changes

Gut microbiome is diverse, varies between individuals, and can fluctuate over time. Western gut microbiome has less species than non-Western gut microbiome.

In addition to several pathological conditions that can alter gut microbiome composition, multiple factors are responsible for the changes in gut microbiome (**Figure 3**) [12, 15–31].

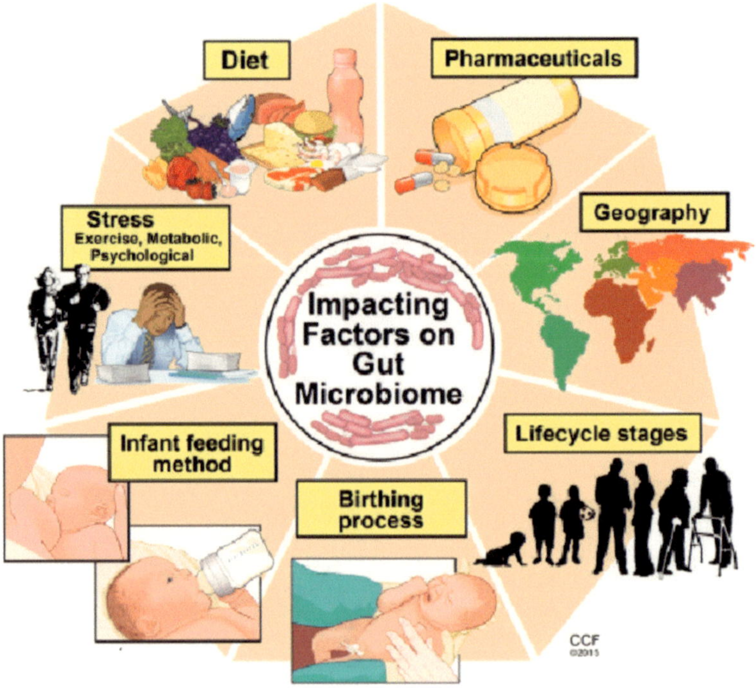

Figure 3.
Multiple factors can impact gut microbiome (Picture downloaded from the Internet).

5.1 Host genetics

There are possible relations between host genetic profile and gut microbiome composition, but additional studies are needed for a better understanding of these relations [15].

5.2 Mode of birth

Mode of birth has an important influence on gut microbiome composition [12, 16]. With vaginal delivery, infants are colonized by maternal vaginal bacteria (dominated by *Lactobacillus* and *Prevotella* genera) while following C-section delivery, infants are colonized by maternal skin bacteria (dominated by *Staphylococcus*, *Corynebacterium*, and *Propionibacterium* genera).

5.3 Age

Age is associated with important changes in gut microbiome [12, 17]. The changes occur mainly before 20 and after 70 years. The diet plays a significant role. In preterm infants, there is a predominance of Proteobacteria phylum. There are marked changes in infants. The choice of diet after birth (breast milk or formula milk) affects the colonization process in the newborn. With age, the introduction of solid food from 2 years and the production of sex hormones from puberty (to menopause in females) bring additional richness and complexity to gut microbiome. There is a relative stability of gut microbiome between 20 and 70 years (predominance of Firmicutes phylum). In elderly subjects, Bacteroidetes phylum is predominant.

5.4 Gender

Gender specificity of gut microbiome appears at puberty with the production of sex hormones [12, 18]. There is a lower abundance of Bacteroidetes phylum in women (role of estrogen).

5.5 Pregnancy

Elevated levels of estrogen and progesterone observed during pregnancy have important impact on gut microbiome [12, 16, 19]. The changes are characterized by a decrease in richness of gut microbiome, a higher abundance of Proteobacteria and Actinobacteria phyla, a decrease in *Faecalibacterium* genus, and an increase in Firmicutes-to-Bacteroidetes phyla ratio.

5.6 BMI

BMI is associated with gut microbiome composition particularly in women [18]. Bacteroidetes phylum is less abundant in subjects with high BMI. The role of estrogen has been proposed.

5.7 Diet

Diet has an important influence on gut microbiome composition [20–25]. However, there is a high interindividual variability. A diet high in fat ($\geq$ 55% of total macronutrients) is associated with increased Firmicutes and Proteobacteria phyla and decreased Bacteroidetes phylum while a diet rich in fiber ($\geq$ 30 g/day) has the opposite effect. The changes in gut microbiome (composition and functionality) induced by diet can be observed as early as 2 days. However, major changes in gut microbiome require long-term change in dietary habits.

Important differences in gut microbiome have been reported in children between Europe and rural African village of Burkina Faso (polysaccharide-rich diet) with Firmicutes-to-Bacteroidetes phyla ratios of 2.8 and 0.5, respectively [26].

Diet may also contribute to the seasonal variations of gut microbiome likely due to different availability of fresh produce containing complex carbohydrates [27].

5.8 Medication

Several medications (e.g., antibiotics, nonsteroidal anti-inflammatory drugs, proton pump inhibitors, and metformin) affect gut microbiome [28–30]. The use of antibiotics is associated with increased Firmicutes phylum, with higher sensitivity in infants.

The impact of prebiotics and probiotics on gut microbiome is presented in Section 8.

5.9 Surgery

Since colon is the main reservoir of gut microbiome, surgical removal of colon may affect gut microbiome [31]. Indeed, right hemicolectomy for colorectal cancer has been reported to be associated with a decrease in diversity and richness of gut microbiome.

The impact of bariatric surgery on gut microbiome is presented in Section 8.

6. Gut microbiome functions

The gut microbiome is involved in multiple physiological functions (**Table 1**) [32, 36–41].

Function of gut microbiome	Mechanism and target
Protection	Killing or inhibiting unwanted organisms competing for nutrients
Immune system	Influencing production of cytokines and antibodies
Metabolism	Regulating energy homeostasis, producing short-chain fatty acids and vitamins, impacting glycemic control, interacting with incretins, regulating metabolism of lipids and bone

Table 1.
Physiological functions of gut microbiome.

6.1 Protection against pathogens

Gut microbiome can protect against pathogens by killing or inhibiting unwanted organisms (e.g., *Clostridium difficile* genera) that are competing for nutrients.

6.2 Regulation of immune system

Gut microbiome regulates immune system by influencing the production of cytokines and antibodies.

6.3 Regulation of metabolism

Gut microbiome is involved in several metabolic processes. These processes include regulation of energy homeostasis and body weight, production of short-chain fatty acids (following fermentation of nondigestible fibers) and vitamins (vitamins B, vitamin K) [32, 36], glycemic control [37, 38], interaction with incretins [39], and metabolism of lipids [40] and bone [41].

7. Gut microbiome in diseases

Dysbiosis is observed in several medical conditions including obesity, malnutrition, type 2 diabetes, inflammatory bowel diseases, neurological disorders, and cancer [33, 42–48]. The dysbiosis can be the cause and/or the consequence of these diseases.

Gut microbiome influences drug pharmacokinetics and bioavailability, and thus, affects the efficacy and safety of several drugs used to treat diseases [49].

8. Gut microbiome and obesity

8.1 Gut microbiome composition in obesity

Although there are some conflicting data, most studies have reported that in obesity, there is a lower gut microbiome diversity, a higher abundance of Firmicutes phylum, a lower abundance of Bacteroidetes phylum, and a higher Firmicutes-to-Bacteroidetes phyla ratio [33, 42–45]. There is also a higher abundance of *Lactobacillus* (genus belonging to Firmicutes phylum).

According to most studies, the low-grade inflammation stimulated by lipopolysaccharide production is the prime mechanism by which gut microbiome induces obesity [50].

8.2 Gut microbiome in obesity management

Gut microbiome can be manipulated for the purpose of obesity management using different tools (**Table 2**) [20, 21, 50–60].

Tool for gut microbiome manipulation	Description
Diet	Low calories, low fat, high fiber
Prebiotics	Inulin, lactulose, resistant starch
Probiotics	Yogurt, cheese, milk
Synbiotics	Combination of prebiotics and probiotics
Bariatric surgery	Roux-en-Y gastric bypass
Fecal microbiota transplantation	Addition of healthy stool

Table 2.
Different tools used for gut microbiome manipulation in obesity management.

8.2.1 Diet

Diet is an important factor for the manipulation of gut microbiome and management of obesity. The amount of daily caloric intake and the content of food significantly affect gut microbiome but with high interindividual variability [20, 21, 51]. A diet that is low in calories, low in fat (< 20% of total macronutrients), and high in fiber (≥ 30 g/day) has a favorable effect on gut microbiome (increase in richness, decrease in Firmicutes-to-Bacteroidetes phyla ratio) and weight control (weight loss).

8.2.2 Prebiotics

Prebiotics are chemicals (nondigestible food ingredients) inducing growth and/or activity of bacteria [50, 52]. Prebiotics must be able to resist gastric acidity, resist enzymatic hydrolysis, resist absorption in the upper gastrointestinal tract, and be fermentable by the gut microbiome. Examples are inulin, lactulose, and resistant starch. Prebiotics can be found in many foods (e.g., leek, asparagus, onion, and soybean).

By modulating gut microbiome and lowering the production of lipopolysaccharide, prebiotics have the potential to manage obesity. In a double-blind, placebo-controlled clinical study, administration of oligofructose-enriched inulin (8 g/day) to overweight/obese children for 16 weeks caused a significant increase in *Bifidobacterium* (genus belonging to Actinobacteria phylum) and significantly slowed the body weight gain compared with placebo [53].

8.2.3 Probiotics

Probiotics are nonpathogenic living microorganisms with direct or indirect effect on gut microbiome [50, 54, 55]. Products containing probiotics should be tested for safety risks before marketing. Probiotics can be found in several foods (e.g., yogurt, cheese, and milk).

Probiotics can manage obesity by reducing the production of lipopolysaccharide through an impact on gut microbiome. In a double-blind, placebo-controlled clinical study, administration of fermented milk containing *Lactobacillus gasseri* species (LG2055) to overweight/obese adults for 12 weeks caused a significant decrease in body weight [56].

8.2.4 Synbiotics

Synbiotics are combination of prebiotics and probiotics. They have the potential to induce more effects on gut microbiome and body weight than prebiotics or probiotics alone.

8.2.5 Bariatric surgery

Bariatric surgery can modify gut microbiome and further affect body weight [57, 58]. The mechanisms include reduced caloric intake, reduced gastric emptying, and alterations in gastric acid production and bile acids.

After Roux-en-Y gastric bypass surgery in obese subjects, there is a decrease in Firmicutes-to-Bacteroidetes phyla ratio and an increase in Proteobacteria phylum [57, 58].

8.2.6 Fecal microbiota transplantation

Fecal microbiota transplantation, which consists of transfer of feces from a healthy donor to a recipient, is an exciting therapy with important potential. It can modify gut microbiome for the purpose of obesity management [59, 60]. The addition of healthy stool can be done through colonoscopy, orogastric tube, esophagogastroduodenoscopy, or oral capsule. It is important to carefully select and screen the donor to avoid risk of infection, aggravation of obesity, or other complications [61, 62].

Available clinical data are very preliminary and limited. Several studies are ongoing. There is no regulatory guidance for the use of fecal microbiota transplantation in the management of obesity.

8.2.7 Cost of gut microbiome manipulation

Cost of gut microbiome manipulation in obesity management is reported in **Table 3**.

Tool for gut microbiome manipulation	Average cost (range)
Diet	Cost of food
Prebiotics	< $100/month
Probiotics	< $100/month
Synbiotics	< $100/month
Bariatric surgery (Roux-en-Y gastric bypass)	$23,000 ($20,000–$30,000)
Fecal microbiota transplantation	$1,800 ($1,600–$2,000) + cost of administration/dose

Table 3.
Cost of different tools used for gut microbiome manipulation in obesity management in the USA.

8.3 Gut microbiome after weight loss

After successful weight loss, there is a decrease in Firmicutes phylum, an increase in Bacteroidetes phylum, and a decrease of Firmicutes-to-Bacteroidetes phyla ratio [45, 51, 57, 58].

9. Clinical study design to assess gut microbiome in obesity

Well-designed clinical studies are urgently needed to better understand the interactions between obesity/obesity treatment and gut microbiome.

Several factors affect the quality of weight-loss studies aimed to assess gut microbiome. A well-calculated sample size allowing subgroup analysis is a key factor. Relevant stratification factors (e.g., race, age, gender, BMI, diet, and medications) at randomization will make the study more informative. Any underestimation of these stratification factors, as it has been the case in several clinical studies, especially in relation to diet and medications, may lead to misleading and conflicting results. The duration of the clinical studies has to be sufficient to allow both short-term and long-term/follow-up assessments. Adequate adjustments should be made during the statistical analysis.

10. Ideal gut microbiome

An ideal gut microbiome should have high diversity. At the level of phyla, the ideal gut microbiome should have low Firmicutes phylum and high Bacteroidetes phylum with a Firmicutes-to-Bacteroidetes phyla ratio < 1.0. At the level of genera, the ideal gut microbiome should be rich in *Prevotella* genus.

The recommended diet to reach the above objectives is a diet adequate in calories (adjusted to the activity), low in fat ($< 20\%$ of total macronutrients), and rich in fiber (≥ 30 g/day).

11. Conclusions

Gut microbiome influences normal physiology and susceptibility to diseases. Profound changes affecting the diversity and the abundance of gut microbiome are associated with obesity. A decrease in microbiome diversity and an increase in the ratio of Firmicutes-to-Bacteroidetes phyla have been reported in obese subjects.

Gut microbiome can be manipulated to change the host metabolism and manage obesity. Potential interventions include diet, prebiotics, probiotics, synbiotics, bariatric surgery, and fecal microbiota transplantation.

A better understanding of the interactions between different diets and gut microbiome should help the development of new guidelines for feeding humans to prevent or manage obesity.

Conflict of interest

The author received honorarium for consultancy from Gelesis, Inc.

Author details

Hassan M. Heshmati
Endocrinology Metabolism Consulting, LLC, Anthem, AZ, USA

*Address all correspondence to: hassanheshmati@yahoo.com

IntechOpen

© 2020 The Author(s). Licensee IntechOpen. This chapter is distributed under the terms of the Creative Commons Attribution License (http://creativecommons.org/licenses/by/3.0), which permits unrestricted use, distribution, and reproduction in any medium, provided the original work is properly cited.

References

[1] Gadde KM, Martin CK, Berthoud HR, Heymsfield SB. Obesity. Pathophysiology and management. Journal of the American College of Cardiology. 2018;**71**:69-84. DOI: 10.1016/j.jacc.2017.11.011

[2] GBD 2015 Obesity Collaborators, Afshin A, Forouzanfar MH, Reitsma MB, et al. Health effects of overweight and obesity in 195 countries over 25 years. The New England Journal of Medicine. 2017;**377**:13-27. DOI: 10.1056/NEJMoa1614362

[3] Shephard RJ. On determining how much obesity is costing society. The Health & Fitness Journal of Canada. 2019;**12**:80-116. DOI: 10.14288/hfjc.v12i1.276

[4] Freedman MR, King J, Kennedy E. Popular diets: A scientific review. Obesity Research. 2001;**9**(Suppl 1): 1S-40S

[5] Onakpoya IJ, Wider B, Pittler MH, Ernst E. Food supplements for body weight reduction: A systematic review of systematic reviews. Obesity. 2011;**19**:239-244. DOI: 10.1038/oby.2010.185

[6] Wadden TA, Butryn ML, Hong PS, Tsai AG. Behavioral treatment of obesity in patients encountered in primary care settings. A systematic review. Journal of the American Medical Association. 2014;**312**:1779-1791. DOI: 10.1001/jama.2014.14173

[7] Saxon DR, Iwamoto SJ, Mettenbrink CJ, et al. Antiobesity medication use in 2.2 million adults across eight large health care organizations: 2009-2015. Obesity. 2019;**27**:1975-1981. DOI: 10.1002/oby.22581

[8] Lee PC, Dixon J. Medical devices for the treatment of obesity. Nature Reviews. Gastroenterology & Hepatology. 2017;**14**:553-564. DOI: 10.1038/nrgastro.2017.80

[9] Radvinsky D, Iskandar M, Ferzli G. Bariatric surgery today: The good, the bad, and the ugly. Annals of Laparoscopic and Endoscopic Surgery. 2017;**2**:52. DOI: 10.21037/ales.2017.02.26

[10] The Human Microbiome Project Consortium. Structure, function and diversity of the healthy human microbiome. Nature. 2012;**486**:207-214. DOI: 10.1038/nature11234

[11] Lozupone CA, Stombaugh JI, Gordon JI, Jansson JK, Knight R. Diversity, stability and resilience of the human gut microbiota. Nature. 2012;**489**:220-230. DOI: 10.1038/nature11550

[12] Kundu P, Blacher E, Elinav E, Pettersson S. Our gut microbiome: The evolving inner self. Cell. 2017;**171**:1481-1493. DOI: 10.1016/j.cell.2017.11.024

[13] Barko PC, McMichael MA, Swanson KS, Williams DA. The gastrointestinal microbiome: A review. Journal of Veterinary Internal Medicine. 2018;**32**:9-25. DOI: 10.1111/jvim.14875

[14] Schmidt TSB, Raes J, Bork P. The human gut microbiome: From association to modulation. Cell. 2018;**172**:1198-1215. DOI: 10.1016/j.cell.2018.02.044

[15] Dąbrowska K, Witkiewicz W. Correlations of host genetics and gut microbiome composition. Frontiers in Microbiology. 2016;7:1357. DOI: 10.3389/fmicb.2016.01357

[16] Nuriel-Ohayon M, Neuman H, Koren O. Microbial changes during pregnancy, birth, and infancy. Frontiers in Microbiology. 2016;7:1031. DOI: 10:3389/fmicb.2016.01031

[17] Odamaki T, Kato K, Sugahara H, et al. Age-related changes in gut microbiota composition from newborn to centenarian: A cross-sectional study. BMC Microbiology. 2016;**16**:90. DOI: 10.1186/s12866-016-0708-5

[18] Dominianni C, Sinha R, Goedert JJ, et al. Sex, body mass index, and dietary fiber intake influence the human gut microbiome. PLoS One. 2015;**10**:e0124599. DOI: 10.1371/journal.pone.0124599

[19] Edwards SM, Cunningham SA, Dunlop AL, Corwin EJ. The maternal gut microbiome during pregnancy. MCN: The American Journal of Maternal/Child Nursing. 2017;**42**:310-317. DOI: 10.1097/NMC.0000000000000372

[20] Wu GD, Chen J, Hoffmann C, et al. Linking long-term dietary patterns with gut microbial enterotypes. Science. 2011;**334**:105-108. DOI: 10.1126/science.1208344

[21] Moschen AR, Wieser V, Tilg H. Dietary factors: Major regulators of the gut's microbiota. Gut and Liver. 2012;**6**:411-416. DOI: 10.5009/gnl.20126.4.411

[22] David LA, Maurice CF, Carmody RN, et al. Diet rapidly and reproducibly alters the human gut microbiome. Nature. 2014;**505**:559-563. DOI: 10.1038/nature12820

[23] Graf D, Di Cagno R, Fåk F, et al. Contribution of diet to the composition of the human gut microbiota. Microbial Ecology in Health and Disease. 2015;**26**:26164. DOI: 10.3402/mehd.v26.26164

[24] Bibbò S, Ianiro G, Giorgio V, et al. The role of diet on gut microbiota composition. European Review for Medical and Pharmacological Sciences. 2016;**20**:4742-4749

[25] Singh RK, Chang HW, Yan D, et al. Influence of diet on the gut microbiome and implications for human health. Journal of Translational Medicine. 2017;**15**:73. DOI: 10.1186/s12967-017-1175-y

[26] De Filippo C, Cavalieri D, Di Paola M, et al. Impact of diet in shaping gut microbiota revealed by a comparative study in children from Europe and rural Africa. PNAS. 2010;**107**:14691-14696. DOI: 10.1073/pnas.1005963107

[27] Davenport ER, Mizrahi-Man O, Michelini K, Barreiro LB, Ober C, Gilad Y. Seasonal variation in human gut microbiome composition. PLoS One. 2014;**9**:e90731. DOI: 10.1371/journal.pone.0090731

[28] Raymond F, Ouameur AA, Déraspe M, et al. The initial state of the human gut microbiome determines its reshaping by antibiotics. The ISME Journal. 2016;**10**:707-720. DOI: 10.1038/ismej.2015.148

[29] Maier L, Pruteanu M, Kuhn M, et al. Extensive impact of non-antibiotic drugs on human gut bacteria. Nature. 2018;**555**:623-628. DOI: 10.1038/nature25979

[30] Le Bastard Q, Al-Ghalith GA, Grégoire M, et al. Systematic review: Human gut dysbiosis induced by non-antibiotic prescription medications. Alimentary Pharmacology & Therapeutics. 2018;**47**:332-345. DOI: 10.1111/apt.14451

[31] Lin XH, Jiang JK, Luo JC, et al. The long term microbiota and metabolic status in patients with colorectal cancer after curative colon surgery. PLoS One. 2019;**14**:e0218436. DOI: 10.1371/journal.pone.0218436

[32] Conrad R, Vlassov AV. The human microbiota: Composition, functions, and therapeutic potential. Medical Science Review. 2015;**2**:92-103. DOI: 10.12659/MSRev.895154

[33] Holmes E, Li JV, Athanasiou T, Ashrafian H, Nicholson JK. Understanding the role of gut microbiome-host metabolic signal disruption in health and disease. Trends in Microbiology. 2011;**19**:349-359. DOI: 10.1016/j.tim.2011.05.006

[34] Ji B, Nielsen J. From next-generation sequencing to systematic modeling of the gut microbiome. Frontiers in Genetics. 2015;**6**:219. DOI: 10.3389/fgene.2015.00219

[35] Magnúsdóttir S, Thiele I. Modeling metabolism of the human gut microbiome. Current Opinion in Biotechnology. 2018;**51**:90-96. DOI: 10.1016/j.copbio.2017.12.005

[36] Ramakrishna BS. Role of the gut microbiota in human nutrition and metabolism. Journal of Gastroenterology and Hepatology. 2013;**28**(Suppl 4):9-17. DOI: 10.1111/jgh.12294

[37] Kovatcheva-Datchary P, Nilsson A, Akrami R, et al. Dietary fiber-induced improvement in glucose metabolism is associated with increased abundance of *Prevotella*. Cell Metabolism. 2015;**22**:971-982. DOI: 10.1016/j.cmet.2015.10.001

[38] Gerard C, Vidal H. Impact of gut microbiota on host glycemic control. Frontiers in Endocrinology. 2019;**10**:29. DOI: 10.3389/fendo.2019.00029

[39] Covasa M, Stephens RW, Toderean R, Cobuz C. Intestinal sensing by gut microbiota: Targeting gut peptides. Frontiers in Endocrinology. 2019;**10**:82. DOI: 10.3389/fendo.2019.00082

[40] Fu J, Bonder MJ, Cenit MC. The gut microbiome contributes to a substantial proportion of the variation in blood lipids. Circulation Research. 2015;**117**:817-824. DOI: 10.1161/CIRCRESAHA.115.306807

[41] Chen YC, Greenbaum J, Shen H, Deng HW. Association between gut microbiota and bone health: Potential mechanisms and prospective. The Journal of Clinical Endocrinology and Metabolism. 2017;**102**:3635-3646. DOI: 10.1210/jc.2017-00513

[42] Hartstra AV, Bouter KEC, Bäckhed F, Nieuwdorp M. Insights into the role of the microbiome in obesity and type 2 diabetes. Diabetes Care. 2015;**38**:159-165. DOI: 10.2337/dc14-0769

[43] Harakeh SM, Khan I, Kumosani T, et al. Gut microbiota: A contributing factor to obesity. Frontiers in Cellular and Infection Microbiology. 2016;**6**:95. DOI: 10.3389/fcimb.2016.00095

[44] Davis CD. The gut microbiome and its role in obesity. Nutrition Today. 2016;**51**:167-174. DOI: 10.1097/0000000000000167

[45] Meijnikman AS, Gerdes VE, Nieuwdorp M, Herrema H. Evaluating causality of gut microbiota in obesity and diabetes in humans. Endocrine Reviews. 2018;**39**:133-153. DOI: 10.1210/er.2017-00192

[46] Lambeth SM, Carson T, Lowe J, et al. Composition, diversity and abundance of gut microbiome in prediabetes and type 2 diabetes. Journal of Diabetes and Obesity. 2015;**2**:1-7. DOI: 10.15436/2376-0949.15.031

[47] Brunkwall L, Orho-Melander M. The gut microbiome as a target for prevention and treatment of hyperglycaemia in type 2 diabetes: From current human evidence to future possibilities. Diabetologia. 2017;**60**:943-951. DOI: 10.1007/s00125-017-4278-3

[48] Hamada T, Nowak JA, Milner DA Jr, Song M, Ogino S. Integration of microbiology, molecular pathology, and epidemiology: A new paradigm to explore the pathogenesis of

microbiome-driven neoplasms. Journal of Pathology. 2019;**247**:615-628. DOI: 10.1002/path.5236

[49] Enright EF, Gahan CGM, Joyce SA, Griffin BT. The impact of the gut microbiota on drug metabolism and clinical outcome. Yale Journal of Biology and Medicine. 2016;**89**:375-382

[50] Dahiya DK, Renuka, Puniya M, et al. Gut microbiota modulation and its relationship with obesity using prebiotics fibers and probiotics: A review. Frontiers in Microbiology. 2017;**8**:563. DOI: 10.3389/fmicb.2017.00563

[51] Voreades N, Kozil A, Weir TL. Diet and the development of the human intestinal microbiome. Frontiers in Microbiology. 2014;**5**:494. DOI: 10.3389/fmicb.2014.00494

[52] Carnahan S, Balzer A, Panchal SK, Brown L. Prebiotics in obesity. Panminerva Medica. 2014;**56**:165-175

[53] Nicolucci AC, Hume MP, Martínez I, Mayengbam S, Walter J, Reimer RA. Prebiotics reduce body fat and alter intestinal microbiota in children who are overweight or with obesity. Gastroenterology. 2017;**153**:711-722. DOI: 10.1053/j.gastro.2017.05.055

[54] Hill C, Guarner F, Reid G, et al. The International Scientific Association for Probiotics and Prebiotics consensus statement on the scope and appropriate use of the term probiotic. Nature Reviews. Gastroenterology & Hepatology. 2014;**11**:506-514. DOI: 10.1038/nrgastro.2014.66

[55] Kobyliak N, Conte C, Cammarota G, et al. Probiotics in prevention and treatment of obesity: A critical view. Nutrition and Metabolism. 2016;**13**:14. DOI: 10.1186/s12986-016-0067-0

[56] Kadooka Y, Sato M, Imaizumi K, et al. Regulation of abdominal adiposity by probiotics (*Lactobacillus gasseri* SBT2055) in adults with obese tendencies in a randomized controlled trial. European Journal of Clinical Nutrition. 2010;**64**:636-643. DOI: 10.1038/ejcn.2010.19

[57] Furet JP, Kong LC, Tap J, et al. Differential adaptation of human gut microbiota to bariatric surgery-induced weight loss. Links with metabolic and low-grade inflammation markers. Diabetes. 2010;**59**:3049-3057. DOI: 10.2337/db10-0253

[58] Sweeney TE, Morton JM. The human gut microbiome. A review of the effect of obesity and surgically induced weight loss. JAMA Surgery. 2013;**148**:563-569. DOI: 10.1001/jamasurg.2013.5

[59] Jayasinghe TN, Chiavaroli V, Holland DJ, Cutfield WS, O'Sullivan JM. The new era of treatment for obesity and metabolic disorders: Evidence and expectations for gut microbiome transplantation. Frontiers in Cellular and Infection Microbiology. 2016;**6**:15. DOI: 10.3389/fcimb.2016.00015

[60] Marotz CA, Zarrinpar A. Treating obesity and metabolic syndrome with fecal microbiota transplantation. Yale Journal of Biology and Medicine. 2016;**89**:383-388

[61] Woodworth MH, Carpentieri C, Sitchenko KL, Kraft CS. Challenges in fecal donor selection and screening for fecal microbiota transplantation: A review. Gut Microbes. 2017;**8**:225-237. DOI: 10.1080/19490976.2017.1286006

[62] Wang S, Xu M, Wang W, et al. Systematic review: Adverse events of fecal microbiota transplantation. PLoS One. 2016;**11**:e0161174. DOI: 10.1371/journal.pone.0161174

Chapter 16

Beneficial Effects of Proanthocyanidins on Intestinal Permeability and Its Relationship with Inflammation

Carlos González-Quilen, Esther Rodríguez-Gallego, Raúl Beltrán-Debón, Montserrat Pinent, Anna Ardévol, Maria Teresa Blay and Ximena Terra

Abstract

The intestinal barrier is constantly exposed to potentially harmful environmental factors including food components and bacterial endotoxins. When the intestinal barrier function and immune homeostasis are compromised, inflammatory conditions may be developed and impact overall health. Evidence from experimental animal and cell-culture studies suggests that exposure of intestinal mucosa to proanthocyanidin-rich plant products may contribute to maintain the barrier function and to ameliorate the inflammation present in prevalent pathologies such as diet-induced obesity and inflammatory bowel disease. In this review, we aim to update the current knowledge on the bioactivity of PACs in experimental models of altered intestinal permeability and in humans, emphasizing the beneficial effects of grape-seed proanthocyanidin extracts in intestinal health and giving insights into the subjacent biochemical and molecular mechanism.

Keywords: gut, permeability, inflammation, metabolic endotoxemia, obesity, IBD, flavonoid, flavan-3-ol, condensed tannin, procyanidin

1. Introduction

The primary function of the intestinal tract is to digest food components and absorb nutrients and water from the lumen to the systemic circulation. The intestine is also a physical barrier that is in contact with the environment. As a result, the intestinal epithelium is constantly exposed to potentially pathogenic microorganisms, toxins, and harmful components of the diet. When there are disturbances in the barrier function and mucosal immune homeostasis, the influx of intestine luminal content triggers barrier dysfunction and an exaggerated mucosal immune response [1]. Ultimately, chronic exposition to these detrimental environmental stimuli may lead to the development of local and systemic inflammatory conditions [2, 3] that contribute to barrier dysfunction.

Natural products have been recognized as a source of therapeutic agents for many years [4]. Some plant-derived phenolic compounds show promising

IntechOpen

anti-inflammatory effects and have been associated with the prevention of certain chronic diseases [5]. Proanthocyanidins (PACs), also known as condensed tannins, are oligo- and polymeric end products of the flavonoid biosynthesis pathway in plants [6]. There has been extensive laboratory research into the effects of both pure PAC molecules and PAC-rich extracts on overall health. These phytochemicals show a wide range of physiological activities [7], including anti-inflammatory and barrier-protective effects in the intestine [8–10], which may be interesting in the context of diet-induced obesity and inflammatory bowel disease (IBD).

We have reported previously that grape-seed PACs and other flavonoids have beneficial effects on inflammation [11–13] and protect the intestine against alterations associated with diet-induced obesity in rats [8, 9, 14, 15]. In addition, research conducted during the last decade with cell culture and animal models has made significant progress in determining the underlying mechanism of the health-promoting properties of PACs in the gastrointestinal tract and peripheral tissues.

2. Altered networks in intestinal dysfunction: barrier integrity and inflammatory response

The intestinal epithelium is a single cell-layer responsible for separating underlying mucosal tissues from the environment and is the largest exposed surface area in the body [16]. As there is a prolific commensal microbial community in the intestinal lumen (intestinal microbiota), epithelial integrity plays a pivotal role in maintaining overall health [16, 17]. The intestinal epithelium is integrated by several cell types with specialized functions. The enterocytes are responsible for the absorptive function and constitute the most abundant epithelial cell lineage. The goblet cells are implicated in the synthesis of secretory mucin glycoproteins that form the mucus layer [18]. Other cellular types integrating the epithelium, microfold (M) [19], Paneth and enteroendocrine cells are specialized in antigen sampling and presentation to dendritic cells, synthesis of antimicrobial peptides, and secretion of hormones, respectively.

The first strategy the host tissue has to maintain its homeostatic relationship with the intestinal microbiota is to minimize the physical interaction with microorganisms, thus limiting microbial translocation and physiological inflammation [20, 21]. The thick mucus layer secreted by goblet cells represents a primary defense line against environmental insults [18]. In addition, the enterocytes are joined together forming an intricately and well-regulated barrier sustained by intercellular junctions linked to the cell cytoskeleton, such as tight junctions (TJs), desmosomes, and adherent junctions. TJs partially seal the paracellular space and prevent passive transport of large molecules, including microbial components and other potentially harmful agents [1, 22].

The paracellular and transcellular pathways are the two major pathways mediating transmembrane transfer of intestinal bacterial substances. Both mechanisms may be involved in intestinal mucosal barrier damage and bacterial translocation. The paracellular pathway is integrated by tight junctions (TJs), consisting of zonulin/zonula occludens (ZO)-1, occludin, claudins, junction adhesion molecules (JAMs), and actin-myosin cytoskeletal proteins. Previous studies have shown that inflammatory cytokines and bacterial antigens can affect the expression level and assembly of these elements, thereby exerting an influence on TJ functions [23]. Immune cells, including neutrophils, dendritic cells, and monocytes, have also been directly implicated in inducing disturbances in TJ barrier function. It has been postulated that pro-inflammatory cytokine-induced opening of the intestinal TJ barrier is an important mechanism contributing to the TJ barrier defects present in various inflammatory conditions of the gut [24]. Previous studies [25–28] have shown that myosin light chain kinase (MLCK) plays a central role in the regulation of intestinal TJ permeability. The activation of MLCK catalyzes the phosphorylation of myosin light chain (MLC), inducing contraction of the peri-junctional actin-myosin filaments and the opening of the TJ barrier. In contrast, inhibition of MLCK activation prevents this effect [27]. It has been suggested that the cytokine-mediated barrier dysfunction could be mediated by an increase in Nuclear Factor (NF)-kB, which, in turn, activates MLCK gene and protein expression [29] (**Figure 1**).

Once intestinal bacteria and endotoxins enter the portal vein and/or lymphatic system, they can reach other tissues and organs, leading to a cascade response modulated by inflammatory mediators. This situation can induce a systemic inflammatory response, which further damages the function of the intestinal barrier [30]. The endotoxin-signaling pathway includes the binding of LPS to LPS-binding protein (LBP) and its subsequent transfer to the CD14 receptor. LBP-bound LPS initiates inflammation via TLRs associated with membrane-anchored CD14 [31]. TLRs are a family of pattern-recognition receptors that play a key role in the innate immune system. Among all, the TLR4 is expressed at high levels in the intestinal tract, and given that LPS is its specific ligand, TLR4 could be considered the first barrier for recognition of bacterial presence in the gastrointestinal tract. NF-kB is the final effector transcription factor of the TLR4 signaling pathway. It promotes the development of many intestinal diseases and also plays a pivotal role in the translation and transcription of inflammatory mediators [30].

In mammals, the NF-kB family comprises five proteins, including p65 (RelA), RelB, c-Rel, p105/p50 (NF-kB1), and p100/p52 (NF-kB2), which associate with each other to form transcriptionally distinct homo- and heterodimeric complexes; the p65:p50 heterodimer is the most abundant and the most relevant for inflammation [32]. In resting cells, the p65:p50 NF-kB heterodimer is sequestered in the cytoplasm by binding to its inhibitory protein, IkappaB (IkB). In response to an inflammatory stimulus, such as LPS, the classical NF-kB activation pathway leads to the activation of the IkB kinase (IkkB), a member of the IKK complex, triggering IkB-a phosphorylation (pIkB-a). Then, pIkB-a is recognized by the ubiquitin ligase machinery, resulting in its polyubiquitination and subsequent proteasomal

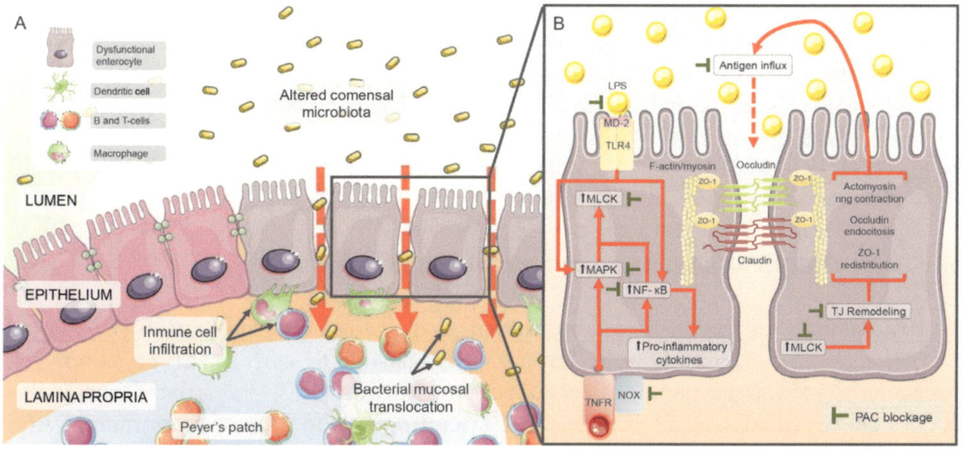

Figure 1.
Protective properties of PACs in the intestinal barrier function. (A) Chronic exposition to detrimental environmental stimuli may lead to dysbiosis, breakdown of the intestinal barrier, influx of bacterial endotoxins and mucosal inflammation. (B) PACs ameliorate loss of barrier function blocking the activation of MLCK mediated by NF-κB and MAPK signaling. See text for details.

degradation. After pIkB-a degradation, the p65:p50 heterodimers are able to translocate to the nucleus, where they bind to the kB motif found in the promoter or enhancer regions of numerous pro-inflammatory genes to induce their expression [33].

NF-kB target genes include cytokines (e.g., tumor necrosis factor (TNF)-α and interleukins), adhesion molecules, acute phase proteins, and inducible enzymes (inducible nitric oxide synthase (iNOS) and cyclooxygenase 2 (COX2)), among others [11]. All of these genes contain verified NF-kB binding sites in their sequences, providing strong experimental evidence for their direct control by NF-kB [34]. Among all of these genes, the expression of iNOS and COX2 has been widely studied in relation to intestinal inflammation. In this regard, sustained high nitric oxide (NO) production by iNOS plays a role in the pathology of chronic inflammatory bowel disease [35, 36]. During the last decade, it has become increasingly clear that NO overproduction by iNOS is deleterious to intestinal function [37], thus contributing significantly to gastrointestinal immunopathology. Cyclooxygenases are enzymes that are responsible for the metabolism of arachidonic acid, converting it into prostaglandins. These products influence a wide variety of biological processes, ranging from homeostasis to inflammation [38]. There are two cyclooxygenase isoforms: the constitutive COX1 isoform and the inducible COX2 isoform [38, 39]. As a result of COX2 induction, prostaglandin E2 levels increase at the site of inflammation and can also be detected systemically.

Multiple environmental factors have been identified as potential triggers of intestinal inflammatory conditions, including Western dietary habits [40]. It has been described that saturated fats play a direct role in inflammatory signaling. Saturated fatty acids (SFA) such as lauric (C12:0) and palmitic (C16:0) directly induce NF-κB activation, acting as non-microbial TLR2 and TLR4 agonists in macrophages [41]. Data suggest that activation of TLRs by SFA is mediated by TLR dimerization and recruitment into lipid rafts [42]. We have reported mild intestinal inflammation and increased permeability in rats feeding on a cafeteria diet consisting of high-saturated fat/high-refined sugar food products [43]. This enhanced permeability has been shown to favor bacterial LPS and other potentially pro-inflammatory molecules entering the systemic circulation, which is known as metabolic endotoxemia [15].

Taken together, these data suggest that HF diet-induced changes in the intestinal microbiota could be responsible for metabolic endotoxemia and for the onset of the corresponding diseases. The causative link between changes in intestinal bacteria populations, endotoxemia, and metabolic disease needs further assessment [44], but the mechanisms likely include altered epithelial permeability, translocation of bacterial products, and upregulation of pro-inflammatory cytokines and hormones produced by gut endocrine cells, mechanisms which might be modulated by PACs.

3. PACs: chemical structure, occurrence, and intake

PACs consist of flavan-3-ol subunits with a degree of polymerization (DP) equal to or greater than 2, mainly linked by $(4 \rightarrow 8)$ or $(4 \rightarrow 6)$ carbon-carbon bonds (B-type PACs) [45]. In some botanical sources an additional $(2 \rightarrow 7)$ ether-linkage also occurs (A-type PACs) [46] (**Figure 2**). Depending on the type of monomers, PACs can be classified into procyanidins, prodelphinidins, and propelargonidins. The most abundant group, procyanidins, consists exclusively of (+)- catechin and (−)- epicatechin monomers [47]. Prodelphinidins and propelargonidins are composed of (−)- gallocatechin/(−)- epigallocatechin and (+)- afzelechin/(−)- epiafzelechin monomers, respectively [45], and have a more limited distribution

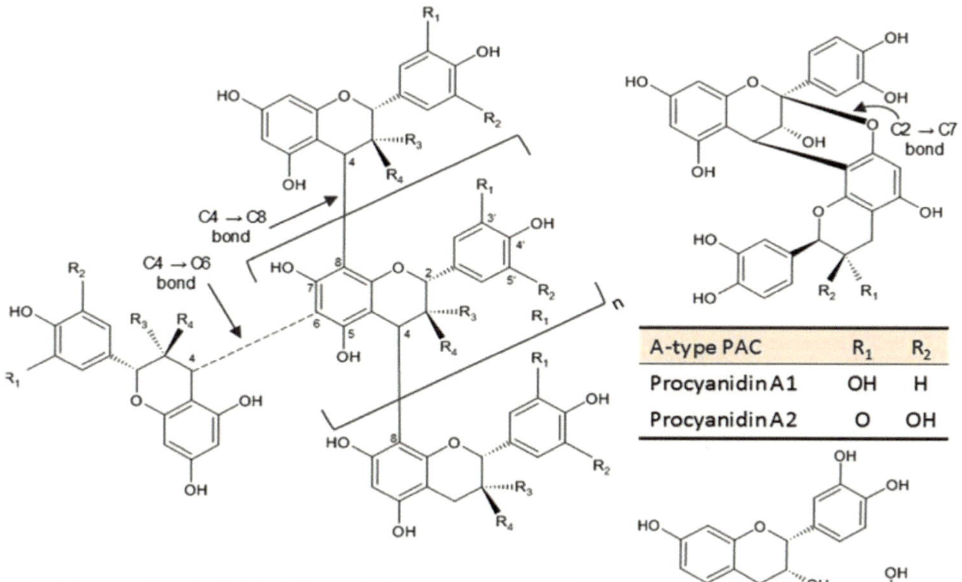

Flavan-3-ol monomer	R_1	R_2	R_3	R_4
(+)-Catechin	H	OH	H	OH
(−)-Epicatechin	H	OH	OH	H
(+)-Gallocatechin	OH	OH	H	OH
(−)-Epigallocatechin	OH	OH	OH	H
(+)-Afzelechin	H	H	H	OH
(−)-Epiafzelechin	H	H	OH	H

A-type PAC	R_1	R_2
Procyanidin A1	OH	H
Procyanidin A2	O	OH

B-type PAC	R_1	R_2
Procyanidin B1	H	OH
Procyanidin B2	OH	H

Figure 2.
Chemical structures of PACs. Flavan-3-ol monomers differ based on the hydroxylation pattern and their cis- or trans-configuration. Dimers A1/A2 and B1/B2 are shown as example of A- and B-type PACs, respectively.

Dietary assessment studies have shown that PACs, especially procyanidins are among the most abundant polyphenols in the human diet [6], as they are present in a variety of botanical sources and plant food products such as tea, fruits, nuts, cacao products, legumes, and cereal grains [1, 2]. However, PAC intake varies widely between geographical regions and cultures and is greatly dependent on eating habits, lifestyle behaviors, and socioeconomic status [48]. The daily PAC (dimers to polymers) intakes in adult populations from Korea, the U.S., Mexico, and EU were estimated as 71 [49], 73 [48], 103 [50], and 123–180 mg [51, 52], respectively, but intakes up to 230 mg d^{-1} have been reported in some regions of Spain and Norway [53].

4. The fate of PACs after ingestion

Flavan-3-ols are remarkably stable during gastric transit in humans [54]. Monomers such as (+)- catechin and (−)- epicatechin are readily absorbed in the upper sections of the small intestine [55, 56], recognized as xenobiotics and then subjected to an extensive phase II metabolism that generates glucuronidated, sulfated, and methylated conjugates [57]. Flavan-3-ol monomers and their conjugated metabolites reach peak plasma concentration 1–4 h after flavan-3-ol-rich food consumption [58–60]. Studies conducted in cultivated epithelial monolayers [61–63], rats [64, 65], and humans [60, 66] indicate that PAC absorption is conversely more limited and is highly dependent on DP, and that the permeation of larger oligomers (DP > 5) and polymers is negligible. No PAC transporter has been identified in the enterocyte membrane in the small intestine. Thus, dimers to tetramers are passively transported across the intestinal epithelium essentially by paracellular diffusion. Although transcellular passive diffusion is not likely to occur due to the hydrophilic nature of PACs conferred by the multiple hydroxyl groups, uptake might be possible by endocytic mechanisms [62].

In humans, a study assessed the contribution of the ingested cocoa flavan-3-ols and procyanidins to the systemic pool, and found that the plasma (−)- epicatechin came from the orally administered cocoa (−)- epicatechin and not from their oligomers or polymers [67]. This is in agreement with the evidence obtained with rats that suggests that PACs from different sources do not depolymerize to monomers after ingestion [68, 69]. Stalmach et al. [56] conducted a study with ileostomized patients who were administered green tea, and found 70% of the ingested flavan-3-ol in the ileal fluid after 24 h. Altogether, these findings suggest that substantial amounts of ingested flavan-3-ol monomers and PACs remain unabsorbed in the small intestine and reach the colon. There, they are efficiently transformed by the colonic microbiota into low molecular weight phenolic compounds that can be absorbed by colonocytes [57].

In vitro fermentation of purified procyanidin dimers with human fecal microbiota has shown to produce mainly 2-(3′,4′-dihydroxyphenyl) acetic acid and 5-(3′,4′-dihydroxyphenyl)-γ-valerolactone [70]. In agreement with this, a randomized cross-over study in healthy humans found that a great portion of the ingested (−)- epicatechin and procyanidin B1 was metabolized by the colonic microbiota to produce phenyl-γ-valerolactones as the major microbial metabolites [60]. In this study, microbial degradation of larger procyanidins was substantially lower, possibly to the inhibition of digesting enzymes or to the antibacterial properties exhibited by these compounds. Other human studies analyzing the bioavailability of flavan-3-ols, reported high levels of phenyl-γ-valerolactones in the circulation and urinary excretion after ingestion of a red grape pomace drink [71] and apple juice [72]. In the colonocytes and hepatocytes, these microbial products undergo further metabolism by phase II enzymes to produce conjugated derivatives. Margalef et al. [73] analyzed the tissue distribution of metabolites derived from a grape-seed proanthocyanidin extract (GSPE) 2 h after ingestion by rats. These authors detected a few microbial metabolites (methyl conjugated phenols) at low concentrations in the colon tissue, while most phase II metabolites (glucuronidated and methyl-glucuronidated forms) were found in the kidneys and liver. In humans, the major contributors to the excretion of phenyl-γ-valerolactones after ingestion of a red grape pomace drink, are sulfated and glucuronidated conjugates of 5-(3′,4′-dihydroxyphenyl)-γ-valerolactone [71].

5. In vitro, in vivo and ex vivo studies on the benefits of PACs for intestinal dysfunction

During the last decade, the beneficial properties of PACs for intestinal function have been reported in several studies performed with cell-culture models and experimental animals (**Tables 1** and **2**). This experimental data indicate that PACs contribute to maintaining the intestinal barrier and improving mucosal inflammation induced by environmental insults. However, there are few studies on the effect of PACs on human intestinal health, although epidemiological studies connect PAC-rich food consumption with a lower risk of colorectal cancer [88].

Extract or compound	Concentration	Time of incubation	Experimental model	Permeability and/or inflammatory inductor	Outcomes		Ref.
					Permeability/integrity	Inflammation/oxidative stress	
Apple procyanidins	13-50 μg mL^{-1}	6 h	Caco-2	PMA (300 ng mL^{-1})	ND	↓ IL-8 release	[82]
Apple procyanidin dimer fraction	50-150 μg mL^{-1}	24 h	Caco-2	LPS (50 μg mL^{-1})	↑ Occludin. ↑ ZO-1.	↓ NF-κB and TNF-α gene expression. ↑GPx, SOD, HO-1.	[10]
Cranberry procyanidins	250 μg mL^{-1}	Preincubation for 24 h	Caco-2/15 cells	Fe/Asc mixture (200 μM/2 mM) or LPS (200 μg mL^{-1}) for 6 h	ND	↓ PGE_2 accretion. ↓ COX-2 protein content. ↓ TNF-α and IL-6 protein content.	[83]
Hexameric procyanidins	20 μM	Preincubation for 30 min	Caco-2	TNF-α (10 ng mL^{-1}) for 60 min	ND	↓ IκBα phosphorylation. ↓ NF-κB p50 and RelA nuclear translocation. ↓ NF-κB-DNA binding. ↓ iNOS mRNA and protein content ↓ ROS.	[84]
Nut polymeric-PAC fraction	4.8-12 (mg cyanidin equivalents mL^{-1})	Preincubation for 1 h followed by co-incubation for 24 h with the inflammation inductor	Caco-2	IL-1β (25 ng mL^{-1})	↑ TEER. ↓ FSA permeation.	↓ IL-6 and IL-8 release. ↓ IκBα phosphorylation. ↓ RelA nuclear translocation.	[85]
Cocoa procyanidin polymers	100 μg mL^{-1}	Preincubation for 24 h	Caco-2	DSS (2% w v^{-1}) for 48 h	ND	↓ IL-8 release.	[86]
			HT-29	TNF-α (5 ng mL^{-1}) for 6 h	↓ FD (4 kD) permeation	ND	
Procyanidin B2	50 μM	Preincubation for 24 h, co-incubation with the inflammation inductor for a further 48h	Caco-2/HT29-MTX co-culture	LPS-activated Raw264.7 medium	≈ TEER. ↑ Claudin-7. ↑ Occludin. ↓ ZO-1.	ND	[76]
Various PAC-rich extracts (apple and avocado peel, cranberry and grape)	12.5-50 μg mL^{-1}	24 h	Caco-2	*p*-Cresol (3.2 mM)	↑ TEER. ↓ FD (4 kD) permeation.	ND	[87]

FSA, fluorescein-5-(and-6)-sulfonic acid trisodium salt. ND, not determined.

Table 1.
Interaction of PACs with intestinal permeability markers in cell culture and animal models [10, 76, 82–87].

Extract or compound	Dose (way of administration)	Time of administration	Experimental model	Permeability and/or inflammatory inductor	Outcomes		Ref.
					Permeability/integrity	Inflammation/oxidative stress	
GSPE	5, 25 or 50 mg kg^{-1} bw (daily oral gavage)	3 weeks (after 15 weeks of cafeteria diet)	Diet-induced obese Wistar rat	Long-term cafeteria diet (18 weeks)	*Ileum:* ↑ ZO-1 gene expression.	*Ileum:* ↓ IL-1β gene expression. ↓ iNOS gene expression. ↓ MPO activity. ↓ ROS.	[14]
GSPE	500 mg kg^{-1} bw (daily oral gavage)	17 weeks every other week or 10 days (before cafeteria diet).	Diet-induced obese Wistar rat	Long-term cafeteria diet (17 weeks)	↓ Plasma OVA *Duodenum, ileum and colon:* ↑ TEER (*ex vivo*). *Ileum:* ↑ Claudin-1 gene expression.	*Ileum:* ↓ MPO activity.	[8]
GSPE	100 or 500 mg kg^{-1} bw (daily oral gavage)	2 weeks (after 15 weeks of cafeteria diet)	Diet-induced obese Wistar rat	Long-term cafeteria diet (17 weeks)	↓ Plasma OVA *Ileum and colon:* ↑ TEER (*ex vivo*). *Ileum:* ↑ Claudin-1 gene expression.	*Duodenum and colon:* ↓ TNF-α release (*ex vivo*). Ileum: ↓ MPO activity.	[15]
Pyracantha fortuneana fruit PAC-rich extract	0.4 or 1 g 100 g^{-1} of dry feed weight (orally)	8 weeks (after second week of high-fat diet).	Diet-induced obese Sprague Dawley rat	High-fat diet (10 weeks)	↓ LMR. ↑ Occludin (segment not specified). ↑ ZO-1 (jejunum).	ND	[88]
GSPE	100, 200 or 400 mg kg^{-1} bw (daily oral gavage)	7 days (after second TNBS-induced colitis)	Wistar rat with TNBS-induced recurrent ulcerative colitis	TNBS (ir. injection of 80 mg kg^{-1}, 30 mg kg^{-1} after 16 days)	ND	*Colon:* ↓ TNF-α. ↓ MPO and iNOS activities. ↓ IKKα/β and IκBα phosphorylation. ↓ NF-κB nuclear translocation. ↓ MDA. ↑ GPx and SOD activities.	[89,90]
GSPE	100, 200 or 400 mg kg^{-1} bw (daily oral gavage)	7 days (after TNBS-induced colitis)	Wistar rat with TNBS-induced ulcerative colitis	TNBS (ir. injection of 100 mg kg^{-1})	ND	*Colon:* ↓ IL-1β. ↓ MPO activity. ↓ IKK activity. ↓ IκBα phosphorylation. ↓ RelA protein content.	[91]

Extract or compound	Dose (way of administration)	Time of administration	Experimental model	Permeability and/or inflammatory inductor	Outcomes		Ref.
					Permeability/integrity	Inflammation/oxidative stress	
Procyanidin B2	10, 20 or 40 mg kg^{-1} (daily oral gavage)	11 days	C57BL/6 mouse with DSS-induced colitis	DSS (2.5 g 100 mL^{-1} of drinking water for 9 days)	ND	*Colon:* ↓ MMP9. ↓ Cleaved caspase-1. ↓ RelA phosphorylation. ↓ TNF-α, IL-1β and IL-6 gene expression.	[92]
GSPE	1 g 100 g^{-1} of dry feed weight (orally)	16 weeks	IL10-deficient mouse prone to colitis	None (spontaneous colitis)	ND	*Colon:* ↓ TNF-α, IL-1β, IL-6 and IFN-γ gene expressions. ↓ MPO protein content and gene expression. ↓ RelA phosphorylation.	[93]
GSPE	0.1 g 100 mL^{-1} of drinking water (orally)	12 weeks	IL10-deficient mouse prone to colitis	None (spontaneous colitis)	ND	*Jejunum:* ↓ TNF-α and IFN-γ. ↑ IκBα protein content. ↑ iNOS gene expression.	[94]
GSPE	75 or 375 mg kg^{-1} bw (daily oral gavage)	15 days (before LPS administration)	Wistar rat with LPS-induced intestinal dysfunction	LPS (ip. injection of 0.3 mg kg^{-1})	↓ Plasma OVA *Duodenum:* ↑ JAM-A gene expression. *Ileum:* ↓ ZO-1, occludin, claudin-2, and JAM-A gene expressions.	*Duodenum:* ↓ COX-2 activity. *Duodenum and ileum:* ↓ MPO activity. Colon: ↓ ROS.	[13]

Bw, body weight. LMR, lactulose to mannitol ratio. Ir., intrarectal. Ip., intraperitoneal. ND, not determined.

Table 2.
Interaction of PACs with permeability and inflammatory markers in animal models of intestinal dysfunction [8, 13–15, 88–94].

In vitro models of inflammation have been fundamental in the comprehension of cellular mechanisms driving physiological effects of bioactive molecules. Studies on intestinal dysfunction have employed human colon carcinoma cell lines, being Caco-2 the most well-established and widely used model of the human intestine barrier ([89] and **Table 1**). Mucus producer [79], macrophages [90], and B cell lines [91] have been employed in co-culture systems to explore the interaction between cell populations. Although there is a strong trend in the industry toward replacing animal experiments with human cell-culture based models [92, 93], there are no in vitro models of the human intestine that replicate the complex interplay between cell types and the regulation of the barrier function by the mucosal innate and adaptive immunity. Therefore, most physiologically relevant data on intestinal dysfunction comes from the animal model. Most in vivo studies testing the effect of PAC supplementation on intestinal health have been performed in diet-induced obesity models and chemical-induced colitis models. The first resemble intestinal alterations seen in humans with metabolic syndrome [43]. The latter closely mimic histopathological features of human colitis and are frequently used to study the pathophysiology of IBD and the effectiveness of novel therapeutic drugs [94]. Notably, PAC-rich grape-seed extracts (GSPE) are among the most studied botanical extracts, mainly by in vivo approaches in rodents (**Table 2**).

5.1 In vitro studies of barrier integrity

The data available on the interaction between PACs and permeability and inflammation markers in cell models of intestinal dysfunction are summarized in **Table 1**. Caco-2-based models have shown to be responsive to pro-inflammatory stimulation, producing a wide range of inflammatory mediators and increasing the paracellular permeability. Pro-inflammatory agents such as LPS, phorbol 12-myristate 13-acetate (PMA), and cytokines (TNF-α and IL-1β) have been used in multiple studies testing the effect of PAC molecules and PAC-rich botanical extracts on Caco-2 cells [10, 74, 77, 78]. Stimulated-Caco-2 cell monolayers incubated with PACs generally show a reduction in gene expression and secretion of TNFα, IL-6, and IL-8 [10, 74, 75, 77], which is often linked to the downregulation of NF-κB signaling at different levels [10, 76, 77]. An increased expression of antioxidant enzymes, such as glutathione peroxidase (GPx), superoxidase dismutase (SOD), and hemeoxygenase 1 (HO-1), has also been reported [10].

When permeable support systems such as transwell or Ussing chamber (UCh) are used, alterations in barrier integrity and paracellular permeability of epithelial cell monolayers are evaluated by transepithelial electrical resistance (TEER), an electrophysiological parameter that measures ion conductance across the monolayer, and by the transepithelial transport of molecular markers such as Lucifer yellow (LY) and fluorescently labeled dextrans (FD) [95, 96]. Some in vitro studies have associated PACs with increased TEER and decreased transport of permeability markers in the context of barrier dysfunction [77, 78, 80]. The expression levels of TJ proteins (claudins, occludins, and ZOs) often correlate, but not always [79], with intestinal permeability and are also considered markers of epithelial integrity. Bitzer et al. [78] found that the dextran sodium sulfate (DSS)-induced loss of barrier function in Caco-2 cells was significantly inhibited by polymeric PACs of cocoa but not by oligomers. Moreover, a higher barrier-protective activity was determined in PACs with DP ≥ 7, which were able to reduce the detrimental effect of DSS in a dose-dependent fashion [78]. Effectiveness of procyanidin B2 ameliorating dextran sodium sulfate (DSS)-induced permeability alterations was examined using a Caco-2/HT29-MTX co-culture model [79]. Although procyanidin B2-incubated cells showed increased levels of the TJ proteins claudin-7, occludin, and ZO-1, these changes did not reduce TEER loss. Altogether, these results suggest that the ability of PACs to strengthen the intestinal barrier integrity depends on the degree of polymerization (DP).

5.2 In vivo studies of diet-induced intestinal permeability

The cafeteria (CAF) diet is a self-selected high-saturated fat/high-refined sugar diet that stimulates hyperphagia and a rapid weight gain in experimental animals [97, 98]. In this feeding regime, highly palatable and energy dense foods commercially available, such as muffins, biscuits, bacon, sausages, and sugared milk, are offered *ad libitum* [15, 99]. A long-term CAF diet (62% carbohydrate (mostly sugar), 23% lipid, and 13% protein) has negative effects on intestinal function in rodents, increasing intestinal permeability, and inducing mucosal inflammation [43]. We have described the beneficial effects of administering GSPE against the intestinal dysfunction induced by a long-term CAF diet (17–18 weeks) in Wistar rats [8, 14, 15]. The composition of the GSPE used in these studies has been analyzed in detail [100]. Both nutritional (5–50 mg kg^{-1} [14]) and pharmacological (100–500 mg kg^{-1} [8, 15]) doses of GSPE administered orally as a preventive [8] or counteractive treatment [14, 15], tended to reduce intestinal inflammatory markers such as TNF-α release or myeloperoxidase (MPO) activity (an indicator of neutrophil infiltration in tissues). The reduction of plasma ovalbumin (OVA), an in vivo marker of intestinal permeability, was supported by (1) the increase in TEER in small and large intestine segments. This parameter is determined *ex vivo* by UCh-based protocols [8, 15]; and (2) by the upregulation of TJ proteins such as ZO-1 [14] and claudin-1 [8, 15]. Notably, the protective effect of GSPE in the intestinal barrier function was linked to the amelioration of metabolic endotoxemia (reduction of plasma LPS) and systemic inflammation (reduction of plasma TNF-α) in obese rats [15, 101]. Other authors have also reported the upregulation of ZO-1 and claudin-1 TJ proteins in high-fat fed rats supplemented with other PAC-rich extracts [81].

5.3 In vivo studies of chemical-induced intestinal dysfunction

Chemical agents administered orally to induce colitis in rodents include trinitrobenzene sulfonic acid (TNBS) and DSS. These agents erode the colonic mucosal lining and produce the loss of the intestinal barrier function and colonic inflammation. In these models, the severity of outcomes depends on the dose of the chemical agent and the frequency of administration. Li et al. [102] found that intragastric administration of GSPE in rats at pharmacological doses (100–400 mg kg^{-1} d^{-1}) prior to TNBS-induced recurrent colitis, reduced weight loss, and attenuated macro- and microscopic tissue damage scores in the colon. This protective effect was accompanied by a reduction in oxidative stress (malondialdehyde; MDA), inflammation (IL-1β), and neutrophil infiltration (MPO activity) in colonic tissues. Remarkably, the beneficial effects of low to high doses of GSPE were comparable to those of sulfasalazine (200 mg kg^{-1} d^{-1}), a potent inhibitor of NF-κB. Subsequent studies carried out by these authors with the same model, confirmed the role of the GSPE down-regulating NF-κB response [83, 84]. A preventive effect of procyanidin B2 was also evidenced in a mouse model of DSS-induced colitis [85]. Administration of procyanidin B2 (10–40 mg kg^{-1} d^{-1}) attenuated the severity of tissue damage in the colon and reduced the levels of matrix metalloproteinase-9 (MMP-9), a marker of macrophage infiltration. In addition, inhibition of the NF-κB signaling and of NLRP3 inflammasome activation was observed, with a concomitant reduction in the gene expression of pro-inflammatory cytokines. Overall, the benefits of procyanidin B2 administration, especially at the highest dosage (40 mg kg^{-1}), were comparable to those of mesalazine (200 mg kg^{-1}), a COX inhibitor. The authors suggest that these effects were largely due to the reduction in activated macrophages infiltrating colonic tissues, probably driven by ROS clearance.

5.4 Other in vivo studies with animal models

The IL-10 deficient mouse is a classic knockout model that develops spontaneous colitis under pathogen-free conditions. Some authors have explored the influence of GSPE in this model, supplementing colitic animals with 0.1–1 g 100 g^{-1} of dry feed weight for 12–16 days [86, 87]. These studies evidenced a reduction of multiple inflammatory markers in the jejunum and colon, such as TNF-α, IL-1β, IL-6, and IFN-γ gene expressions, as well as MPO activity. This anti-inflammatory effect was associated with the inhibition of the NF-κB signaling. Interestingly, GSPE supplementation also increased the density of goblet cells in the jejunum of treated animals, suggesting that there is an alternative mechanism by which inflammation is attenuated.

Cardoso et al. [13] recently tested both dietary (75 mg kg^{-1}) and pharmacological doses of GSPE (375 mg kg^{-1}) in a rat model of mild intestinal dysfunction induced by intraperitoneal injection of LPS. GSPE was administered daily by oral gavage for 15 days prior to LPS-induced intestinal dysfunction. LPS enhanced intestinal permeability and induced both oxidative stress and inflammation. GSPE-treated animals reduced OVA permeation to the circulation, MPO activity and COX-2 in the small intestine tissues, and reactive oxygen species (ROS) levels in the colon. Furthermore, a gene expression analysis with a low-density microarray technique revealed that unlike the dietary dose of GSPE, the pharmacological dose had a striking effect on the LPS-gene expression profile, showing a strong modulation of multiple genes associated with chemokines and ILs, including upregulation of the anti-inflammatory cytokine IL-13.

5.5 Human ex vivo studies

Although the use of animal models is the predominate approximation at preclinical stages for testing novel therapies in intestinal permeability, there is a strong trend in the industry towards replacing animal experiments with human cell-culture based models [92, 93]. Nevertheless, advantages related to the usefulness of in vitro models for screening of bioactives and exploring action mechanisms, are offset by limitations regarding the mimicking of the in vivo situation and translation to the human [103]. Thus, some human ex vivo models have been proposed to test immunomodulatory properties of drug candidates in intestinal explants from IBD patients [104, 105]. Intestinal function can also be studied with UCh-based protocols. The UCh system consists of two halves with an opening between them, where mucosal tissue is adapted, thus isolating the apical and basolateral sides of the tissue. This technique has been applied for studying drug absorption [106] and secretion of enterohormones [107] in human endoscopic biopsies. An advantage of UCh models over explant-based models is that UCh models make it possible to measure the electrophysiological parameters, including TEER [106]. All these set-ups permit analyzing the cytokine profiling of intestinal explants or biopsies retaining their in situ conditioning in a polarized fashion [105, 108]. We have employed the UCh to determine TEER and cytokine release (TNF-α) in intestinal tissues from cafeteria diet-induced obese rats treated with GSPE [8, 15]. It could also be useful for testing the effect of bioactives on dysfunctional human intestine.

A feature of ex vivo models is that screening of drug effects does not compromise the patients by exposing them to unknown outcomes.

5.6 Clinical trials

Translation of doses of PAC-rich extracts used in rodent models of intestinal dysfunction to human equivalent doses (HED) indicates that pharmacological doses (up to 5 g d^{-1} for a 60 kg person) could be required to achieve beneficial effects in clinical trials [14, 15]. Thus, the first uncertainty involved in assessing the use of PACs as therapy agents in humans, is safety. Grape seed and skin proanthocyanidin-rich extracts have been subjected to toxicological tests in rats to determine their safety for use in functional foods [109–111]. In these studies, the median lethal dose (LD50) was found to be greater than 5000 mg kg^{-1} bw (HED of ≈50 g) when administered once by oral gavage, and 1400–2000 mg kg^{-1} d^{-1} (HED of ≈14–20 g d^{-1}) was found to be the no-observed-adverse-effect level (NOAEL) for systemic toxicity in sub-chronic administration. A recent study evaluated the safety and tolerability of GSPE intake (up to 2.5 g d^{-1}) in a small number of healthy adults for a 4-week period and found a good tolerability without adverse effects on hematological or biochemical parameters [47].

To date, there are few clinical studies that evaluate the influence of PACs on intestinal inflammatory conditions. A clinical study revealed that the postprandial increase of plasma LPS associated with the intake of a high-fat meal was significantly reduced in obese subjects who consumed 1 g of GSPE [112]. As translocation of LPS to the circulation is considered an indicator of intestinal permeability and a critical factor in the appearance of systemic low-grade inflammation in patients with metabolic syndrome [113], reduction of postprandial endotoxemia could be particularly interesting from a therapeutic perspective. Large double-blind clinical studies need to be conducted to provide more information on PAC clinical efficacy in intestinal dysfunction so that these phytochemicals can be used therapeutically to improve intestinal health in obese and IBD individuals.

6. Biochemical and molecular mechanisms underlying the barrier-protective and anti-inflammatory properties of PAC in the intestine

PACs were often considered to be nutritionally undesirable due to their ability to form complexes with macronutrients and reduce the activity of virtually any enzyme implicated in digestion [114, 115]. Nevertheless, based on the anti-cancerous, anti-mutagenic, and anti-microbial activities these phytochemicals elicited in laboratory experiments, a role in the modulation of the metabolism and immune system was suggested [115]. The ability of PACs to form cross-links with biomolecules can be attributed to the hydroxyl groups and aromatic rings in their structure that can establish hydrogen bonds and hydrophobic interactions [116]. PACs have a significant affinity for proline-rich proteins and peptides [117]. In general, binding to proteins seems to increase with the DP as larger PAC molecules have more potential binding sites for the associations with proline residues [117]. The interaction results in effects determined by the biological function of the target protein. Thus, PACs not only alter enzymatic activity, but they may also prevent ligand-receptor interactions and the binding of transcription factors to their specific sites in DNA. In addition, some PAC molecules can be adsorbed non-specifically onto biomembrane surfaces [118], affecting their physical characteristics, such as fluidity and density, and potentially altering membrane-dependent processes, including protein receptor activity [119]. Altogether, these effects lead ultimately to the alteration of cell signaling pathways and the modulation of gene expression.

6.1 Modulation of TJ integrity

The precise mechanisms underlying the improvement in intestine paracellular permeability due to PACs in inflammation are not yet completely elucidated; however, it is known that they lead ultimately to the upregulation (e.g., ZO-1 and claudin-1 [8, 13]) or downregulation (e.g., claudin-2 [86]) of TJ protein expression. Loss of TJ integrity in the pro-inflammatory state is mediated by the NF-κB signaling pathway and by the activation of protein kinases MAPKs, PI3Ks, AMPK, and MLCK [120]. MLCK is particularly crucial in actomyosin-based cytoskeletal functions and multiple studies highlight its important role in intestinal TJ remodeling [121, 122]. PACs reduce the production of pro-inflammatory mediators (e.g., TNF-α) and reactive oxygen species (i.e., iNOS activity) associated with enhancing intestinal permeability by antagonizing the NF-κB signaling pathway. In addition, PACs are potent inhibitors of kinases including MLCK [120, 123]. Contreras et al. [124] also suggested that there is an upstream novel mechanism associated with flavan-3-ols that leads to the prevention of TNF-α-induced intestinal permeability. In this study, TNF-α-stimulated Caco-2 monolayers incubated with (−)-epicatechin showed a reduction of NOX activity, an enzyme that also facilitates activation of TNF-α signaling. This effect was directly associated with the inhibition of ERK1/2 MAPK activity of IκB phosphorylation and of MLCK activation.

6.2 Interaction with bacterial endotoxins

Delehanty et al. [125] demonstrated that naturally occurring A- and B-type cranberry PACs were able to bind the lipid A moiety of LPS, exhibiting an affinity similar to that of polymyxin B, a potent LPS-binding molecule. In this study, PACs efficiently blocked endocytosis of bacterial LPS in a dose-dependent manner in HEK 293 (human embryonic kidney cells) that expressed receptors TLR4/MD-2 and CD14, thus preventing the induction of the NF-κB signaling pathway without any interaction with cellular components. However, other authors reported that PACs isolated from cocoa beans did not abrogate the binding of LPS to TLR4 in cultivated human dendritic cells [126]. PAC-LPS binding has been linked to the reduction of the post prandial increase in blood LPS associated with the ingestion of a high-fat meal in obese subjects ingesting an oral dose of GSPE [112].

7. PACs modulation of intestinal microbiota

Diet plays an important role in the composition of intestine microbiota, promoting or inhibiting growth of microorganisms [127]. Alterations in the composition and metabolism of the intestinal microbiota (dysbiosis) have also been associated with the consumption of high-saturated fat diets in rodents and humans [128, 129]. In fact, metagenomic analysis of the intestinal microbiome in Western populations has shown a reduction not only of microbial diversity, but also of functional potential [130]. Dysbiosis is linked to obesity-associated intestinal inflammation, although the "egg or hen" question related to the cause-effect relationship is not answered yet [131]. High-fat intake in rodents often decreases overall diversity of microbiota and the abundance of Bacteroidetes, and increases the relative abundance of Firmicutes [132, 133]. Several human studies have described similar associations [134, 135], but the importance of the ratio Firmicutes to Bacteroidetes remains controversial [136, 137], and some authors state that the experimental results are not sufficiently consistent [138]. Interestingly, the existence of a colitogenic microbiota was demonstrated in T-bet−/− × RAG2−/− deficient mice whose spontaneous ulcerative colitis was horizontally transmissible to wild-type individuals when co-housed [139]. Although mechanisms by which dysbiosis trigger intestinal dysfunction are not fully understood, it is known that they involve the loss of immune tolerance due to local immune homeostasis disruption and continuous abnormal activation of TLRs [140].

Several authors have suggested that both dietary PACs, which are the substrates of intestinal bacteria, and the metabolites produced during PACs degradation in the colon may modulate and induce oscillations in the composition of the microbiota populations by means of prebiotic and antimicrobial effects against gut pathogenic microorganisms [141–144]. Dietary PACs, specifically longer polymers, reach the distal intestine nearly intact, where they become fermentable substrates for the commensal microbiota [145]. PACs have been associated with prebiotic properties, boosting the composition of several kinds of probiotics such as *Bifidobacterium* spp., *Lactobacillus* spp. [146] and the stimulator of mucus production *Akkermansia muciniphila* [147, 148]. Nevertheless, current evidence is somewhat controversial as effects described in different in vivo studies mainly performed with rodents, do not always agree. This suggests that interactions between PACs and microbiota depend largely on the botanical source, the types of molecules present in the extracts tested and the animal model [149].

A recent study by Casanova-Marti et al. [150] found that oral administration of GSPE in Wistar rats for 8 days resulted in profound changes in the cecal microbiota composition, reducing diversity indices and the ratio of *Firmicutes* to *Bacteroidetes*. Similar results were found in diet-induced obese Sprague Dawley rats supplemented with a PAC-rich extract of the *Pyracantha fortuneana* fruit, although in this study an increase in microbiota diversity was also reported [81]. GSPE supplementation in IL-10 deficient mice resulted in an increased abundance of *Bacteroides* and *Lactobacilli* [86]. Xing et al. [148] reported that the administration of procyanidin B2 in rabbits feeding a high-fat-cholesterol diet, promoted an increase in the relative abundance of *Akkermansia*. These authors proposed that the reduction of metabolic endotoxemia found in animals treated with procyanidin B2 was attributed to the ability of *Akkermansia* to retain the thickness of the intestinal mucus layer, thus reducing intestinal permeability and the leakage of LPS into the circulation [151].

Cueva et al. [146] found that in vitro fermentation of grape-seed monomers and PACs in human feces resulted in a reduced abundance of *Clostridium histolyticum*. Inhibition of the growth of some infectious microorganisms, such as the mentioned *C. histolyticum* in the intestine and *Helicobacter pylori* in the stomach [152], may be related to the anti-adherence activity that PACs have demonstrated in in vitro studies [153], as adherence to the epithelium is a prerequisite for colonization and infection of the intestinal gastrointestinal mucosa.

Finally, phenolic acids and phenyl-γ-valerolactones resulting from the colonic fermentation of PACs also exhibit a significant bioactivity in cell models and experimental animals [154]. They therefore may partially account for the beneficial anti-inflammatory effects reported in intestinal and peripheral tissues in vivo. Further research is needed to clarify the importance of these microbial products in health-promoting properties associated with the intake of PACs.

8. Conclusions and future perspectives

The health-promoting properties of PACs in the intestine are attributed not only to the antioxidant activity inherent to phenolic compounds, but also to the capacity of these phytochemicals to interact with multiple biomolecules, including proteins, biomembrane lipids, and endotoxins. Bioactivity of PACs is highly structure-dependent and enriched botanical extracts composed by a large variety of molecular structures exert a wide range of unrelated physiological effects. In this way, PAC-rich extracts can modulate kinase activity, several signal transduction pathways implicated in the inflammatory response and the remodeling of TJs. Flavan-3-ol monomers and short PAC oligomers are absorbed by enterocytes and immune cells and exert a direct action on kinases and transcription factors. Bioactivity of larger oligomers and polymeric PACs do not require direct intestinal absorption and are able to bind protein receptors on the enterocyte and immune cell surfaces as well as luminal bacterial endotoxins, thus inhibiting pro-inflammatory signaling and improving barrier integrity. Due to the negligible absorption of large PAC molecules in the small intestine, phenyl-γ-valerolactones and phenolic acids produced by the microbiota metabolism in the colon are thought to play an important role in these health-promoting effects, and thus need to be further researched.

The barrier-protective properties of PACs are emerging as a potential adjunctive support to current therapies for managing obesity related intestinal dysfunction and IBD. However, there have been no large, well-designed clinical trials establishing the efficacy of these phytochemicals in chronic conditions. At preclinical stages, the use of animal models is the predominant approach for testing novel therapies for intestinal dysfunction, although several strategies for replacing animal experiments have been proposed. As there are still no studies on the impact of PACs on human intestinal health, ex vivo models of the human intestine could be a more physiologically reliable alternative to human cell lines and an alternative to animal experimentation in preclinical development.

Acknowledgements

C. González-Quilen has received financial support through a FI-AGAUR grant from the Generalitat de Catalunya. M. Pinent and X. Terra are Serra-Húnter fellows at the Universitat Rovira i Virgili, Tarragona, Spain.

Conflicts of interest

The authors declare no conflict of interest.

Funding

This work was funded by the Spanish Ministerio de Economía y Competitividad (Grant: AGL2017-83477-R).

Author details

Carlos González-Quilen, Esther Rodríguez-Gallego, Raúl Beltrán-Debón, Montserrat Pinent, Anna Ardévol, Maria Teresa Blay and Ximena Terra*
MoBioFood Research Group, Departament de Bioquímica i Biotecnologia, Universitat Rovira i Virgili, Tarragona, Spain

*Address all correspondence to: ximena.terra@urv.cat

IntechOpen

© 2020 The Author(s). Licensee IntechOpen. This chapter is distributed under the terms of the Creative Commons Attribution License (http://creativecommons.org/licenses/by/3.0), which permits unrestricted use, distribution, and reproduction in any medium, provided the original work is properly cited.

References

[1] Chelakkot C, Ghim J, Ryu SH. Mechanisms regulating intestinal barrier integrity and its pathological implications. Experimental & Molecular Medicine. 2018;**50**:103

[2] Fukui H. Increased intestinal permeability and decreased barrier function: Does it really influence the risk of inflammation? Inflammatory Intestinal Diseases. 2016;**1**:135-145. DOI: 10.1159/000447252

[3] Clemente-Postigo M, Oliva-Olivera W, Coin-Aragüez L, Ramos-Molina B, Giraldez-Perez RM, Lhamyani S, et al. Metabolic endotoxemia promotes adipose dysfunction and inflammation in human obesity. American Journal of Physiology-Endocrinology and Metabolism. 2019;**316**:E319-E332. DOI: 10.1152/ajpendo.00277.2018

[4] Harvey A. Strategies for discovering drugs from previously unexplored natural products. Drug Discovery Today. 2000;**5**:294-300

[5] Costa C, Tsatsakis A, Mamoulakis C, Teodoro M, Briguglio G, Caruso E, et al. Current evidence on the effect of dietary polyphenols intake on chronic diseases. Food and Chemical Toxicology. 2017;**110**:286-299

[6] Smeriglio A, Barreca D, Bellocco E, Trombetta D. Proanthocyanidins and hydrolysable tannins: Occurrence, dietary intake and pharmacological effects. British Journal of Pharmacology. 2017;**174**:1244-1262. DOI: 10.1111/bph.13630

[7] Bladé C, Aragonès G, Arola-Arnal A, Muguerza B, Bravo FI, Salvadó MJ, et al. Proanthocyanidins in health and disease. BioFactors. 2016;**42**:5-12. DOI: 10.1002/biof.1249

[8] Gil-Cardoso K, Ginés I, Pinent M, Ardévol A, Blay M, Terra X. The co-administration of proanthocyanidins and an obesogenic diet prevents the increase in intestinal permeability and metabolic endotoxemia derived to the diet. The Journal of Nutritional Biochemistry. 2018;**62**:35-42. DOI: 10.1016/J.JNUTBIO.2018.07.012

[9] Gil-Cardoso K, Ginés I, Pinent M, Ardévol A, Blay M, Terra X. Effects of flavonoids on intestinal inflammation, barrier integrity and changes in gut microbiota during diet-induced obesity. Nutrition Research Reviews. 2016;**29**:1-15. DOI: 10.1017/S0954422416000159

[10] Wu H, Luo T, Li YM, Gao ZP, Zhang KQ, Song JY, et al. Granny Smith apple procyanidin extract upregulates tight junction protein expression and modulates oxidative stress and inflammation in lipopolysaccharide-induced Caco-2 cells. Food & Function. 2018;**9**:3321-3329. DOI: 10.1039/c8fo00525g

[11] Terra X, Valls J, Vitrac X, Mérrillon J-M, Arola L, Ardèvol A, et al. Grape-seed procyanidins act as antiinflammatory agents in endotoxin-stimulated RAW 264.7 macrophages by inhibiting NFkB signaling pathway. Journal of Agricultural and Food Chemistry. 2007;**55**:4357-4365. DOI: 10.1021/jf0633185

[12] Martinez-Micaelo N, González-Abuín N, Pinent M, Ardévol A, Blay M. Procyanidin B2 inhibits inflammasome-mediated IL-1β production in lipopolysaccharide-stimulated macrophages. Molecular Nutrition & Food Research. 2015;**59**:262-269. DOI: 10.1002/mnfr.201400370

[13] Gil-Cardoso K, Comitato R, Ginés I, Ardévol A, Pinent M, Virgili F, et al. Protective effect of proanthocyanidins in a rat model of mild intestinal inflammation and impaired intestinal

permeability induced by LPS. Molecular Nutrition & Food Research. 2019;**63**: 1800720. DOI: 10.1002/mnfr.201800720

[14] Gil-Cardoso K, Ginés I, Pinent M, Ardévol A, Arola L, Blay M, et al. Chronic supplementation with dietary proanthocyanidins protects from diet-induced intestinal alterations in obese rats. Molecular Nutrition & Food Research. 2017;**61**:1601039. DOI: 10.1002/mnfr.201601039

[15] González-Quilen C, Gil-Cardoso K, Ginés I, Beltrán-Debón R, Pinent M, Ardévol A, et al. Grape-seed proanthocyanidins are able to reverse intestinal dysfunction and metabolic endotoxemia induced by a cafeteria diet in wistar rats. Nutrients. 2019;**11**:pii: E979. DOI: 10.3390/nu11050979

[16] Allaire JM, Crowley SM, Law HT, Chang SY, Ko HJ, Vallance BA. The intestinal epithelium: Central coordinator of mucosal immunity. Trends in Immunology. 2018;**39**: 677-696

[17] Bischoff SC, Barbara G, Buurman W, Ockhuizen T, Schulzke J-D, Serino M, et al. Intestinal permeability—A new target for disease prevention and therapy. BMC Gastroenterology. 2014;**14**:189. DOI: 10.1186/s12876-014-0189-7

[18] Birchenough GMH, Johansson MEV, Gustafsson JK, Bergström JH, Hansson GC. New developments in goblet cell mucus secretion and function. Mucosal Immunology. 2015;**8**:712-719. DOI: 10.1038/mi.2015.32

[19] Nakamura Y, Kimura S, Hase K. M cell-dependent antigen uptake on follicle-associated epithelium for mucosal immune surveillance. Inflammation and Regeneration. 2018; **38**:15. DOI: 10.1186/s41232-018-0072-y

[20] Fiocchi C. What is "physiological" intestinal inflammation and how does it differ from "pathological" inflammation? Inflammatory Bowel Diseases. 2008;**14**:S77-S78. DOI: 10.1097/00054725-200810001-00040

[21] Belkaid Y, Harrison OJ. Homeostatic immunity and the microbiota. Immunity. 2017;**46**:562-576

[22] Ulluwishewa D, Anderson RC, McNabb WC, Moughan PJ, Wells JM, Roy NC. Regulation of tight junction permeability by intestinal bacteria and dietary components. The Journal of Nutrition. 2011;**141**:769-776. DOI: 10.3945/jn.110.135657

[23] Luo H, Guo P, Zhou Q. Role of TLR4/NF-κB in damage to intestinal mucosa barrier function and bacterial translocation in rats exposed to hypoxia. PLoS One. 2012;**7**:e46291. DOI: 10.1371/journal.pone.0046291

[24] Suzuki T. Regulation of intestinal epithelial permeability by tight junctions. Cellular and Molecular Life Sciences. 2013;**70**:631-659. DOI: 10.1007/s00018-012-1070-x

[25] Suzuki M, Nagaishi T, Yamazaki M, Onizawa M, Watabe T, Sakamaki Y, et al. Myosin light chain kinase expression induced via tumor necrosis factor receptor 2 signaling in the epithelial cells regulates the development of colitis-associated carcinogenesis. PLoS One. 2014;**9**: e88369. DOI: 10.1371/journal.pone.0088369

[26] Barreau F, Hugot JP. Intestinal barrier dysfunction triggered by invasive bacteria. Current Opinion in Microbiology. 2014;**17**:91-98. DOI: 10.1016/j.mib.2013.12.003

[27] Al-Sadi R, Ye D, Dokladny K, Ma TY. Mechanism of IL-1beta-induced increase in intestinal epithelial tight junction permeability. Journal of

Immunology. 2008;**180**:5653-5661. DOI: 180/8/5653 [pii]

[28] Al-Sadi R, Guo S, Ye D, Dokladny K, Alhmoud T, Ereifej L, et al. Mechanism of IL-1β modulation of intestinal epithelial barrier involves p38 kinase and activating transcription factor-2 activation. Journal of Immunology. 2013;**190**:6596-6606. DOI: 10.4049/jimmunol.1201876

[29] Ye D, Ma TY. Cellular and molecular mechanisms that mediate basal and tumour necrosis factor-alpha-induced regulation of myosin light chain kinase gene activity. Journal of Cellular and Molecular Medicine. 2008;**12**: 1331-1346. DOI: 10.1111/j.1582-4934.2008.00302.x

[30] Luo H, Guo P, Zhou Q. Role of TLR4/NF-kappaB in damage to intestinal mucosa barrier function and bacterial translocation in rats exposed to hypoxia. PLoS One. 2012;7:e46291. DOI: 10.1371/journal.pone.0046291

[31] Laugerette F, Furet J-P, Debard C, Daira P, Loizon E, Geloen a, et al. Oil composition of high-fat diet affects metabolic inflammation differently in connection with endotoxin receptors in mice. American Journal of Physiology-Endocrinology and Metabolism. 2012; **302**:E374-E386. DOI: 10.1152/ajpendo.00314.2011

[32] Li Q, Verma IM. NF-kappaB regulation in the immune system. Nature Reviews. Immunology. 2002;**2**: 725-734. DOI: 10.1038/nri910

[33] Hayden MS, West AP, Ghosh S. NF-kappaB and the immune response. Oncogene. 2006;**25**:6758-6780. DOI: 10.1038/sj.onc.1209943

[34] Pahl HL. Activators and target genes of Rel/NF-kappaB transcription factors. Oncogene. 1999;**18**:6853-6866. DOI: 10.1038/sj.onc.1203239

[35] Toumi R, Soufli I, Rafa H, Belkhelfa M, Biad A, Touil-Boukoffa C. Probiotic bacteria *Lactobacillus* and *Bifidobacterium* attenuate inflammation in dextran sulfate sodium-induced experimental colitis in mice. International Journal of Immunopathology and Pharmacology. 2014;**27**:615-627

[36] Wang W, Xia T, Yu X. Wogonin suppresses inflammatory response and maintains intestinal barrier function via TLR4-MyD88-TAK1-mediated NF-κB pathway in vitro. Inflammation Research. 2015;**64**:423-431. DOI: 10.1007/s00011-015-0822-0

[37] Kolios G, Valatas V, Ward SG. Nitric oxide in inflammatory bowel disease: A universal messenger in an unsolved puzzle. Immunology. 2004;**113**:427-437. DOI: 10.1111/j.1365-2567.2004.01984.x

[38] Martinez-Micaelo N, Gonzalez-Abuin N, Terra X, Richart C, Ardevol A, Pinent M, et al. Omega-3 docosahexaenoic acid and procyanidins inhibit cyclo-oxygenase activity and attenuate NF-kappaB activation through a p105/p50 regulatory mechanism in macrophage inflammation. The Biochemical Journal. 2012;**441**:653-663. DOI: 10.1042/BJ20110967

[39] Du CYQ, Choi RCY, Dong TTX, Lau DTW, Tsim KWK. Yu Ping Feng San, an ancient Chinese herbal decoction, regulates the expression of inducible nitric oxide synthase and cyclooxygenase-2 and the activity of intestinal alkaline phosphatase in cultures. PLoS One. 2014;**9**:e100382. DOI: 10.1371/journal.pone.0100382

[40] Ananthakrishnan AN, Bernstein CN, Iliopoulos D, Macpherson A, Neurath MF, Ali RAR, et al. Environmental triggers in IBD: A review of progress and evidence. Nature Reviews. Gastroenterology & Hepatology. 2018;**15**:39-49

[41] Huang S, Rutkowsky JM, Snodgrass RG, Ono-Moore KD, Schneider DA, Newman JW, et al. Saturated fatty acids activate TLR-mediated proinflammatory signaling pathways. Journal of Lipid Research. 2012;**53**:2002-2013. DOI: 10.1194/jlr.D029546

[42] Wong SW, Kwon MJ, Choi AMK, Kim HP, Nakahira K, Hwang DH. Fatty acids modulate toll-like receptor 4 activation through regulation of receptor dimerization and recruitment into lipid rafts in a reactive oxygen species-dependent manner. The Journal of Biological Chemistry. 2009;**284**: 27384-27392. DOI: 10.1074/jbc.M109.044065

[43] Gil-Cardoso K, Ginés I, Pinent M, Ardévol A, Terra X, Blay M. A cafeteria diet triggers intestinal inflammation and oxidative stress in obese rats. The British Journal of Nutrition. 2017;**117**:218. DOI: 10.1017/S0007114516004608

[44] Cani PD, Bibiloni R, Knauf C, Waget A, Neyrinck AM, Delzenne NM, et al. Changes in gut microbiota control metabolic endotoxemia-induced inflammation in high-fat diet-induced obesity and diabetes in mice. Diabetes. 2008;**57**:1470-1481. DOI: 10.2337/db07-1403

[45] Serrano J, Puupponen-Pimiä R, Dauer A, Aura AM, Saura-Calixto F. Tannins: Current knowledge of food sources, intake, bioavailability and biological effects. Molecular Nutrition & Food Research. 2009;**53**: 310-329. DOI: 10.1002/mnfr.200900039

[46] Bittner K, Rzeppa S, Humpf H-U. Distribution and quantification of flavan-3-ols and procyanidins with low degree of polymerization in nuts, cereals, and legumes. Journal of Agricultural and Food Chemistry. 2013; **61**:9148-9154. DOI: 10.1021/jf4024728

[47] Rue EA, Rush MD, van Breemen RB. Procyanidins: A comprehensive review encompassing structure elucidation via mass spectrometry. Phytochemistry Reviews. 2018;**17**:1-16. DOI: 10.1007/s11101-017-9507-3

[48] Wang Y, Chung S-J, Song WO, Chun OK. Estimation of daily proanthocyanidin intake and major food sources in the U.S. diet. The Journal of Nutrition. 2011;**141**:447-452. DOI: 10.3945/jn.110.133900

[49] Jun S, Shin S, Joung H. Estimation of dietary flavonoid intake and major food sources of Korean adults. The British Journal of Nutrition. 2016;**115**:480-489. DOI: 10.1017/S0007114515004006

[50] Zamora-Ros R, Biessy C, Rothwell JA, Monge A, Lajous M, Scalbert A, et al. Dietary polyphenol intake and their major food sources in the Mexican Teachers' Cohort. The British Journal of Nutrition. 2018;**120**:353-360. DOI: 10.1017/S0007114518001381

[51] Vogiatzoglou A, Mulligan AA, Luben RN, Lentjes MAH, Heiss C, Kelm M, et al. Assessment of the dietary intake of total flavan-3-ols, monomeric flavan-3-ols, proanthocyanidins and theaflavins in the European Union. The British Journal of Nutrition. 2014;**111**:1463-1473. DOI: 10.1017/S0007114513003930

[52] Zamora-Ros R, Knaze V, Rothwell JA, Hémon B, Moskal A, Overvad K, et al. Dietary polyphenol intake in Europe: The European Prospective Investigation into Cancer and Nutrition (EPIC) Study. European Journal of Nutrition. 2016;**55**:1359-1375. DOI: 10.1007/s00394-015-0950-x

[53] Knaze V, Zamora-Ros R, Luján-Barroso L, Romieu I, Scalbert A, Slimani N, et al. Intake estimation of total and individual flavan-3-ols,

proanthocyanidins and theaflavins, their food sources and determinants in the European Prospective Investigation into Cancer and Nutrition (EPIC) study. The British Journal of Nutrition. 2012; **108**:1095-1108. DOI: 10.1017/S0007114511006386

[54] Rios LY, Bennett RN, Lazarus SA, Remesy C, Scalbert A, Williamson G. Cocoa procyanidins are stable during gastric transit in humans. The American Journal of Clinical Nutrition. 2002;**76**: 1106-1110

[55] Donovan JL, Crespy V, Manach C, Morand C, Besson C, Scalbert A, et al. Catechin is metabolized by both the small intestine and liver of rats. The Journal of Nutrition. 2001;**131**:1753-1757. DOI: 10.1093/jn/131.6.1753

[56] Stalmach A, Mullen W, Steiling H, Williamson G, Lean MEJ, Crozier A. Absorption, metabolism, and excretion of green tea flavan-3-ols in humans with an ileostomy. Molecular Nutrition & Food Research. 2010;**54**:323-334. DOI: 10.1002/mnfr.200900194

[57] Thilakarathna SH, Vasantha Rupasinghe HP. Flavonoid bioavailability and attempts for bioavailability enhancement. Nutrients. 2013;**5**:3367-3387. DOI: 10.3390/nu5093367

[58] Rein D, Lotito S, Holt RR, Keen CL, Schmitz HH, Fraga CG. Epicatechin in human plasma: In vivo determination and effect of chocolate consumption on plasma oxidation status. The Journal of Nutrition. 2000;**130**:2109S-2114S. DOI: 10.1093/jn/130.8.2109S

[59] Ullmann U, Haller J, Decourt JP, Girault N, Girault J, Richard-Caudron AS, et al. A single ascending dose study of epigallocatechin gallate in healthy volunteers. The Journal of International Medical Research. 2003;**31**:88-101. DOI: 10.1177/147323000303100205

[60] Wiese S, Esatbeyoglu T, Winterhalter P, Kruse HP, Winkler S, Bub A, et al. Comparative biokinetics and metabolism of pure monomeric, dimeric, and polymeric flavan-3-ols: A randomized cross-over study in humans. Molecular Nutrition & Food Research. 2015;**59**:610-621. DOI: 10.1002/mnfr.201400422

[61] Deprez S, Mila I, Huneau J-F, Tome D, Scalbert A. Transport of proanthocyanidin dimer, trimer, and polymer across monolayers of human intestinal epithelial Caco-2 cells. Antioxidants & Redox Signaling. 2001; **3**:957-967. DOI: 10.1089/152308601317203503

[62] Zumdick S, Deters A, Hensel A. In vitro intestinal transport of oligomeric procyanidins (DP 2 to 4) across monolayers of Caco-2 cells. Fitoterapia. 2012;**83**:1210-1217. DOI: 10.1016/j.fitote.2012.06.013

[63] Mendoza-Wilson AM, Carmelo-Luna FJ, Astiazarán-García H, Mata-Haro V, Espinosa-Plascencia A, del Carmen Bermúdez-Almada M, et al. Absorption of dimers, trimers and tetramers of procyanidins present in apple skin by IEC-18 cell monolayers. Journal of Functional Foods. 2016;**27**:386-391. DOI: 10.1016/J.JFF.2016.09.020.

[64] Shoji T, Masumoto S, Moriichi N, Akiyama H, Kanda T, Ohtake Y, et al. Apple procyanidin oligomers absorption in rats after oral administration: Analysis of procyanidins in plasma using the porter method and high-performance liquid chromatography/tandem mass spectrometry. Journal of Agricultural and Food Chemistry. 2006; **54**:884-892. DOI: 10.1021/jf052260b

[65] Serra A, MacI A, Romero MP, Valls J, Bladé C, Arola L, et al. Bioavailability of procyanidin dimers and trimers and matrix food effects in in vitro and in vivo models. The British Journal of Nutrition. 2010;**103**:944-952. DOI: 10.1017/S0007114509992741

[66] Sano A, Yamakoshi J, Tokutake S, Tobe K, Kubota Y, Kikuchi M. Procyanidin B1 is detected in human serum after intake of proanthocyanidin-rich grape seed extract. Bioscience, Biotechnology, and Biochemistry. 2003; **67**:1140-1143

[67] Ottaviani JI, Kwik-Uribe C, Keen CL, Schroeter H. Intake of dietary procyanidins does not contribute to the pool of circulating flavanols in humans. The American Journal of Clinical Nutrition. 2012;**95**:851-858. DOI: 10.3945/ajcn.111.028340

[68] Tsang C, Auger C, Mullen W, Bornet A, Rouanet J-M, Crozier A, et al. The absorption, metabolism and excretion of flavan-3-ols and procyanidins following the ingestion of a grape seed extract by rats. The British Journal of Nutrition. 2005;**94**:170-181

[69] Gu L, House SE, Rooney L, Prior RL. Sorghum bran in the diet dose dependently increased the excretion of catechins and microbial-derived phenolic acids in female rats. Journal of Agricultural and Food Chemistry. 2007; **55**:5326-5334. DOI: 10.1021/jf070100p

[70] Appeldoorn MM, Vincken JP, Aura AM, Hollman PCH, Gruppen H. Procyanidin dimers are metabolized by human microbiota with 2-(3,4-dihydroxyphenyl)acetic acid and 5-(3,4-dihydroxyphenyl)-γ-valerolactone as the major metabolites. Journal of Agricultural and Food Chemistry. 2009; **57**:1084-1092. DOI: 10.1021/jf803059z

[71] Castello F, Costabile G, Bresciani L, Tassotti M, Naviglio D, Luongo D, et al. Bioavailability and pharmacokinetic profile of grape pomace phenolic compounds in humans. Archives of Biochemistry and Biophysics. 2018;**646**: 1-9. DOI: 10.1016/j.abb.2018.03.021

[72] Trošt K, Ulaszewska MM, Stanstrup J, Albanese D, De Filippo C, Tuohy KM, et al. Host: Microbiome co-metabolic processing of dietary polyphenols—An acute, single blinded, cross-over study with different doses of apple polyphenols in healthy subjects. Food Research International. 2018;**112**: 108-128. DOI: 10.1016/j.foodres. 2018.06.016

[73] Margalef M, Pons Z, Bravo FI, Muguerza B, Arola-Arnal A. Tissue distribution of rat flavanol metabolites at different doses. The Journal of Nutritional Biochemistry. 2015;**26**: 987-995. DOI: 10.1016/j.jnutbio.2015. 04.006

[74] Yoshioka Y, Akiyama H, Nakano M, Shoji T, Kanda T, Ohtake Y, et al. Orally administered apple procyanidins protect against experimental inflammatory bowel disease in mice. International Immunopharmacology. 2008;**8**: 1802-1807. DOI: 10.1016/j.intimp. 2008.08.021

[75] Denis M-C, Desjardins Y, Furtos A, Marcil V, Dudonné S, Montoudis A, et al. Prevention of oxidative stress, inflammation and mitochondrial dysfunction in the intestine by different cranberry phenolic fractions. Clinical Science. 2015;**128**:197-212. DOI: 10.1042/CS20140210

[76] Erlejman AG, Jaggers G, Fraga CG, Oteiza PI. TNFα-induced NF-κB activation and cell oxidant production are modulated by hexameric procyanidins in Caco-2 cells. Archives of Biochemistry and Biophysics. 2008;**476**: 186-195. DOI: 10.1016/j.abb.2008. 01.024

[77] Gentile C, Perrone A, Attanzio A, Tesoriere L, Livrea MA. Sicilian pistachio (*Pistacia vera* L.) nut inhibits expression and release of inflammatory mediators and reverts the increase of paracellular permeability in IL-1β-exposed human intestinal epithelial cells. European Journal of Nutrition. 2015;**54**:811-821. DOI: 10.1007/ s00394-014-0760-6

[78] Bitzer ZT, Glisan SL, Dorenkott MR, Goodrich KM, Ye L, O'Keefe SF, et al. Cocoa procyanidins with different degrees of polymerization possess distinct activities in models of colonic inflammation. The Journal of Nutritional Biochemistry. 2015;**26**: 827-831. DOI: 10.1016/j.jnutbio.2015.02.007

[79] Bianchi MG, Chiu M, Taurino G, Brighenti F, Del Rio D, Mena P, et al. Catechin and Procyanidin B2 modulate the expression of tight junction proteins but do not protect from inflammation-induced changes in permeability in human intestinal cell monolayers. Nutrients. 2019;**11**:2271. DOI: 10.3390/nu11102271

[80] Wong X, Carrasco-Pozo C, Escobar E, Navarrete P, Blachier F, Andriamihaja M, et al. Deleterious effect of p-cresol on human colonic epithelial cells prevented by proanthocyanidin-containing polyphenol extracts from fruits and proanthocyanidin bacterial metabolites. Journal of Agricultural and Food Chemistry. 2016;**64**:3574-3583. DOI: 10.1021/acs.jafc.6b00656

[81] Xu H, Zhao C, Li Y, Liu R, Ao M, Li F, et al. The ameliorative effect of the: *Pyracantha fortuneana* (Maxim.) H. L. Li extract on intestinal barrier dysfunction through modulating glycolipid digestion and gut microbiota in high fat diet-fed rats. Food & Function. 2019;**10**: 6517-6532. DOI: 10.1039/c9fo01599j

[82] Wang Y-H, Yang X-L, Wang L, Cui M-X, Cai Y-Q, Li X, et al. Effects of proanthocyanidins from grape seed on treatment of recurrent ulcerative colitis in rats. Canadian Journal of Physiology and Pharmacology. 2010;**898**:888-898. DOI: 10.1139/Y10-071

[83] Wang Y-H, Ge B, Yang X-L, Zhai J, Yang L-N, Wang X-X, et al. Proanthocyanidins from grape seeds modulates the nuclear factor-kappa B signal transduction pathways in rats with TNBS-induced recurrent ulcerative colitis. International Immunopharmacology. 2011;**11**: 1620-1627. DOI: 10.1016/j.intimp.2011.05.024

[84] Li X, Yang X, Cai Y, Qin H, Wang L, Wang Y, et al. Proanthocyanidins from grape seeds modulate the NF-κB signal transduction pathways in rats with TNBS-induced ulcerative colitis. Molecules. 2011;**16**:6721-6731. DOI: 10.3390/molecules16086721

[85] Chen L, You Q, Hu L, Gao J, Meng Q, Liu W, et al. The antioxidant procyanidin reduces reactive oxygen species signaling in macrophages and ameliorates experimental colitis in mice. Frontiers in Immunology. 2018;**8**:1910. DOI: 10.3389/fimmu.2017.01910

[86] Wang H, Xue Y, Zhang H, Huang Y, Yang G, Du M, et al. Dietary grape seed extract ameliorates symptoms of inflammatory bowel disease in IL10-deficient mice. Molecular Nutrition & Food Research. 2013;**57**:2253-2257. DOI: 10.1002/mnfr.201300146

[87] Bibi S, Kang Y, Yang G, Zhu M-J. Grape seed extract improves small intestinal health through suppressing inflammation and regulating alkaline phosphatase in IL-10-deficient mice. Journal of Functional Foods. 2016;**20**: 245-252. DOI: 10.1016/J.JFF.2015.10.021

[88] He X, Sun LM. Dietary intake of flavonoid subclasses and risk of colorectal cancer: Evidence from population studies. Oncotarget. 2016;**7**: 26617-26627. DOI: 10.18632/oncotarget.8562

[89] Sambuy Y, De Angelis I, Ranaldi G, Scarino ML, Stammati A, Zucco F. The Caco-2 cell line as a model of the intestinal barrier: Influence of cell and culture-related factors on Caco-2 cell functional characteristics. Cell Biology and Toxicology. 2005;**21**:1-26

[90] Kämpfer AAM, Urbán P, Gioria S, Kanase N, Stone V, Kinsner-Ovaskainen A. Development of an in vitro co-culture model to mimic the human intestine in healthy and diseased state. Toxicology in Vitro. 2017;**45**:31-43. DOI: 10.1016/j.tiv.2017.08.011

[91] Chassaing B, Rolhion N, De Vallée A, Salim SY, Prorok-Hamon M, Neut C, et al. Crohn disease-associated adherent-invasive *E. coli* bacteria target mouse and human Peyer's patches via long polar fimbriae. The Journal of Clinical Investigation. 2011;**121**:966-975. DOI: 10.1172/JCI44632.

[92] Goh JY, Weaver RJ, Dixon L, Platt NJ, Roberts RA. Development and use of in vitro alternatives to animal testing by the pharmaceutical industry 1980–2013. Toxicology Research (Cambridge). 2015;**4**:1297-1307. DOI: 10.1039/c5tx00123d

[93] Kang TH, Kim HJ. Farewell to animal testing: Innovations on human intestinal microphysiological systems. Micromachines. 2016;7:107

[94] Randhawa PK, Singh K, Singh N, Jaggi AS. A review on chemical-induced inflammatory bowel disease models in rodents. The Korean Journal of Physiology & Pharmacology. 2014;**18**: 279-288. DOI: 10.4196/kjpp.2014.18.4.279

[95] Hidalgo IJ, Raub TJ, Borchardt RT. Characterization of the human colon carcinoma cell line (Caco-2) as a model system for intestinal epithelial permeability. Gastroenterology. 1989; **96**:736-749. DOI: 10.1016/S0016-5085(89)80072-1

[96] Srinivasan B, Kolli AR, Esch MB, Abaci HE, Shuler ML, Hickman JJ. TEER measurement techniques for in vitro barrier model systems. Journal of Laboratory Automation. 2015;**20**: 107-126. DOI: 10.1177/2211068214561025

[97] Sampey BP, Vanhoose AM, Winfield HM, Freemerman AJ, Muehlbauer MJ, Fueger PT, et al. Cafeteria diet is a robust model of human metabolic syndrome with liver and adipose inflammation: Comparison to high-fat diet. Obesity (Silver Spring). 2011;**19**:1109-1117. DOI: 10.1038/oby.2011.18

[98] Ginés I, Gil-Cardoso K, Serrano J, Casanova-Martí À, Blay M, Pinent M, et al. Effects of an intermittent grape-seed proanthocyanidin (GSPE) treatment on a cafeteria diet obesogenic challenge in rats. Nutrients. 2018;**10**:315. DOI: 10.3390/nu10030315

[99] Baselga-Escudero L, Pascual-Serrano A, Ribas-Latre A, Casanova E, Salvadó MJ, Arola L, et al. Long-term supplementation with a low dose of proanthocyanidins normalized liver miR-33a and miR-122 levels in high-fat diet-induced obese rats. Nutrition Research. 2015;**35**:337-345. DOI: 10.1016/j.nutres.2015.02.008

[100] Margalef M, Pons Z, Iglesias-Carres L, Arola L, Muguerza B, Arola-Arnal A. Gender-related similarities and differences in the body distribution of grape seed flavanols in rats. Molecular Nutrition & Food Research. 2016;**60**: 760-772. DOI: 10.1002/mnfr.201500717

[101] Terra X, Pallarés V, Ardèvol A, Bladé C, Fernández-Larrea J, Pujadas G, et al. Modulatory effect of grape-seed procyanidins on local and systemic inflammation in diet-induced obesity rats. The Journal of Nutritional Biochemistry. 2011;**22**:380-387. DOI: 10.1016/j.jnutbio.2010.03.006

[102] Li X-L, Cai Y-Q, Qin H, Wu Y-J. Therapeutic effect and mechanism of proanthocyanidins from grape seeds in rats with TNBS-induced ulcerative colitis. Canadian Journal of Physiology and Pharmacology. 2008;**86**:841-849. DOI: 10.1139/Y08-089

[103] Hollman PCH, Cassidy A, Comte B, Heinonen M, Richelle M, Richling E, et al. The biological relevance of direct antioxidant effects of polyphenols for cardiovascular health in humans is not established. The Journal of Nutrition. 2011;**141**:989S-1009S. DOI: 10.3945/jn.110.131490

[104] Tsilingiri K, Sonzogni A, Caprioli F, Rescigno M. A novel method for the culture and polarized stimulation of human intestinal mucosa explants. Journal of Visualized Experiments. 2013: e4368. DOI: 10.3791/4368

[105] Vadstrup K, Galsgaard ED, Gerwien J, Vester-Andersen MK, Pedersen JS, Rasmussen J, et al. Validation and optimization of an ex vivo assay of intestinal mucosal biopsies in Crohn's disease: Reflects inflammation and drug effects. PLoS One. 2016;**11**:e0155335. DOI: 10.1371/journal.pone.0155335

[106] Sjöberg Å, Lutz M, Tannergren C, Wingolf C, Borde A, Ungell A-L. Comprehensive study on regional human intestinal permeability and prediction of fraction absorbed of drugs using the Ussing chamber technique. European Journal of Pharmaceutical Sciences. 2013;**48**:166-180. DOI: 10.1016/J.EJPS.2012.10.007

[107] Geraedts MCP, Troost FJ, De Ridder RJ, Bodelier AGL, Masclee AAM, Saris WHM. Validation of Ussing chamber technology to study satiety hormone release from human duodenal specimens. Obesity. 2012;**20**:678-682. DOI: 10.1038/oby.2011.104

[108] Wood MW, Breitschwerdt EB, Nordone SK, Linder KE, Gookin JL. Uropathogenic *E. coli* promote a paracellular urothelial barrier defect characterized by altered tight junction integrity, epithelial cell sloughing and cytokine release. Journal of Comparative Pathology. 2012;**147**:11-19. DOI: 10.1016/j.jcpa.2011.09.005

[109] Ray S, Bagchi D, Lim PM, Bagchi M, Gross SM, Kothari SC, et al. Acute and long-term safety evaluation of a novel IH636 grape seed proanthocyanidin extract. Research Communications in Molecular Pathology and Pharmacology. 2001;**109**: 165-197

[110] Yamakoshi J, Saito M, Kataoka S, Kikuchi M. Safety evaluation of proanthocyanidin-rich extract from grape seeds. Food and Chemical Toxicology. 2002;**40**:599-607. DOI: 10.1016/s0278-6915(02)00006-6

[111] Lluís L, Muñoz M, Rosa Nogués M, Sánchez-Martos V, Romeu M, Giralt M, et al. Toxicology evaluation of a procyanidin-rich extract from grape skins and seeds. Food and Chemical Toxicology. 2011;**49**:1450-1454. DOI: 10.1016/j.fct.2011.03.042

[112] Wong X, Madrid AM, Tralma K, Castillo R, Carrasco-Pozo C, Navarrete P, et al. Polyphenol extracts interfere with bacterial lipopolysaccharide in vitro and decrease postprandial endotoxemia in human volunteers. Journal of Functional Foods. 2016;**26**:406-417. DOI: 10.1016/J.JFF.2016.08.011

[113] Cani PD, Osto M, Geurts L, Everard A. Involvement of gut microbiota in the development of low-grade inflammation and type 2 diabetes associated with obesity. Gut Microbes. 2012;**3**:279-288

[114] Butler LG. Effects of condensed tannin on animal nutrition. In: Chemistry and Significance of Condensed Tannins. US: Springer; 1989. pp. 391-402

[115] Chung KT, Wong TY, Wei CI, Huang YW, Lin Y. Tannins and human health: A review. Critical Reviews in Food Science and Nutrition. 1998;**38**: 421-464. DOI: 10.1080/1040869989 1274273

[116] Brás NF, Gonçalves R, Fernandes PA, Mateus N, Ramos MJ, De Freitas V. Understanding the binding of procyanidins to pancreatic elastase by experimental and computational methods. Biochemistry. 2010;**49**: 5097-5108. DOI: 10.1021/bi100410q

[117] De Freitas V, Mateus N. Structural features of procyanidin interactions with salivary proteins. Journal of Agricultural and Food Chemistry. 2001; **49**:940-945. DOI: 10.1021/jf000981z

[118] Zhu W, Xiong L, Peng J, Deng X, Gao J, Li CM. Molecular insight into affinities of gallated and nongallated proanthocyanidins dimers to lipid bilayers. Scientific Reports. 2016;**6**: 37680. DOI: 10.1038/srep37680

[119] Verstraeten SV, Jaggers GK, Fraga CG, Oteiza PI. Procyanidins can interact with Caco-2 cell membrane lipid rafts: Involvement of cholesterol. Biochimica et Biophysica Acta, Biomembranes. 2013;**1828**:2646-2653. DOI: 10.1016/j.bbamem.2013.07.023

[120] Yang G, Bibi S, Du M, Suzuki T, Zhu MJ. Regulation of the intestinal tight junction by natural polyphenols: A mechanistic perspective. Critical Reviews in Food Science and Nutrition. 2017;**57**:3830-3839. DOI: 10.1080/10408398.2016.1152230

[121] Cunningham KE, Turner JR. Myosin light chain kinase: Pulling the strings of epithelial tight junction function. Annals of the New York Academy of Sciences. 2012;**1258**:34-42. DOI: 10.1111/j.1749-6632.2012.06526.x

[122] Marchiando AM, Shen L, Graham WV, Edelblum KL, Duckworth CA, Guan Y, et al. The epithelial barrier is maintained by in vivo tight junction expansion during pathologic intestinal epithelial shedding. Gastroenterology. 2011;**140**:1208. e2-1218.e2. DOI: 10.1053/j.gastro.2011. 01.004

[123] Wang BH, Lai Yeap F, Polya GM. Differential inhibition of eukaryote protein kinases by condensed tannins. Phytochemistry. 1996;**43**:359-365. DOI: 10.1016/0031-9422(96)00259-2

[124] Contreras TC, Ricciardi E, Cremonini E, Oteiza PI. (−)-Epicatechin in the prevention of tumor necrosis alpha-induced loss of Caco-2 cell barrier integrity. Archives of Biochemistry and Biophysics. 2015;**573**: 84-91. DOI: 10.1016/j.abb.2015.01.024

[125] Delehanty JB, Johnson BJ, Hickey TE, Pons T, Ligler FS. Binding and neutralization of lipopolysaccharides by plant proanthocyanidins. Journal of Natural Products. 2007;**70**:1718-1724. DOI: 10.1021/np0703601

[126] Williams AR, Klaver EJ, Laan LC, Ramsay A, Fryganas C, Difborg R, et al. Co-operative suppression of inflammatory responses in human dendritic cells by plant proanthocyanidins and products from the parasitic nematode *Trichuris suis*. Immunology. 2017;**150**:312-328. DOI: 10.1111/imm.12687

[127] Zmora N, Suez J, Elinav E. You are what you eat: Diet, health and the gut microbiota. Nature Reviews. Gastroenterology & Hepatology. 2019; **16**:35-56

[128] Guirro M, Costa A, Gual-Grau A, Herrero P, Torrell H, Canela N, et al. Effects from diet-induced gut microbiota dysbiosis and obesity can be ameliorated by fecal microbiota transplantation: A multiomics approach. PLoS One. 2019;**14**:e0218143. DOI: 10.1371/journal.pone.0218143

[129] Wan Y, Wang F, Yuan J, Li J, Jiang D, Zhang J, et al. Effects of dietary fat on gut microbiota and faecal metabolites, and their relationship with cardiometabolic risk factors: A 6-month randomised controlled-feeding trial.

Gut. 2019;**68**:1417-1429. DOI: 10.1136/gutjnl-2018-317609

[130] Segata N. Gut microbiome: Westernization and the disappearance of intestinal diversity. Current Biology. 2015;**25**:R611-R613

[131] Buttó LF, Haller D. Dysbiosis in intestinal inflammation: Cause or consequence. International Journal of Medical Microbiology. 2016;**306**: 302-309

[132] Ley RE, Bäckhed F, Turnbaugh P, Lozupone CA, Knight RD, Gordon JI. Obesity alters gut microbial ecology. Proceedings of the National Academy of Sciences of the United States of America. 2005;**102**:11070-11075. DOI: 10.1073/pnas.0504978102

[133] Lee SM, Kim N, Yoon H, Nam RH, Lee DH. Microbial changes and host response in F344 rat colon depending on sex and age following a high-fat diet. Frontiers in Microbiology. 2018;**9**:2236. DOI: 10.3389/fmicb.2018.02236

[134] Ley RRE, Turnbaugh PJP, Klein S, Gordon JIJ. Microbial ecology: Human gut microbes associated with obesity. Nature. 2006;**444**:1022-1023. DOI: 10.1038/4441022a

[135] Koliada A, Syzenko G, Moseiko V, Budovska L, Puchkov K, Perederiy V, et al. Association between body mass index and *Firmicutes/Bacteroidetes* ratio in an adult Ukrainian population. BMC Microbiology. 2017;**17**:120. DOI: 10.1186/s12866-017-1027-1

[136] Duncan SH, Lobley GE, Holtrop G, Ince J, Johnstone AM, Louis P, et al. Human colonic microbiota associated with diet, obesity and weight loss. International Journal of Obesity. 2008; **32**:1720-1724. DOI: 10.1038/ijo.2008.155

[137] Schwiertz A, Taras D, Schäfer K, Beijer S, Bos NA, Donus C, et al. Microbiota and SCFA in lean and overweight healthy subjects. Obesity. 2010;**18**:190-195. DOI: 10.1038/oby.2009.167

[138] Castaner O, Goday A, Park YM, Lee SH, Magkos F, Shiow SATE, et al. The gut microbiome profile in obesity: A systematic review. International Journal of Endocrinology. 2018;**2018**:1-9. DOI: 10.1155/2018/4095789

[139] Garrett WS, Lord GM, Punit S, Lugo-Villarino G, Mazmanian SKK, Ito S, et al. Communicable ulcerative colitis induced by T-bet deficiency in the innate immune system. Cell. 2007; **131**:33-45. DOI: 10.1016/j.cell.2007.08.017

[140] Karczewski J, Poniedziałek B, Adamski Z, Rzymski P. The effects of the microbiota on the host immune system. Autoimmunity. 2014;**47**: 494-504

[141] Etxeberria U, Fernández-Quintela A, Milagro FI, Aguirre L, Martínez JA, Portillo MP. Impact of polyphenols and polyphenol-rich dietary sources on gut microbiota composition. Journal of Agricultural and Food Chemistry. 2013; **61**:9517-9533. DOI: 10.1021/jf402506c

[142] Tzounis X, Rodriguez-Mateos A, Vulevic J, Gibson GR, Kwik-Uribe C, Spencer JPE. Prebiotic evaluation of cocoa-derived flavanols in healthy humans by using a randomized, controlled, double-blind, crossover intervention study. The American Journal of Clinical Nutrition. 2011;**93**: 62-72. DOI: 10.3945/ajcn.110.000075. Diet.

[143] Queipo-Ortuño MI, Boto-Ordóñez M, Murri M, Gomez-Zumaquero JM, Clemente-Postigo M, Estruch R, et al. Influence of red wine polyphenols and ethanol on the gut microbiota ecology and biochemical biomarkers. The American Journal of Clinical Nutrition. 2012;**95**:1323-1334. DOI: 10.3945/ajcn.111.027847

[144] Hervert-Hernández D, Goñi I. Dietary polyphenols and human gut microbiota: A review. Food Review International. 2011;**27**:154-169. DOI: 10.1080/87559129.2010.535233

[145] Cardona F, Andrés-Lacueva C, Tulipani S, Tinahones FJ, Queipo-Ortuño MI. Benefits of polyphenols on gut microbiota and implications in human health. The Journal of Nutritional Biochemistry. 2013;**24**:1415-1422. DOI: 10.1016/j.jnutbio.2013.05.001

[146] Cueva C, Sánchez-Patán F, Monagas M, Walton GE, Gibson GR, Martín-Álvarez PJ, et al. In vitro fermentation of grape seed flavan-3-ol fractions by human faecal microbiota: Changes in microbial groups and phenolic metabolites. FEMS Microbiology Ecology. 2013;**83**:792-805. DOI: 10.1111/1574-6941.12037

[147] Anhê FF, Pilon G, Roy D, Desjardins Y, Levy E, Marette A. Triggering Akkermansia with dietary polyphenols: A new weapon to combat the metabolic syndrome? Gut Microbes. 2016;**7**:146-153. DOI: 10.1080/19490976.2016.1142036

[148] Xing Y-W, Lei G-T, Wu Q-H, Jiang Y, Huang M-X. Procyanidin B2 protects against diet-induced obesity and non-alcoholic fatty liver disease via the modulation of the gut microbiota in rabbits. World Journal of Gastroenterology. 2019;**25**:955-966. DOI: 10.3748/wjg.v25.i8.955

[149] Tao W, Zhang Y, Shen X, Cao Y, Shi J, Ye X, et al. Rethinking the mechanism of the health benefits of proanthocyanidins: Absorption, metabolism, and interaction with gut microbiota. Comprehensive Reviews in Food Science and Food Safety. 2019;**18**: 971-985. DOI: 10.1111/1541-4337.12444

[150] Casanova-Martí À, Serrano J, Portune KJ, Sanz Y, Blay MT, Terra X, et al. Grape seed proanthocyanidins influence gut microbiota and enteroendocrine secretions in female rats. Food & Function. 2018;**9**: 1672-1682. DOI: 10.1039/c7fo02028g

[151] Everard A, Belzer C, Geurts L, Ouwerkerk JP, Druart C, Bindels LB, et al. Cross-talk between *Akkermansia muciniphila* and intestinal epithelium controls diet-induced obesity. Proceedings of the National Academy of Sciences of the United States of America. 2013;**110**:9066-9071. DOI: 10.1073/pnas.1219451110

[152] Gotteland M, Andrews M, Toledo M, Muñoz L, Caceres P, Anziani A, et al. Modulation of *Helicobacter pylori* colonization with cranberry juice and *Lactobacillus johnsonii* La1 in children. Nutrition. 2008;**24**:421-426. DOI: 10.1016/j.nut.2008.01.007

[153] Pastene E, Parada V, Avello M, Ruiz A, García A. Catechin-based procyanidins from *Peumus boldus* Mol. aqueous extract inhibit *Helicobacter pylori* urease and adherence to adenocarcinoma gastric cells. Phytotherapy Research. 2014;**28**: 1637-1645. DOI: 10.1002/ptr.5176

[154] Mena P, Bresciani L, Brindani N, Ludwig IA, Pereira-Caro G, Angelino D, et al. Phenyl-γ-valerolactones and phenylvaleric acids, the main colonic metabolites of flavan-3-ols: Synthesis, analysis, bioavailability, and bioactivity. Natural Product Reports. 2019;**36**: 714-752

Chapter 17

Artificial Sweeteners

Kanagamani Krishnasamy

Abstract

Nowadays, sugar*free food is very popular because of its low calorie value. So food industries make use of various artificial sweeteners of low calorie as an alternative to high calorie sugars and they provide low glycemic response. The U.S. Food and Drug Administration has approved artificial sweeteners such as saccharin, acesulfame-K, sucralose, aspartame, etc. as per acceptable daily intake value (ADI) value, but these artificial sweeteners that breakdown products during metabolism in turn are known to have health and metabolic effects. Hence, in this work, we will discuss about artificial sweeteners, types, and their metabolic and health effects.

Keywords: artificial sweeteners, adverse effects, potential toxicity

1. Introduction

In the recent scenario, the people are more concerned about health and better quality of life and so they avoid consumption of food rich in sugars, salt or fat so as to protect themselves from obesity and other non-communicable diseases. With the concern of reducing energy intake, food products containing artificial sweeteners other than simple sugars (monosaccharides and disaccharides) have become increasingly popular. Natural sweeteners add to more of nutritional value so they are called nutritive sweeteners. However, synthetic (artificial) sweeteners do not contain nutritional value so they are known as non- nutritive sweeteners On the contrary, artificial sweeteners are gaining very popular because they help reduce calories, control weight, manage diabetes, and prevent cavities. However, their safety has been controversial. In general, artificial sweeteners undergo a safety evaluation to assess their benefits and risks before using them. A health organization such as FDA evaluating all scientific studies and determines the maximum amount that can be eaten on a day without causing any adverse effects for each sweetener. The aim of this paper is to give an idea about the sweeteners, artificial sweetener, their chemical structure and properties and their potential health effects in humans.

2. Sweeteners

A sugar substitute is a food additive that provides a sweet taste like that of sugar is called sweeteners and classification of sweeteners based on calorific value was shown in **Figure 1**.

IntechOpen

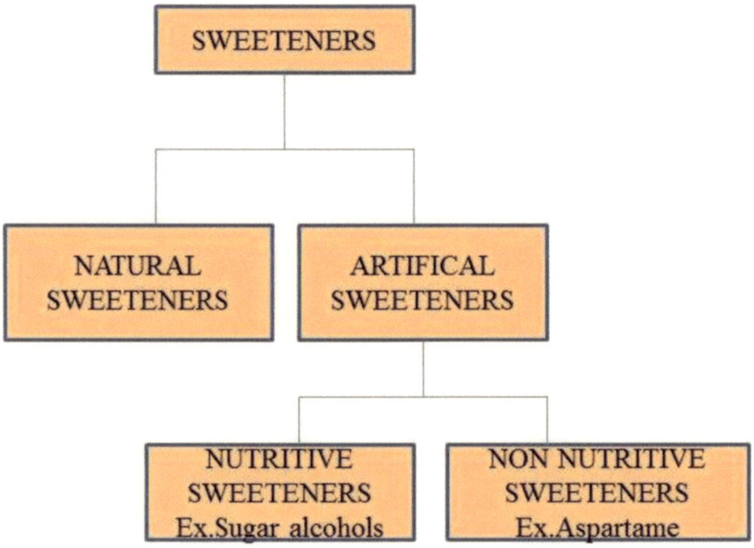

Figure 1.
Classification of sweeteners.

2.1 Nutritive sweeteners

Nutritive sweeteners are otherwise called as carbohydrate sweeteners (caloric). These sweeteners provide high-quality sweet taste and have an acceptable texture and shape and therefore remain as the most popular sweetener. Example for nutritive sweeteners are:

2.1.1 Monosaccharide polyols

Monosaccharide alcohol is the general term for the chain – like polyalcohol obtained by reducing the carboxyl group of sugars.

2.1.1.1 Sorbitol (D-glucitol)

Sorbitol occurs naturally in cherries, plums, apples, many berries, seaweeds and algae. It is moderately sweet, relatively inexpensive and has less shelf life because of hygroscopic property.

2.2 Non-nutritive sweeteners

These are low-calorie sweeteners (referred to as non-nutritive sweeteners, artificial sweeteners or sugar calories) added to foods, yogurt, medicinal preparation, dentifrices, mouthwash and beverages to provide sweetness without adding a calorie. The non-caloric sweeteners are generally much sweeter than sucrose and can, therefore, be used in small amounts.

2.2.1 Requirements for an ideal artificial sweetener

- It should provide sweetness with no unpleasant after taste.

- It should not contain any calories.

- More economical in productivity.
- Should be resistant to heat when cooked.
- It should not be carcinogenic (causing cancer) or mutagenic (change in genetic material in organism)

2.3 Artificial sweeteners

2.3.1 Aspartame

Aspartame is an artificial non saccharide sweetener of molecular formula.

$C_{14}H_{18}N_2O_5$ and finds its use in food and beverages as sugar substitute. Aspartame is a methyl ester of aspartic acid/phenylalanine dipeptide and marketed under the name NutraSweet, Equal and Canderel. In 1965, Aspartame was reported and U.S. Food and Drug Administration (FDA) in 1981 approved its use in the food products (**Figure 2**).

2.3.1.1 Metabolism and health aspect

Aspartame is one of the low calorie sweetener used in low, reduced calorie foods and also used in beverages. It is also a low calorie table top sweetener used in gums, breakfast cereals and dry foods. Upon breaking Aspartame produces about 4 calories of energy per gram. On prolonged heating aspartame decomposes and therefore it cannot be used for food items involving cooking and also converts into liquid on storage. The breakdown products upon ingestion are aspartic acid, phenylalanine, methanol and further breakdown products including formaldehyde, formic acid and diketopiperazine. FDA insisted that food products with aspartame should have warning in the label that the person with the rare genetic disorder phenylketonuria should avoid ingesting aspartame. Phenylketonuria is an inborn disease associated with error of metabolism that leads to attenuated metabolism of the amino acid phenylalanine. Phenylketonuria leads to behavioral problems and mental disorders. Peoples suffering from phenylketonuria will have insufficient level of enzyme phenylalanine hydroxylase which is required for the breakdown of phenylalanine [1] and as a result phenyl alanine accumulates in case of people affected with phenylketonuria. The breakdown products of aspartame like methanol, phenylalanine and aspartic acid leads to headache, blurred vision, brain tumors, eye problems, memory loss and nausea [2]. The aspartic acid one of the breakdown products of aspartame leads to excitotoxin. The aspartic acid acts like neurotransmitters

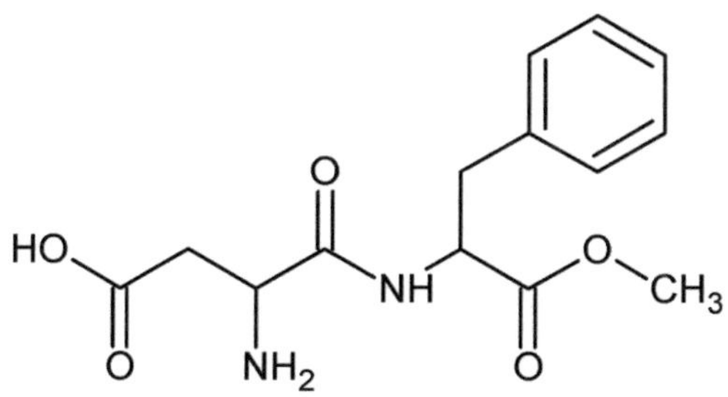

Figure 2.
Structure of aspartame.

stimulating the nerve cells to either damage or kills and may lead to spinal cord injury, stroke and hearing loss [3].

2.3.2 Acesulfame-K

Acesulfame potassium also known as Acesulfame-K is a calorie-free sugar substitute (artificial sweetener) marketed as Sunett and Sweet One. Acesulfame potassium is the potassium salt of 6-methyl-1,2,3-oxathiazine-4(3*H*)-one 2,2-dioxide. Acesulfame-K is a white crystalline powder having molecular formula of $C_4H_4KNO_4S$ and molecular weight 201.24 g/mol. It is approximately 120 times sweeter than sucrose and has high water solubility. Acesulfame-K is heat stable and can be used in cooking and baking. Ace-K is often blended with other sweeteners (Sucralose or Aspartame) (**Figure 3**).

2.3.2.1 Metabolism and health aspect

Acesulfame-K is not metabolized in the body and excreted in urine without undergoing any modification and not stored in the body. Pharmaco kinetic studies show that 95% of the consumed sweeteners basically excreted in the urine. It does not influence potassium in take despite of its potassium content. In 1988 UFDA approved to use Ace-K as a general purpose sweetener in a variety of dry products and in alcoholic beverages [4]. The breakdown product of Ace-K is acetoacetamide known to be toxic if consumed in very large doses but human exposure to breakdown products is negligible. Acesulfame-K contains methylene chloride and may lead to headache, depression, nausea, mental confusion, liver and kidney effects [5].

2.3.3 Sucralose

Sucralose is an artificial sweetener and sugar substitute having the molecular formula of $C_{12}H_{19}Cl_3O_8$ and molecular mass 397.64 g/mol. In the European Union it is known with the E number E955 and marketed under the name Splenda. Chlorination of sucrose leads to formation of sucralose. Sucralose is approximately 320–1000 times sweeter than sucrose and three times as sweet as aspartame and acesulfame potassium, and twice than sodium saccharin (**Figure 4**).

2.3.3.1 Metabolism and health aspect

Although sucralose is made from sugar, the human body does not recognize it as a sugar and does not metabolize. It does not produce any calories [6]. Sucralose is responsible for the shrunken thymus glands with diets of 5% sucralose, and also it causes diarrhea and dizziness on prolonged exposure.

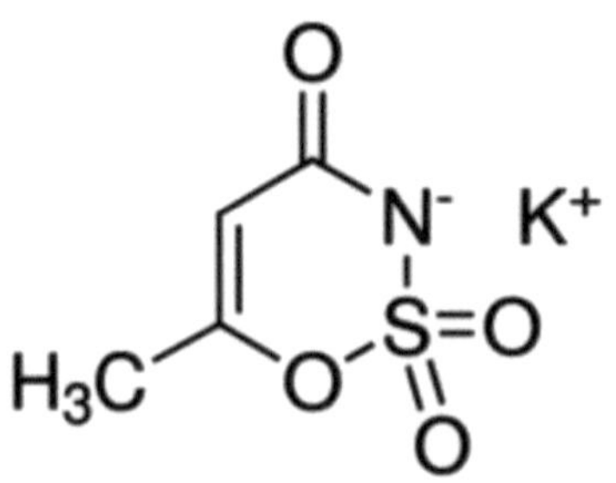

Figure 3.
Structure of Acesulfame-K.

2.3.4 Saccharin

Sodium saccharin of molecular formula $C_7H_5NO_3S$ (benzoic sulfimide) is an artificial sweetener with no calories. It is about 300–400 times as sweet as sucrose but has a bitter after taste at higher amount of intake. Saccharin finds use in products such as drinks, candies, cookies, and medicines. Saccharin is often blended with other artificial sweeteners because of taste purpose and when used in such combinations reduced sugar levels are preferred. In case of oral hygiene products, saccharin masks undesired tastes of other ingredients. Saccharin when used as a starter feed for livestock reduces feed intake after weaning. Besides its applications as an artificial sweetener, saccharin also finds application in electrolytic nickel deposition. Addition of saccharin to the nickel salt solutions increases the hardness and brightness of the nickel plate. This effect is important characteristic feature of saccharin compared to other sweeteners (**Figure 5**).

2.3.4.1 Metabolism and health aspect

The FDA tried to ban saccharin in 1977 because animal studies have revealed that it caused cancer in rat. But there is no supportive evidence to show the carcinogenic effect of saccharin at lower doses. Saccharin is now permitted to use in beverages, processed food and sugar substitutes and level of saccharin is to be indicated in the label [7]. Saccharin causes a headache, breathing difficulties, skin eruptions and diarrhea.

2.3.5 Sodium cyclamate

Sodium cyclamate is an artificial sweetener of molecular formula $C_6H_{12}NNaO_3S$. It is 30–50 times sweeter than sucrose (table sugar) and because of this it is least potent of the commercially used artificial sweeteners. It is always blended with

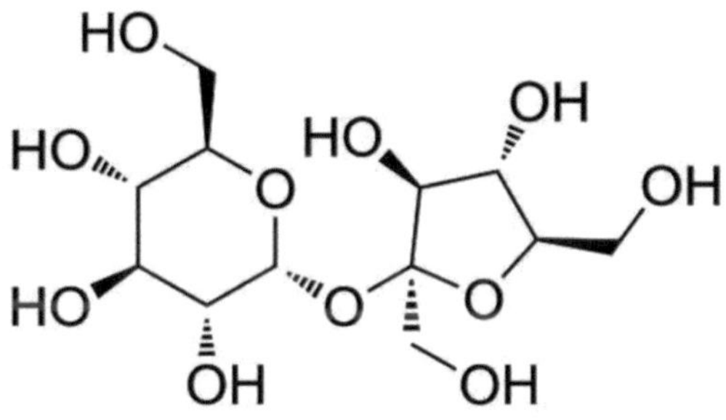

Figure 4.
Structure of sucralose.

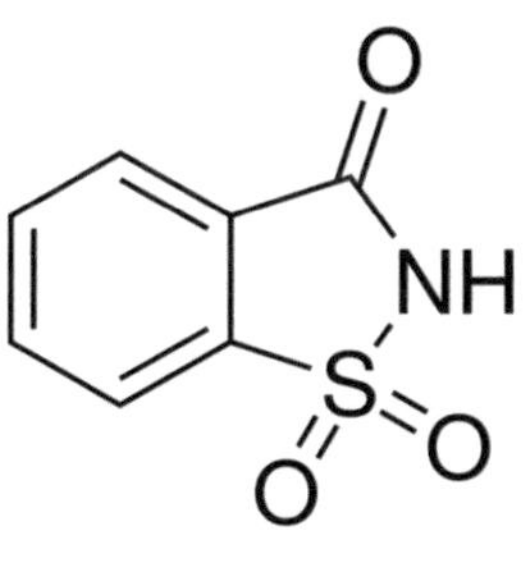

Figure 5.
Structure of saccharin.

other artificial sweeteners; especially saccharin in the ratio of 10:1 that is 10 parts of cyclamate to 1 part of saccharin. It is less expensive than most sweeteners including sucralose and stable under heat. Cyclamates are being banned in the United States and other countries due to safety reasons. But European Union considers them as safe (**Figure 6**).

2.3.5.1 Metabolism and health aspects

Cyclamate itself shows very slow toxicity but it is metabolized to cyclohexylamine which shows greater toxicity because of the nature of the cyclamate metabolism [8]. The possible exposure to cyclahexylamine from cyclamate metabolism in humans over a period is relevant to the establishment of ADI for cyclamate.

2.3.6 Neotame

Neotame is the low calorie artificial sweetener of molecular formula $C_{20}H_{30}N_2O_5$ and molecular mass 378.469 g mol^{-1} and it is the derivative of aspartame. A t-butyl group is added to the free amine group of aspartic acid. It is 8000 times sweetener than sucrose. It can be used alone or often blended with other sweeteners especially saccharin. Neotame is used in carbonated soft drinks, cakes, drink powders, table top sweetener and bubble gums. The neotame was approved in 2002 as a general purpose sweetener, excluding in meat and poultry by FDA (**Figure 7**).

2.3.6.1 Metabolism and health aspects

Neotame is rapidly metabolized by esterase present throughout the body into methyl ester and also forms a minor amount of methanol. This metabolic process yields de-esterified neotame which is completely eliminated from the body in urine and feces within 72 h. It is safer to use with people suffering from phenylketonuria because t-butyl group is added to the free amine group of aspartic acid breaks the peptide bond between the aspartic acid and phenylalanine, thus reduce the availability of phenylalanine which is responsible for phenylketonuria [9]. Neotame causes some of the toxic effects at high doses in the human such as it to reveal changes in body weight and food consumption and headache.

2.3.7 Alitame

Alitame of molecular formula $C_{14}H_{25}N_3O_4S$ is an aspartic acid-containing dipeptide sweetener. It was developed by Pfizer in the early 1980s and currently marketed in some countries under the brand name Aclame. It is an intense sweetener with sweetness potency 200 times greater than that of sucrose (**Figure 8**).

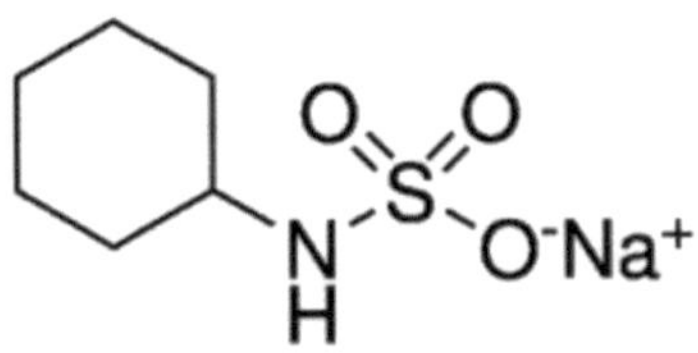

Figure 6.
Structure of sodium cyclamate.

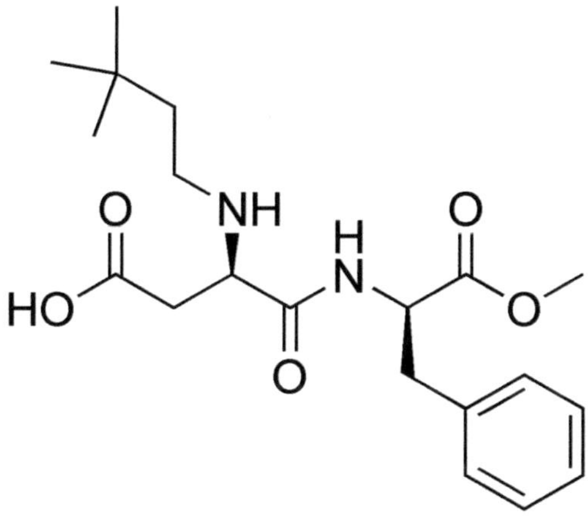

Figure 7.
Structure of neotame.

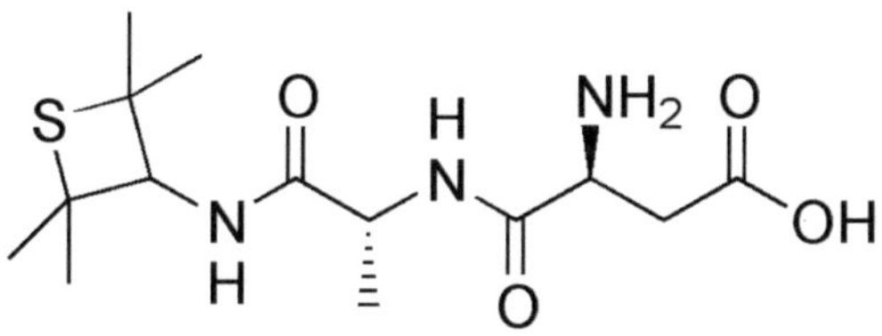

Figure 8.
Structure of alitame.

2.3.7.1 Metabolism and health aspects

Alitame is readily absorbed in gastrointestinal tract and then rapidly metabolized and excreted [10]. Alitame consists of two main components namely aspartic acid and alanine amide. The aspartic acid component is metabolized normally and alanine amide passes through the body with minimal changes.

3. Conclusion

The increased concern about obesity and the associated metabolic comorbidities have led to a reduced consumption of simple sugars and an increase in the intake of artificial sweeteners. These sweeteners, which appear as sugar alternatives, have been critically evaluated by the FDA and EFSA. Artificial sweeteners are not carbohydrates and so they will not increase blood sugar levels leading to diabetics but instead every gram of table sugar contains four calories and contributes to obesity [11]. The artificial sweeteners like saccharin, acesulfame-K and aspartame induces DNA damage in human peripheral lymphocytes [11]. The degradation products of acesulfame-K under basic conditions such as acetoacetic acid and acetoacetamide-N-sulfonic acid may cause DNA strand breaks [5]. Aspartame leads to gastrointestinal problems. The toxic potential of various artificial sweeteners for the human body was shown in **Table 1**. Therefore artificial sweeteners provide some potential health benefits. In addition they are toxic at high concentrations for the long time exposure. Artificial sweeteners consumption has been shown to cause mild to serious side effects including life threatening brain damages at high concentrations. But however low concentrations of these sweeteners does not cause threat to human health.

Common name	Brand names	FDA approval	Number of times sweeter than sucrose	kcal/g	Commercial uses
Acesulfame-K	Sunett, Sweet One	1988—tabletop	200	0	Baked goods, frozen desserts, candies, beverages, cough drops, breath mints
		1993—beverages			
		2003—general use, but not in meat or poultry			
Alitame	Aclame	Pending	2000	1.4	Baked goods, hot and cold beverages, milk products, frozen desserts and mixes, fruit preparations, chewing gums and candies, tabletop sweeteners, toiletries, pharmaceuticals
Aspartame	NutraSweet, Equal	1981—tabletop	200	4	General-purpose foods
		1996—general purpose			
Cyclamate	SugarTwin, Sucaryl	GRAS until banned in 1970	30	0	Tabletop sweetener, beverages
Neotame		2002	7000–13,000	0	Baked goods, soft drinks, chewing gum, frosting, frozen desserts, jams, jellies, gelatins, puddings, processed fruit and fruit juices, toppings, syrups
Saccharin	Sweet'N Low, Sweet Twin, Necta Sweet	GRAS	200–700	0	Tabletop sweetener, baked goods, soft drinks, jams, chewing gum
Sucralose	Splenda	1998—in 15 food categories	~600	0	Tabletop sweetener, beverages, chewing gum, frozen desserts, fruit juices, gelatins
		1999—general-purpose sweetener			

FDA, Food and Drug Administration; GRAS, generally recognized as safe.

Table 1.
List of few artificial sweeteners, ADI value and uses.

DOI: http://dx.doi.org/10.5772/intechopen.93199

Author details

Kanagamani Krishnasamy
Department of Chemistry, SNS College of Technology, Coimbatore, India

*Address all correspondence to: kanagamanichem@gmail.com

IntechOpen

© 2020 The Author(s). Licensee IntechOpen. This chapter is distributed under the terms of the Creative Commons Attribution License (http://creativecommons.org/licenses/by/3.0), which permits unrestricted use, distribution, and reproduction in any medium, provided the original work is properly cited.

References

[1] Magnuson BA, Burdock GA, Doull J, Kroes RM, Marsh GM, Pariza MW, et al. Aspartame: A safety evaluation based on current use levels, regulations, and toxicological and epidemiological studies. Critical Reviews in Toxicology. 2007;**37**(8):629-727

[2] Stegink LD, Filer LJ, Baker GL. Effect of aspartame and aspartate loading upon plasma and erythrocyte free amino acid levels in normal adult volunteers. Journal of Nutrition. 1997;**107**(10):1837-1845

[3] Olney JW. Excitotoxins in foods. Neurotoxicology. 1994;**15**(3):535-544

[4] Clauss J, Schmidt RK, Spiss HW. Determination of domain sizes in heterogeneous polymers by solid state NMR. Acta Polymerica. 1993;**44**:1-17

[5] Findikli Z, Turkoglu S. Determination of the effects of some artificial sweeteners on human peripheral lymphocytes using the comet assay. Journal of Toxicology and Environmental Health Sciences. 2014;**6**(8):147-153

[6] Knight I. The development and applications of sucralose: A new high intensity sweetener. Canadian Journal of Physiology and Pharmacology. 1993;**72**:435-439

[7] Kroger M, Meister K, Kava R. Low calorie sweeteners and other sugar substitutes: A review of the safety issues. Comprehensive Reviews in Food Science and Food Safety. 2006;**5**:35-47

[8] Bopp BA, Sonders RC, Keterson JW. Toxicological aspects of cyclamate and cyclohexylamine. Critical Reviews in Toxicology. 1986;**16**:213-306

[9] Sweeteners Holdings, Inc. Neotame [Internet]. 2002. Available from: www.neotame.com [Accessed: 08 July 2007]

[10] Chattopadhyay S, Raychaudhari U, Chakraborthy R. Artificial sweeteners—A review. Journal of Food Science and Technology. 2006;**51**(4):611-621

[11] Whitehouse CR, Boullata J, Mccauley L. The potential toxicity of artificial sweeteners. AAOHN Journal. 2008;**56**(6):251-259

Chapter 18

Long-Term Weight Loss Maintenance

Martin Fischer, Nadine Oberänder and Arved Weimann

Abstract

Weight maintenance can be considered a challenge for all patients who are in a reduced obese state. In this chapter, we first provide an overview of the chances for maintaining weight loss, how physiological adaptations and psychological dynamics lead to weight regain in the long-term, and of the factors that have been associated with long-term success. Then we review what is known about the patient perspective on that critical time period following weight loss, focusing on the experience of barriers and facilitators as well as attempted strategies. Finally, we introduce an approach for providing a targeted and individualized support at this stage.

Keywords: obesity, weight loss, weight loss maintenance, weight regain, lifestyle intervention, behavior change

1. Introduction: is weight maintenance a losing battle?

The importance of weight loss for people in the western world is reflected by a growing diet industry that is providing easier, faster, and more powerful products. In addition to public demand, the diet industry keeps growing because many of their products simply work, i.e., they do enable customers to reduce their body weight short-term. Socio-cultural ideals of beauty and attractiveness are major motivators for reducing body weight even if it already falls within a healthy norm. However, for approximately 20% of adults in western societies, losing weight has become a health-related issue as they are suffering from obesity. It has been shown that comorbidities of obesity such as cardiovascular diseases, joint damage, or diabetes as well as quality of life significantly improve when weight is reduced [1]. However, the same way it has been shown that short-term weight loss is achievable for many people, it has become clear that only few are successful in the long-term [2, 3]. The authors of a recent systematic review concluded that substantial weight loss cannot be sustained by the average person in the absence of a continued follow-up intervention [4]. Moreover, behavioral treatments have been questioned ethically with respect to the claim of permanent weight loss [5]. However, recent data suggest that treatment programs comprising of intensified lifestyle interventions with continued support can lead to longer-term weight loss [6]. Therefore, a better understanding of the interaction between physiological and psychological barriers to weight maintenance has been recommended as well as the development of more individualized and targeted strategies.

2. What makes weight loss maintenance challenging?

A number of physiological and psychological factors have to be emphasized in order to understand the challenge of weight loss maintenance. Physiologically, weight loss induces metabolic adaptations that favor weight regain by creating an energy gap [7–9]. These comprise the hormonal regulation of appetite, satiety, and satiation as well as resting energy expenditure. Energy expenditure is lowered beyond what changes of body composition predict and this might be due to adaptive thermogenesis, that is, the capability of the human body to reduce energy expenditure by producing less body heat [10]. Moreover, there is evidence that at least some of these changes can last over several years, even after partial weight regain [11, 12].

Psychologically, it is known that the effect of health behavior interventions generally diminishes over time, and that behavior maintenance has to be regarded as a separate challenge [13]. Five overarching themes have been associated with behavior maintenance and may explain why it is difficult to achieve, i.e., maintenance motives [...], self-regulation, resources, habits, and contextual influences [13]. With respect to weight maintenance, it has to be considered that adherence not just to a single but to a whole set of behavior is required in order to balance and regulate energy intake and expenditure [14]. These changes comprise areas such as meal structure, eating behavior, food shopping, calorie counting, alcohol consumption, exercise, stress management, sleep, leisure activities, and vacation. Although they are referred to as a single change of lifestyle, the difficulties to maintain each associated behavior change may rather accumulate than complement. In accordance with this is the observation that even after several years of successful weight maintenance, its execution is still experienced as a burden [15].

Taken together, weight loss maintenance is a challenge because it requires actively counteracting a possibly infinite physiological resistance against weight reduction as well as the psychological tendency to relapse from health behavior changes of which many are necessary for long-term maintenance. Therefore, after successful weight loss, obese patients should not be treated as cured, normal-weight people, but rather as reduced obese individuals [16].

3. Factors associated with weight loss maintenance

Despite its physiological and psychological challenges, a considerable number of patients are able to minimize weight regain [17]. This has been attributed to personal characteristics such as internal motivation, social support, self-efficacy, novelty seeking, or sleep chronotype, as well as to a set of specific behaviors observed in successful maintainers such as high levels of physical activity, compliance to a low-energy diet with a regular meal rhythm, flexible eating restraint, portion control, control of over-eating, self-monitoring, immediate regulation of weight gain, and active problem solving [18–23].

Notably, successful maintenance practices seem to differ from successful weight loss practices [24]. In recent reviews, energy intake on one side and energy expenditure on the other have been used as a framework to explain how different determinants may affect weight maintenance [8, 20]. According to this view, any factor or strategy that enables a weight-reduced patient to permanently reduce calorie intake will support weight maintenance. Similarly, any strategy that enables a patient to permanently increase energy expenditure will support maintenance as well. It has to be noted that none of these determinants are believed to alter the physiological adaptations associated with weight loss but rather help to minimize their impact. In other words, it is assumed that a cognitive control of energy regulation is an inevitable necessity.

Although several determinants of successful weight loss maintenance have been observed, intervention studies reported mainly disappointing results [17, 25, 26]. An increase of physical activity and exercise, for example, is clearly predictive of weight loss maintenance, but when applied as a clinical intervention in randomized controlled trials, its effectiveness remains questionable, especially in the long-term [27, 28]. The reason for this is still not clear but an important factor could be adherence. Therefore, additional mediators need to be identified that may explain why some patients continue pursuing weight maintenance behaviors and some others are not [22]. For example, the contribution of novel neuropsychological factors such as executive functioning and neurocognitive control to weight loss maintenance have been recently discussed [16, 29]. Another important approach for improving long-term adherence might be the provision of more tailored and multidisciplinary weight loss maintenance strategies [14]. This requires a deeper understanding of the patient perspective [30].

4. The patient perspective

In order to provide a tailored support after weight loss, it is crucial to understand the patient perspective on weight loss maintenance. What do patients experience during this time? How do the physiological and psychological challenges translate into the individual's perception and what measures do they undertake in response to that and with what kind of perceived success? These questions can be answered by identifying factors that patients perceive as threats and factors that they perceive as facilitators during weight loss maintenance. It might also be useful to identify the different maintenance strategies patients rely on and their experience with them. Most studies have used qualitative designs to explore how patients experience and explain their success or failure during weight maintenance, respectively. Although the transferability of a single qualitative study may be limited, a more valid view can be generated by thematically synthesizing many of them [31]. To expand insights gathered by qualitative studies, it could also be helpful to utilize quantitative designs in future studies of patient perspective [30, 32].

4.1 Barriers

A great variety of barriers to weight maintenance have been revealed by reviews of qualitative studies on patient perspective (**Table 1**). For example, in one review, the identified barriers included bad weather conditions such as extreme winters, poor health and sickness, lack of motivation (e.g., due to previous failure, body image, or eating for reasons other than hunger), lack of time management, problems at home (e.g., due to the inability to afford a healthy lifestyle), festivities, and past stigmatizing experiences [33]. Additional barriers, identified in another review included maladaptive habits, poor self-regulation skills, emotional problems, social-cultural factors (e.g., pressure, saboteurs, and social commitments), and environmental limitations (e.g., feeling unsafe to exercise in the neighborhood) [34]. Identity conflicts and negative beliefs about weight management are two more barriers patients experience during weight loss maintenance [31]. It is possible that a considerable overlap between some of these barriers exists and that they can be reduced to a small number of main barriers [30]. It is also noteworthy that the perception of barriers and their relevance for actual weight regain could change over time and there might even be moments when some patients are not experiencing

Barriers	Facilitators	Strategies
• Bad weather conditions • Poor health and sickness • Lack of motivation • Lack of time management • Problems at home • Festivities • Past stigmatizing experiences • Maladaptive habits • Poor self-regulation skills • Emotional problems • Social-cultural factors • Environmental factors • Identity conflict • Negative beliefs about weight management	• Identity shift • Psychological commitment and preparedness to integrate weight management strategies into everyday life • Environmental factors • Socio-cultural factors • Improved self-perception	• Self-motivation/ self-reinforcement • Self-monitoring • Adoption of a food choice system • Establishing a non-food reward system • Habit formation • Restructuring the environment • Accepting and committing to weight loss maintenance as a lifelong challenge • Balancing eating restraint and flexibility • Being open for building new relationships

[a]*Main themes according to recent reviews of qualitative studies [31, 33, 34].*

Table 1.
Main barriers, facilitators, and strategies of weight loss maintenance from patient perspective.[a]

any barriers to weight loss maintenance [30, 35]. Also, despite the experience of external barriers and facilitators, many patients may still take mostly personal responsibility for weight maintenance as excess weight is oftentimes attributed to unhealthy, modifiable behaviors [34].

In one of our studies, we found that patients who had been successfully treated for severe obesity were experiencing four main barriers to weight loss maintenance during the first 3 years after treatment completion [30]. The first barrier, 'Hedonic Hunger', reflected difficulties arising from food-related pleasure and the struggle with availability of highly palatable foods. The second barrier, 'mental distress', reflected difficulties arising from stress, emotional eating, and mental issues. The third barrier, 'Binge Eating', reflected difficulties arising from subclinical loss of control eating, binge episodes, boredom, and craving. The last barrier, 'Demoralization', reflected several difficulties arising from an implicit demoralized state, a low self-efficacy and helplessness such as lacking social support, finances, health, and motivation. Each barrier was found to be relevant for weight regain, but also that time could be a mediator. In particular, "Binge Eating" was found to be most critical at the beginning of weight loss maintenance and 'Mental Distress" at later stages.

4.2 Facilitators

Perceived facilitators of weight maintenance that have been revealed by reviews of qualitative studies include an identity shift (e.g., living healthily became a need), a psychological commitment, and preparedness to integrate weight management strategies into everyday life, environmental factors (e.g., healthy choices are visible, available and attractive), socio-cultural factors (e.g., support and engagement by friends, family, colleagues, and professionals), and an improved self-perception due to successful weight loss (**Table 1**) [8, 31, 33, 34]. However, the experience of facilitation can differ inter-individually. For example, for some patients, social support seems to be irrelevant [36], and past stigmatizing experiences seem to inhibit some patients for a long time, whereas others are rather motivated by them in the short- and long-term [33].

4.3 Strategies

Patients who are able to maintain weight loss report several strategies to explain their success including self-motivating and reinforcing strategies (e.g., consciously enjoying physical activity as a new quality of a weight-reduced life; intentionally turning dieting and exercise into meaningful hobbies), self-monitoring (e.g., app-based monitoring of food intake, physical activity, and body weight), adoption of a food choice system to reduce energy intake (e.g., preferring high-grade, unprocessed foods), establishing a nonfood reward system for weight maintenance (e.g., buying clothes), habit formation (e.g., avoiding the candy isle; parking faraway), restructuring the environment (e.g., food storage at home; avoiding high-risk situations), accepting and committing to weight loss maintenance as a lifelong challenge, balancing eating restraint and flexibility (e.g., having a slightly relaxed mind-set, faith in the process, testing limits, and consciously plan for occasional treats and even lapses), and being open for building new relationships (e.g., when former relationships loosen due to an incompatibility with the new lifestyle) (**Table 1**) [15, 36–38]. It should be noted though that successful weight maintainers may not use these strategies consistently, and the differences to unsuccessful patients could therefore be less pronounced than previously assumed [36]. Also, the burden patients associate with implementing weight maintenance strategies seems to remain much higher compared to lifetime weight stable persons who are relying on comparable strategies [15].

So far, mainly strategies that successful patients employ have been explored. In contrast, it is less clear which strategies less successful patients try to employ and how that relates to their weight regain and failed recovery attempts. For example, less successful patients oftentimes end up not eating breakfast, a strategy consistently reported by weight maintainers [23]. Is that because they have never managed to eat breakfast on a regular basis, because they discontinued it prior to regain, or because they discontinued it after weight began to regain? In other words, is it a lack of behavior change, behavior maintenance, or self-efficacy?

4.4 The experience of tension as a psychological core issue

According to a recent psychological model that integrated findings from 26 qualitative studies on perceived barriers, facilitators, and strategies, the core issue for patients during weight loss maintenance is the experience of tension [31]. This tension is a conceptualization of the aforementioned burden that patients associate with adhering to the strategies required for long-term success. However, the novelty of this model is that it (a) assumes variability of the tension, (b) suggests that barriers, facilitators, and strategies are relevant to the degree they are affecting a patients' individual tension, and (c) classifies all of these factors with respect to one of four key concepts, that is, "sources of tension", "modifiers of tension", strategies for "managing tension", and strategies for "reducing the tension":

- "Sources of tension" are comprised of psychological factors such as old habits and impulses, beliefs about identity, beliefs about weight management, and unmet needs.

- "Modifiers of tensions" are comprised of barriers and facilitators such as environmental and social factors, as well as health, finances, and other personal circumstances.

- Strategies for "reducing the tension" are comprised of developing automaticity, meeting needs more healthily, and changing beliefs and self-concept.
- Strategies for "managing the tension" are comprised of learning and insight, self-regulation, managing internal and external influences, and willpower or motivation.

Most of the patient experience revealed by qualitative studies can be explained by using this framework, and therefore, the introduction of this model could be an important step to shift the research focus forward. Particularly, there is a need for prospective studies to evaluate the predictive value of patient perspective ensuring that it does not reflect merely post-hoc rationalizations. Furthermore, the contribution of physiological adaptations, probably as a "source of tension", to the psychological dynamics of weight maintenance should be evaluated.

5. Providing support during weight loss maintenance

With respect to the available findings on patient perspective as well as our own experience, we suggest that an ideal weight loss maintenance treatment program comprises of two components, one provided during and immediately after weight loss in a structured manner, and one provided and tailored as part of a longer-term follow-up care.

5.1 Structured component of a weight loss maintenance program

The structured component of a weight loss maintenance program should promote early (i.e., already at the weight loss stage) cognitive-behavioral changes such as habit formation that will later help reduce the tension of weight loss maintenance. Additionally, during the transition from weight loss to maintenance, this component should support the development of strategies for managing the tension (**Table 2**) [31]. An important cognitive goal of this component is to help patients accept the challenge of weight loss maintenance early, so they have time to make a psychological commitment and be prepared for integrating weight management strategies into everyday life (facilitator of WLM). Therefore, weight loss maintenance treatment ideally begins during the last weeks of the weight loss stage, when weight reduction is just starting to level off. Ways to support early acceptance include psychoeducation, cognitive restructuring (e.g., by increasing awareness of already achieved improvements), and introduction of former patients as role models. This acceptance also requires acceptance of the end of the current weight loss episode. The latter is not easy for many patients because they are experiencing weight loss as a rather euphoric state with rapid success and regular reinforcement due to social adoration, improved quality of life, and health. Also, they are feeling in control of their disease and some might even feel cured, expecting to continue until some far-away ideal weight is being reached. Therefore, it is essential for them to gain insight into the fact that weight loss is going to cease, largely due to physiological adaptations, and that it is psychologically healthier, easier, and more functional to start focusing on maintenance than further weight loss. For this purpose, it can be helpful to emphasize differences between the two (**Table 3**).

5.2 Tailored longer-term follow-up care

The second component of an ideal weight loss maintenance treatment program should provide tailored interventions as part of a longer-term follow-up care.

Strategy[a]	Interventional tools	Examples
Reducing the tension		
Developing automaticity	Stimulus control Habit formation Nudging Model learning	• Eating before food shopping • Parking further away from the office • Move the TV out of the living room • Joining a fitness tracker community
Meeting needs more healthily	Cognitive restructuring Problem solving Mindfulness-based stress reduction Social skills training Physical activity Exercise	• Identify pleasant aspects of vacations that are not food related • Feeling healthy by eating healthy food • Learning to say 'no' • Using exercise performance as an indicator of success
Changing identity	Cognitive restructuring	• Showing others who you were and who you want to be • Associate personal values with healthy choices • Photo shoot • Joining a Nordic walking group
Changing beliefs about weight management	Psychoeducation Cognitive restructuring Model learning	• Appreciating the weight loss outcome • Accepting the weight maintenance challenge • Getting to know successful maintainers
Managing the tension		
Self-regulation, learning and insight	Psychoeducation Diaries, protocols, Apps	• Self-monitoring • Using social accountability • Becoming aware of personal risk factors • Flexible eating restraint • Recognizing lapses and relapses • Owning up to and growing from lapses • Relapse recovery
Managing internal and external influences	Psychoeducation Acceptance-based treatment	• Anticipating, planning, and avoiding at-risk situations • Defusing food cravings
Willpower or motivation	Buddying Self-help	• Patient-led workshops • Sharing success with new patients

[a]Strategies adopted from a conceptual model of the dynamics of weight loss maintenance [31].

Table 2.
Approach to a structured weight loss maintenance treatment.

The time frame should be at least 3 years after weight loss, as these years are most critical with respect to weight regain [39]. During this time, a continuous assessment of body weight change, cognitive-behavioral changes, emergence of barriers, and loss of facilitators should be performed to allow immediate intervention. To get a more valid picture, data can be recorded by patients prior to a consultation [36]. With respect to the different barriers patients are experiencing, at least five tailored interventions may need to be offered.

A first intervention should be targeted towards patients who are primarily experiencing difficulties due to festivities, environmental factors such as food availability, social-cultural factors such as peer pressure, and old habits. Practicing

	Weight loss period	Weight loss maintenance period
Main goal	Body weight reduction (fat mass reduction)	Identity change ("healthily living person")
Time frame	3–6 months	3+ years
Dietary focus	Calorie reduction ("less") Rigid adherence	High-grade ("better") Planning & remaining flexible
Physical activity Focus	Decreasing sedentary times Adhere to exercise plans	Habitual physical activity Enjoying physical activity/exercise
Motivation	Continuous success due to weight loss (improvements of health, quality of life, self-perception) Group support Compliments	Improved mobility, new choices, new freedom Healthy lifestyle as a hobby (experiences, insights, exchange, role model) Continuous success due to exercise (improvements of physical fitness, body composition)
Required Willpower	Very high at beginning Later context dependent	High at beginning Later intermittently
Help & support	Regular external monitoring Multi-professional treatment Exchange with others	Like-minded people and groups Professional consultation

Table 3.
Example for how weight loss maintenance can be emphasized as a separate challenge to patients.

stimulus control techniques, social skills, and mindfulness eating might help these patients to gain back control over externally triggered hedonic eating motives.

A second intervention should be targeted towards patients who primarily report emotional problems, lack of time management, or negative beliefs about weight management. Stress prevention and reduction trainings might help these patients to free the resources necessary to pursue healthy behaviors again and to not rely on emotional eating as a coping mechanism. Of note, some of these patients may need to be referred to psychotherapy to treat an underlying affective disorder.

A third intervention should be made available to patients who primarily experience a lack of control over eating in the absence of clear external or emotional causes. A training comprising of acceptance-based and cognitive-behavioral techniques, proven effective for the treatment of binge eating disorder, might be helpful.

A fourth intervention should be made available for patients whose primary issue is a directly experienced lack of motivation or who are demoralized by the experience of barriers seemingly out of their control such as bad weather conditions, poor health and sickness, financial problems at home, a lack of social support, or poor body image. Training these patients in problem-solving might enable them to find solutions for their respective issues and more importantly, may increase their self-efficacy and beliefs in long-term success. Self-efficacy can be further promoted by applying methods such as mentoring, adequate goal setting, action planning, and motivational interviewing. With respect to body weight, it should be considered that stabilization of a partly regained weight is a more realistic goal for recovery than anew weight loss [40].

A fifth intervention should be made available for patients who are experiencing identity conflicts as their primary issue such as discomfort with the new body, social insecurities, or inhibition by past stigmatizing experiences. Cognitive-behavioral techniques can be used to dispute potentially idealizing of the former obese self or an exaggerated significance of body image to self-worth. They can also be used to help patients seek and build on self-esteem fostering situations. Psychoeducation about optional plastic surgery after weight loss might be offered as well.

As described before, it is likely that patients are experiencing several of the barriers in parallel or intermittently during weight maintenance. However, we think it is still beneficial to treat one barrier at a time in order to focus on behavior and cognition instead of weight loss to achieve long-term improvements.

6. Conclusion

Weight loss maintenance is a complex physiological and psychological challenge associated with a high risk of failure. Studies on patient perspective have revealed valuable information on how this process is experienced. Although generally experienced as an ongoing burden, the underlying psychological tension is variable and moderated by a number of now well-defined barriers, facilitators, and strategies. With this novel information, a more tailored long-term support can be provided which may help improve weight loss maintenance.

Author details

Martin Fischer[1*], Nadine Oberänder[2] and Arved Weimann[2]

1 St. George Obesity Treatment Study Group, Klinikum St. Georg, Leipzig, Germany

2 Klinikum St. Georg, Leipzig, Germany

*Address all correspondence to: martin.fischer@sanktgeorg.de

IntechOpen

© 2020 The Author(s). Licensee IntechOpen. This chapter is distributed under the terms of the Creative Commons Attribution License (http://creativecommons.org/licenses/by/3.0), which permits unrestricted use, distribution, and reproduction in any medium, provided the original work is properly cited.

References

[1] Bischoff SC, Boirie Y, Cederholm T, Chourdakis M, Cuerda C, Delzenne NM, et al. Towards a multidisciplinary approach to understand and manage obesity and related diseases. Clinical Nutrition. 2017;**36**:917-938. DOI: 10.1016/j.clnu.2016.11.007

[2] Wing RR, Phelan S. Long-term weight loss maintenance. The American Journal of Clinical Nutrition. 2005;**82**:222S-225S. DOI: 10.1093/ajcn/82.1.222S

[3] Anderson JW, Konz EC, Frederich RC, Wood CL. Long-term weight-loss maintenance: A meta-analysis of US studies. The American Journal of Clinical Nutrition. 2001;**74**:579-584. DOI: 10.1088/1751-8113/44/8/085201

[4] Nordmo M, Danielsen YS, Nordmo M. The challenge of keeping it off, a descriptive systematic review of high-quality, follow-up studies of obesity treatments. Obesity Reviews. 2020;**21**:1-15. DOI: 10.1111/obr.12949

[5] Cooper Z, Doll HA, Hawker DM, Byrne S, Bonner G, Eeley E, et al. Testing a new cognitive behavioural treatment for obesity: A randomized controlled trial with three-year follow-up. Behaviour Research and Therapy. 2010;**48**:706-713. DOI: 10.1016/j.brat.2010.03.008

[6] Weimann A, Fischer M, Oberänder N, Prodehl G, Weber N, Andrä M, et al. Willing to go the extra mile: Prospective evaluation of an intensified non-surgical treatment for patients with morbid obesity. Clinical Nutrition. 2019;**38**:1773-1781. DOI: 10.1016/j.clnu.2018.07.027

[7] Sumithran P, Proietto J. The defence of body weight: A physiological basis for weight regain after weight loss. Clinical Science. 2013;**124**:231-241. DOI: 10.1042/CS20120223

[8] Melby CL, Paris HL, Foright RM, Peth J. Attenuating the biologic drive for weight regain following weight loss: Must what goes down always go back up? Nutrients. 2017;**9**:pii:E468. DOI: 10.3390/nu9050468

[9] Keesey RE, Hirvonen MD. Obesity: Common symptom of diverse gene-based metabolic dysregulations. The Journal of Nutrition. 1997;**127**:1875S-1883S

[10] Camps SGJA, Verhoef SPM, Westerterp KR. Weight loss, weight maintenance, and adaptive thermogenesis. The American Journal of Clinical Nutrition. 2013;**97**:990-994. DOI: 10.3945/ajcn.112.050310

[11] Fothergill E, Guo J, Howard L, Kerns JC, Knuth ND, Brychta R, et al. Persistent metabolic adaptation 6 years after "the biggest loser" competition. Obesity. 2016;**24**:1612-1619. DOI: 10.1002/oby.21538

[12] Sumithran P, Proietto J. Maintaining weight loss: An ongoing challenge. Current Obesity Reports. 2016;**5**:383-385. DOI: 10.1007/s13679-016-0230-y

[13] Kwasnicka D, Dombrowski SU, White M, Sniehotta F. Theoretical explanations for maintenance of behaviour change: A systematic review of behaviour theories. Health Psychology Review. 2016;**10**:277-296. DOI: 10.1080/17437199.2016.1151372

[14] MacLean PS, Wing RR, Davidson T, Epstein L, Goodpaster B, Hall KD, et al. NIH working group report: Innovative research to improve maintenance of weight loss. Obesity. 2015;**23**:7-15. DOI: 10.1002/oby.20967

[15] Kruseman M, Schmutz N, Carrard I. Long-term weight maintenance strategies are experienced as a burden by persons who have lost

weight compared to persons with a lifetime normal, stable weight. Obesity Facts. 2017;**10**:373-385. DOI: 10.1159/000478096

[16] Poulimeneas D, Yannakoulia M, Anastasiou CA, Scarmeas N. Weight loss maintenance: Have we missed the brain? Brain Sciences. 2018;**8**:174. DOI: 10.3390/brainsci8090174

[17] Dombrowski SU, Knittle K, Avenell A, Araújo-Soares V, Sniehotta FF. Long term maintenance of weight loss with non-surgical interventions in obese adults: Systematic review and meta-analyses of randomised controlled trials. BMJ. 2014;**348**:1-12. DOI: 10.1136/bmj.g2646

[18] Elfhag K, Rössner S. Who succeeds in maintaining weight loss? A conceptual review of factors associated with weight loss maintenance and weight regain. Obesity Reviews. 2005;**6**:67-85. DOI: 10.1111/j.1467-789X.2005.00170.x

[19] Teixeira PJ, Carraça EV, Marques MM, Rutter H, Oppert J-MM, De Bourdeaudhuij I, et al. Successful behavior change in obesity interventions in adults: A systematic review of self-regulation mediators. BMC Medicine. 2015;**13**:84. DOI: 10.1186/s12916-015-0323-6

[20] Varkevisser RDM, van Stralen MM, Kroeze W, Ket JCF, Steenhuis IHM. Determinants of weight loss maintenance: A systematic review. Obesity Reviews. 2019;**20**:171-211. DOI: 10.1111/obr.12772

[21] Ross KM, Graham Thomas J, Wing RR. Successful weight loss maintenance associated with morning chronotype and better sleep quality. Journal of Behavioral Medicine. 2016;**39**:465-471. DOI: 10.1007/s10865-015-9704-8

[22] Montesi L, El Ghoch M, Brodosi L, Calugi S, Marchesini G, Grave RD. Long-term weight loss maintenance for obesity: A multidisciplinary approach. Diabetes, Metabolic Syndrome and Obesity: Targets and Therapy. 2016;**9**:37-46. DOI: 10.2147/DMSO.S89836

[23] Paixão C, Dias CM, Jorge R, Carraça EV, Yannakoulia M, de Zwaan M, et al. Successful weight loss maintenance: A systematic review of weight control registries. Obesity Reviews. 2020:2008-2011. DOI: 10.1111/obr.13003

[24] Sciamanna CN, Kiernan M, Rolls BJ, Boan J, Stuckey H, Kephart D, et al. Practices associated with weight loss versus weight-loss maintenance: Results of a national survey. American Journal of Preventive Medicine. 2011;**41**:159-166. DOI: 10.1016/j.amepre.2011.04.009

[25] Berk KA, Buijks HIM, Verhoeven AJM, Mulder MT, Özcan B, van't Spijker A, et al. Group cognitive behavioural therapy and weight regain after diet in type 2 diabetes: Results from the randomised controlled POWER trial. Diabetologia. 2018;**61**:790-799. DOI: 10.1007/s00125-017-4531-9

[26] Sniehotta FF, Evans EH, Sainsbury K, Adamson A, Batterham A, Becker F, et al. Behavioural intervention for weight loss maintenance versus standard weight advice in adults with obesity: A randomised controlled trial in the UK (NULevel trial). PLoS Medicine. 2019;**16**:1-18. DOI: 10.1371/journal.pmed.1002793

[27] Foright RM, Presby DM, Sherk VD, Kahn D, Checkley LA, Giles ED, et al. Is regular exercise an effective strategy for weight loss maintenance? Physiology & Behavior. 2018;**188**:86-93. DOI: 10.1016/j.physbeh.2018.01.025

[28] Johansson K, Neovius M, Hemmingsson E. Effects of anti-obesity drugs, diet, and exercise on weight-loss

maintenance after a very-low-calorie diet or low-calorie diet: A systematic review and meta-analysis of randomized controlled trials. The American Journal of Clinical Nutrition. 2014;**99**:14-23. DOI: 10.3945/ajcn.113.070052

[29] Gettens KM, Gorin AA. Executive function in weight loss and weight loss maintenance: A conceptual review and novel neuropsychological model of weight control. Journal of Behavioral Medicine. 2017;**40**:687-701. DOI: 10.1007/s10865-017-9831-5

[30] Fischer M, Oberänder N, Weimann A. Four main barriers to weight loss maintenance? A quantitative analysis of difficulties experienced by obese patients after successful weight reduction. European Journal of Clinical Nutrition. 2020. DOI: 10.1038/s41430-020-0559-x

[31] Greaves C, Poltawski L, Garside R, Briscoe S. Understanding the challenge of weight loss maintenance: A systematic review and synthesis of qualitative research on weight loss maintenance. Health Psychology Review. 2017;**11**:145-163. DOI: 10.1080/17437199.2017.1299583

[32] Hartmann-Boyce J, Aveyard P, Piernas C, Koshiaris C, Velardo C, Salvi D, et al. Cognitive and behavioural strategies for weight management in overweight adults: Results from the Oxford Food and Activity Behaviours (OxFAB) cohort study. PLoS One. 2018;**13**:e0202072. DOI: 10.1371/journal.pone.0202072

[33] Gupta H. Barriers to and facilitators of long term weight loss maintenance in adult UK people: A thematic analysis. International Journal of Preventive Medicine. 2014;**5**:1512-1520

[34] Garip G, Yardley L. A synthesis of qualitative research on overweight and obese people's views and experiences of weight management. Clinical Obesity. 2011;**1**:110-126. DOI: 10.1111/j.1758-8111.2011.00021.x

[35] Karfopoulou E, Mouliou K, Koutras Y, Yannakoulia M. Behaviours associated with weight loss maintenance and regaining in a Mediterranean population sample. A qualitative study. Clinical Obesity. 2013;**3**:141-149. DOI: 10.1111/cob.12028

[36] Kwasnicka D, Dombrowski SU, White M, Sniehotta FF. 'It's not a diet, it's a lifestyle': A longitudinal, data-prompted interview study of weight loss maintenance. Psychology and Health. 2019;**34**:963-982. DOI: 10.1080/08870446.2019.1579913

[37] Natvik E, Råheim M, Andersen JR, Moltu C. An experientially derived model of flexible and intentional actions for weight loss maintenance after severe obesity. Frontiers in Psychology. 2019;**10**:2503. DOI: 10.3389/fpsyg.2019.02503

[38] Natvik E, Råheim M, Andersen JR, Moltu C. Living a successful weight loss after severe obesity. International Journal of Qualitative Studies on Health and Well-Being. 2018;**13**:1487762. DOI: 10.1080/17482631.2018.1487762

[39] Coughlin JW, Brantley PJ, Champagne CM, Vollmer WM, Stevens VJ, Funk K, et al. The impact of continued intervention on weight: Five-year results from the weight loss maintenance trial. Obesity. 2016;**24**:1046-1053. DOI: 10.1002/oby.21454

[40] Phelan S, Hill JO, Lang W, Dibello JR, Wing RR. Recovery from relapse among successful weight maintainers. The American Journal of Clinical Nutrition. 2003;**78**:1079-1084. DOI: 10.1093/ajcn/78.6.1079